HELPING BEREAVED CHILDREN

Second Edition

HELPING BEREAVED CHILDREN

A Handbook for Practitioners

Second Edition

Edited by

NANCY BOYD WEBB, DSW

Fordham University
Graduate School of Social Service

Foreword by Kenneth J. Doka, PhD

THE GUILFORD PRESS
New York   London

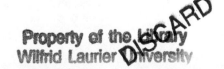

© 2002 The Guilford Press
A Division of Guilford Publications, Inc.
72 Spring Street, New York, NY 10012
www.guilford.com

Printed in the United States of America

This book is printed on acid-free paper.

Last digit is print number: 9 8 7 6 5 4 3 2 1

Library of Congress Cataloging-in-Publication Data

Helping bereaved children : a handbook for practitioners / edited by Nancy Boyd Webb; foreword by Kenneth J. Doka.—2nd ed.
   p. cm.
   Includes bibliographical references and index.
   ISBN 1-57230-632-7 (hardcover : alk. paper)
   1. Bereavement in children. 2. Grief in children. 3. Children and death. 4. Children—Counseling of. 5. Children—Counseling of—Case studies. I. Webb, Nancy Boyd.

BF723.G75 H34 2002
155.9'37'083—dc21   2001053190

TO KEMPTON
For Love, Support, and Jokes
Past, Present, and Future

N. B. W.

About the Editor

Nancy Boyd Webb, DSW, BCD, RPT-S, is a leading authority on play therapy with children who have experienced loss and traumatic bereavement. Her bestselling books are considered essential references for clinical courses and with agencies that work with children. These include *Play Therapy with Children in Crisis* (2nd edition): *Individual, Group, and Family Treatment* (Guilford Press), *Culturally Diverse Parent–Child and Family Relationships* (Columbia University Press), and *Social Work Practice with Children* (Guilford Press). In addition, she has published widely in professional journals and produced a video, *Techniques of Play Therapy: A Clinical Demonstration,* which won a bronze medal at the New York Film Festival's International Non-Broadcast Media Competition. Dr. Webb is the editor of The Guilford Press book series Social Work Practice with Children and Families, and serves as a consulting editor for *Children and Schools.* She is a board member of the New York Association for Play Therapy and on the editorial advisory board for the journal *Trauma and Loss: Research Interventions.*

A board-certified diplomate in clinical social work and a registered play therapy supervisor, Dr. Webb presents frequently at play therapy, social work, and bereavement conferences in the United States and abroad. She has been a professor on the faculty of the Fordham University School of Social Service since 1979, and in October 1997 was named University Distinguished Professor of Social Work. In 1985, she founded Fordham's Post-Master's Certificate Program in Child and Adolescent Therapy to meet the need in the New York metropolitan area for training in play therapy. In April 2000, she appeared as a panelist in a satellite teleconference *Living with Grief: Children, Adolescents, and Loss,* sponsored by the Hospice Foundation of America. Hosted by Cokie Roberts, the conference was beamed to more than 2,100 sites.

In addition to teaching, writing, and consulting, Dr. Webb maintains a clinical practice and supervises and consults with schools and agencies. She lectures and conducts workshops throughout the United States, Canada, Australia, Europe, Hong Kong, and Taiwan on play therapy, trauma, and bereavement.

Contributors

Teresa Bevin, MA, Professor, Mental Health Program, Montgomery College, Takoma Park, Maryland; formerly, School Based Mental Health Program, Children's Hospital, National Medical Center, Washington, DC, and Montgomery County Crisis Center, Bethesda, Maryland. Her published work includes one novel, *Havana Split* (1998), and a collection of short stories, *Dreams and Other Ailments* (2001) in English and Spanish.

Barbara O. Dane, PhD, Professor, Shirley Ehrenkranz School of Social Work at New York University. She directs and teaches in the School's Post-Master's Certificate Program, in addition to teaching core courses in the MSW curriculum and an elective on acute, chronic, and life-threatening illness, spirituality, and social work practice. Dr. Dane has published three books and 23 articles and book chapters, many related to HIV-related grief, loss, spirituality, and survivorship.

Betty Davies, RN, PhD, FANN, Professor and Chair, School of Nursing, Department of Family Health Care Nursing, University of California, San Francisco. She helped to establish North America's first free-standing hospice for children in Vancouver, Canada. In addition to over 100 articles and chapters pertaining to palliative care and bereavement, she is the author of *Fading Away: The Experience of Transition in Families Facing Terminal Illness* (1995) and *Shadows in the Sun: Experiences of Sibling Bereavement in Childhood* (1999).

Kenneth J. Doka, PhD, Professor of Gerontology, The College of New Rochelle (New York), and Senior Consultant to the Hospice Foundation of America. He has been both past president of the Association of Death Education and Counseling and past chair of the International Work Group on Dying, Death and Bereavement. He is the editor of *Journeys*, a newsletter for the bereaved, and of *Living with Grief: Children, Adolescents and Loss* (1990), both published by the Hospice Foundation of America. In addition, he has edited or authored 14 books and over 60 book chapters or articles. For the past 8 years he has organized an annual National Bereavement Teleconference that is beamed to more than 2,000 sites in the United States and Canada. Dr. Doka is also a Lutheran clergyman.

Sandra L. Elder, PhD, formerly, Instructor, Department of Educational and Leadership Studies, University of Victoria, British Columbia, Canada, and coordinator, developer and facilitator of the Living & Learning Through Loss Program, Brentwood Bay, British Columbia, Canada. She also maintained a private practice, the major focus of which was on working with clients dealing with grief and loss. Dr. Elder died suddenly in December 2000, shortly after completing her coauthored chapter.

Sarah J. Gamble, PhD, Staff Psychologist, Traumatic Stress Institute/ Center for Adult & Adolescent Psychotherapy, South Windsor, Connecticut. She presents frequently at professional conferences, and with her colleagues K. W. Saakvitne, Laurie Pearlman, and Beth Tabor Lev, is a coauthor of *Risking Connection* (2000).

Robin F. Goodman, PhD, ATR-BC, Clinical Associate Professor in Psychiatry, New York University School of Medicine. She established the first Child Life Program in Pediatric Hematology/Oncology at Mount Sinai Hospital in New York. At the New York University Child Study Center, she is director of a child mental health and parenting web site, AboutOurKids.org, and Director of Public Education Programs, including activities for the *Childhood Revealed* exhibit project and the National Child Mental Health Initiative. She is past president of the American Art Therapy Association, and has published *Childhood Revealed: Art Expressing Pain, Discovery and Hope* (1999) and *Turbulent Times, Prophetic Dreams: Art of Israeli and Palestinian Children* (2000).

Don Knowles, PhD, formerly, Professor, Department of Educational and Leadership Studies, University of Victoria, British Columbia, Canada, where he served as Associate Dean and Department Chair. He also published many research articles and books. He died in March 2001.

Kathleen Nader, DSW, has worked nationally and internationally in the field of posttraumatic stress and related fields since 1974. Between 1985 and 1994, Dr. Nader served as Director of Evaluations for the UCLA Trauma, Violence, and Sudden Bereavement Program. Her work has included the provision of consultation, training, and specialized interventions for children and adults following catastrophic events. Dr. Nader has written and coauthored a variety of publications, screening instruments, and videotapes regarding childhood trauma and school intervention. Her book, *Honoring Differences: Cultural Issues in the Treatment of Trauma and Loss* (coedited with Nancy Dubrow and B. Hudnall Stamm), was published in 1999.

Donna O'Toole, MA, is a counselor, author, trainer, and storyteller. She is Founding Director of Compassion Books, Inc., an international resource center distributing a variety of written and electronic materials related to loss and grief. She is a working member of IWG, the International Work Group on Death, Dying and Bereavement, and the winner of state and national awards for her written and training work in bereavement.

Robert G. Stevenson, EdD, has been an educator/counselor for over 35 years. Currently he works in a reentry program for New Jersey parolees and teaches graduate counseling courses at Mercy College in New York. Dr. Stevenson has published numerous articles and books on loss and grief. He is an active member of both the International Work Group on Death, Dying and Bereavement and the Association for Death Education and Counseling.

Nancy Boyd Webb, DSW, BCD, RPT-S. See "About the Editor."

Foreword

Robert Kastenbaum (1972) wrote an article entitled "The Kingdom Where Nobody Dies." His point in that piece is that we often like to think of childhood as a kingdom where nobody dies. We attempt then to protect children from death. In fact, we are only protecting ourselves.

Children are no strangers to loss and death. They may experience deaths of grandparents, neighbors, and pets. They may even experience the deaths of friends, parents, and siblings. I teach a graduate course on Children and Death at The College of New Rochelle. As the class meets, I ask each student to recount his or her first death experience. Most experiences occur prior to the students' being 6 years old. Rarely has a student had a first encounter when he or she was older than 12. Even if children never have suffered a death, they are not strangers to loss. Many of them have had loss experiences such as divorce, separation, or relocation.

Children, then, do grieve. But their grief is often disenfranchised. They have little opportunity to publicly mourn, to express their grief, and to receive support. Their grief becomes manifest in indirect ways—sleep disturbances, physical complaints, acting-out behaviors, and regressive behaviors.

We need to find ways to help children deal with their grief. Yet helping grieving children is not easy. It is both difficult and different from helping adults cope with grief for a number of reasons. First, children do not usually have the opportunity to choose counseling. The adults in their lives—parents, guardians, and teachers—often make that choice for them. This violation of the counseling contract—the assumption that the individual has reached out for assistance—is further complicated by the triangulated approaches to confidentiality that need to be negotiated between the child, counselor, and guardian.

Methods and approaches to helping grieving children have to be different as well. Nothing strikes more terror into the heart of many children than when an adult, especially an unknown adult, sits them in a room and says, "Let's talk." Children speak in their own language—a language of play, art, and story. This is why expressive methods are far better approaches for working with children. Yet these methods also have to be intentional and prescriptive. Different children will each have their own special modality. There is a need then to be "eclectically expressive" when working with these children.

Children, too, are at different developmental levels. As they get older, they are developing cognitively, gaining a more mature and richer conception of the meanings of loss and death. Children develop in other ways as well. They grow in affect. Very young children may find it difficult to identify the emotions that they are experiencing. They may have a "short feeling span," unable to sustain strong emotions for long periods of time. Their sense of empathy develops as well. Young children tend to see loss only from their perspective, only responding to the personal implications, while older children can see how the loss affects others, offering support even within the family system.

Children also grow spiritually. From the earliest ages, children explore questions of meaning ("Why did he have to die?"). At very young ages, children still may be exploring their beliefs, trying to figure out answers to their questions, attempting to make sense of the world. As they get older, they may develop spiritual constructs, beliefs that can be applied to various crises that they face.

So children are in a paradoxical situation. They do face death and loss. Yet it is not always easy to approach and assist them as they encounter loss.

That is one reason why this timely second edition of *Helping Bereaved Children* is so welcome. Dr. Webb brings three great gifts to the task. Two are personal. She is a superb and sensitive therapist who is a pioneer in play therapy. But there is a third gift. She has assembled a wonderful group of colleagues who contribute their own, very special expertise.

In my reading, the book offers four contributions to the task of helping grieving children. First, it offers solid theory and concepts. This work is on the cutting edge of grief theory, incorporating insights such as the importance of retaining continuing bonds with the deceased, the value of narrative approaches, and the possibility of growth in loss. Dr. Webb continues to develop here one of her significant conceptual contributions, disabling grief. To Dr. Webb, one of the critical factors in assessing grief reactions is the degree to which these reactions are disabling—that is, how much they impair the individual's ability to function. This idea is a welcome alternative to fruitless debates about pathological grief.

A second contribution is the book's sensitivity to the world of the child. Children live in families and go to schools. The sensitivity of the school and the ability of the family to support the grieving child will be critical factors in the eventual outcome, the implication of the loss in the child's ongoing life. Therapists will find in the book useful tools for empowering the natural support systems in the child's life.

A third contribution lies in the grounded methodologies and diverse modalities offered. As stated earlier, children are different; the therapist will need to select an approach(es) that will best suit the needs of each child. Some children will prosper with art therapy. Others will respond well to play. Still others will benefit from the use of story. Ultimately, readers will find an eclectic array of methodologies so that they can prescribe the most effective approach for their clients.

There is a final contribution: In her early remarks, Dr. Webb notes that students often want formulas—what to do in each situation and circumstance. She wisely notes that this is an impossible, and in fact dangerous, approach. There is no one formula that can substitute for sensitivity and skill. But in the place of one standard formula she and the book's contributors offer much else—tools, case vignettes, and clear methodological approaches. This will do much to assist those who wish to help bereaved children. Most important, though, the frequent use of methodological examples should spur the reader's creativity. And that is the book's greatest gift.

KENNETH J. DOKA

REFERENCE

Kastenbaum, R. (1972, December 23). The kingdom where nobody dies. *Saturday Review of Literature*, 33–38.

Preface

Nine years ago I edited the first edition of this book as an outgrowth of *Play Therapy with Children in Crisis*, which was published in 1991. Because of the comprehensiveness of that book, it could not present sufficient attention to the topic of bereaved children. As a child therapist, I have worked with many children who experienced a death during the time I was in contact with them, as well as with others who had been bereaved previously. Death, unlike many other crisis situations, is inevitable and universal. Therefore, anyone who works with children must be prepared to offer help to a child who can become bereaved suddenly, traumatically, or naturally.

Like other crisis situations, the bereaved child's reactions and need for professional intervention differ depending on the child's personal background, availability of supports, and the circumstances of the event. Although there is a growing body of children's psychoeducational literature dealing with fictionalized death situations, detailed guidance for counselors and therapists working with bereaved children is still scanty. My intention in this book is to present not only the theoretical principles that guide intervention with bereaved children but also detailed case examples of the helping process.

There have been many refinements and some new approaches to counseling children who have suffered losses associated with death since the first edition of *Helping Bereaved Children* was published in 1993. In particular, the increased occurrence of violent deaths has had an impact on children (as well as adults) and requires specialized helping methods. Schools and communities are now more aware of the need to help children following incidents of murder, bombings, and terrorist attacks.

This second edition contains a number of follow-up reports on the cases previously discussed. In addition, it includes new chapters on child bereavement following urban terrorist attacks, on the use of art therapy, storytelling, and bereavement groups, and on self-care for bereavement counselors. All the chapters have been revised to include recent literature and new approaches for helping bereaved children.

As a professor of social work, I appreciate the needs of students who want specifics about what to say and what not to say. Although there are, of course, no formulas to plug in, I have tried to include as much dialogue as possible to make the work come alive through the actual interchanges between the therapist/counselor and the client. The discussion questions at the end of each chapter offer opportunities to evaluate the dynamic features of the case and to consider alternative interventions.

The book is divided into five major sections.

Part I presents the theoretical framework for understanding the child's views about death and for assessing the bereaved child. Chapter 2, on assessment of the bereaved child, includes several forms that can be used to record significant information about the child's background as well as particulars about the death situation and the family, social, and religious supports. Each death occurs in a context that affects survivors uniquely. Therefore, it is essential to consider this context thoroughly to understand the nature of the child's bereavement and the appropriate helping role of the therapist/counselor.

Part II focuses on deaths occurring in families, including a range of situations from the anticipated, timely death of a grandparent to the traumatic murder–suicide of both parents. Included also are chapters on sibling death and on helping children following suicidal deaths, as well as on situations of complicated bereavement when a death occurs at the same time as a parental divorce. The treatment modalities reflect a range of interventions, including family therapy, individual play therapy, and groups for bereaved children.

Part III deals with death situations when these have occurred in the community and when groups of school children have been affected by the shared loss of a peer, a counselor, or a teacher, or by random, violent deaths. Several of these chapters demonstrate the need for multilevel interventions, including individual, small-group, and large-group approaches to helping bereaved children. As always, the age of the children and their unique personal histories affect their responses to death. Often the school-based counselor must identify children who require individual follow-up and possible referral to mental health practitioners.

Part IV presents specific methods of intervention with bereaved children. These include individual counseling and therapy, bereavement groups, and the special methods of art therapy and storytelling. A separate chapter deals with the importance of self-care for bereavement counselors.

The terrorist attacks on September 11 led to the addition of Part V, after the manuscript had already been submitted to the publisher. The uniqueness and magnitude of these tragic events required separate consideration related to the combination of national outrage and support that they generated. An entire nation was in mourning, with all the attendant feelings of sadness, anger, and anxiety about the future. Adults' reactions, both in the family and in the community, inevitably influenced the nature of children's responses to their individual losses. Although Part II of the book deals with deaths in families and Part III deals with deaths occurring in schools and communities, the overlay of trauma and the undercurrent of fear associated with deaths from terrorist attacks makes this situation a special kind of bereavement that requires great sensitivity and attention by adults to children's special needs, while simultaneously dealing with their own troubled feelings.

The Appendix is a resource for those seeking further training and information about play therapy, grief counseling, and trauma/crisis counseling. It also provides a list of references to different religious/cultural/ ethnic practices related to death.

This book serves two major groups of professionals who work and come in contact with bereaved children: those who are trained in the mental health fields of psychology, psychiatry, psychiatric nursing, and clinical social work, and those who are trained in counseling fields such as pastoral counseling and educational counseling. School-based personnel have extensive contact with children. They can provide bereavement counseling in the school and refer "at-risk" children to mental health specialists when the grief is traumatic or complicated. As will be discussed, a timely referral places initial focus on the trauma in order to permit subsequent grief work.

The preface of a book is always written after it is completed. As a contributing author and the editor, I can use this opportunity to evaluate the book's strengths and shortcomings. I am pleased with the range of approaches presented here to help children bereaved in a variety of situations. We have presented bereavement counseling during and after the crisis of death. The important "unfinished business" at the completion of this book is to emphasize the advisability of helping children *before* a death occurs. I would be very happy if this book leads to the routine inclusion of death education units at the elementary school level. This would serve in a primary prevention model to educate and prepare children before they have to deal with the pain of a loss. Death touches children's lives in many ways, and we must do everything we can to help them before, during, and after their inevitable death experiences.

NANCY BOYD WEBB

Acknowledgments

I knew that this book needed to be written when a former student with many years' post-MSW experience in hospice told me that, as a father with young children, he could not bear the pain of working with bereaved children. I hope that he and others who counsel bereaved families now will be more knowledgeable and comfortable when circumstances bring them in contact with a bereaved child.

As in the first edition, the evolution of this second edition depended heavily on the 10 contributing authors who carefully followed my detailed outline and completed the necessary revisions in keeping with my deadline. My circle of personal and professional contacts has continued to widen in the course of seeking out and working with the skilled practitioners who have written about their direct interventions with bereaved children. Sadly, two authors died shortly after finishing their chapter. Sandra L. Elder, from British Columbia, died suddenly in December 2000, and Don Knowles, who was terminally ill, died the following March. Three days before her death, Sandra wrote to me about how pleased she was to have had the opportunity to work together with Dr. Knowles, who had been her dissertation advisor at the University of Victoria. Both devoted their life's work to counseling and teaching related to children's and adolescents' death concerns. I am grateful to them, and to all the authors, as well as to their child and adolescent clients, who proudly and eagerly agreed to share their counseling/therapy experiences for the benefit of others.

Jill Krementz was especially open and generous about permitting me to quote excerpts from her wonderful book *How It Feels When a Parent Dies,* and for putting me in contact with Amira Thoran, who enthusiastically agreed to provide an update of her early childhood bereavement.

My own child clients and their families have also been open in granting me permission to write about our work together. I value the trust they have accorded me and hope they will take deserved pride in knowing that their experiences of loss can train therapists/counselors to help other bereaved children. Except for the examples noted otherwise, all the clinical cases have been disguised to protect the confidentiality of the children and their families. The situations and the dynamics are based on reality, but the identities of the individuals have been altered.

Time is a serious pressure in producing a book such as this. I especially appreciate the help and support of my husband, who has witnessed the full range of both the satisfactions and the difficulties entailed in such a project. He has helped in numerous ways, both substantive and logistically, always managing to buoy me up and move me ahead.

Once again, my former Dean, Mary Ann Quaranta, and the current Dean of the Fordham University Graduate School of Social Service, Peter Vaughn, have supported my efforts and understood my time pressures. They both appreciate the importance of educating students and practitioners to serve children and families. I am grateful for their support.

It has again been a pleasure to work with the editors of The Guilford Press. I would like to recognize both Seymour Weingarten, Editor-in-Chief, and Rochelle Serwator, Editor. Over the past 10 years of my association with The Guilford Press, I have been impressed and pleased by the high professional standards of the entire staff. I also want to acknowledge and thank the support staff and student assistants at Fordham's Graduate School of Social Service who have helped in various ways. These include (in alphabetical order) Roxia Bullock, Kieran Delamere, Marla Mendillo, Nivia Pelicier, and C. K. Sample.

I also thank all the dozens of individuals who have been involved in the production of this book. I hope that they will take pride in participating in this effort to break through the taboo surrounding the topic of children and death. Bereaved children *can* be helped, and this book is dedicated to that helping process.

NANCY BOYD WEBB

Contents

Part IV. Interventions with Bereaved Children

Part V. Helping Children Bereaved by Terrorism

Appendix

PART I

🐚

Introduction

1

❧

The Child and Death

NANCY BOYD WEBB

A simple child
That lightly draws its breath
And feels its life in every limb
What should it know of death?
—WORDSWORTH (1798/1928, pp. 74–75)

What, indeed, should the child know about death, and when should he/
she know it and by what means should he/she find out? The notion of
childhood innocence as portrayed by the poet conveys the wish that
children's knowledge about death could be avoided or postponed. Edna
St. Vincent Millay said that "childhood is the kingdom where nobody
dies" (1934/1969), and Becker refers to adults' "ever-present fear of death"
as well as to their "utter obliviousness to this fear" (1973, p. 17). If adults
cannot confront and make peace with their own fears about the end of
life, how can they possibly consider the reality of death in the lives of
children? Many adults refrain from discussing death with children because of their own anxiety about the subject. In addition, they may inadvertently want to avoid distressing the child and having to respond to
questions for which they have no answers. Many parents and other adults
find it easier to talk to children about sex than about death. As in both
Wordsworth's and Millay's eras, discussion about death today still represents a powerful taboo.

This taboo contradicts the reality of the contemporary child's life,
however, since most children, through television, view hundreds of
deaths, both real and fictionalized, in the daily course of watching car-

3

toons, news, and G/PG-rated dramatizations and movies. Images of all types of deaths make imprints on the minds and psyches of the watching children, but different children respond differently to what they see and hear. Does familiarity bring desensitization as to death and/or easy acceptance of it? Obviously, children must take a huge leap from knowing that death occurs to fantasy creatures on television to awareness that it occurs to everyone, including family members, and that in real life, unlike on television, the dead person does not return.

CHILDREN'S PROGRESSION TOWARD MATURE UNDERSTANDING ABOUT DEATH

The necessary truth about death that we all eventually come to know is that it is irreversible, inevitable, and universal. Most children achieve this knowledge by approximately 7 or 8 years of age due to their normal cognitive development and life experience. Some may achieve a mature conception at younger ages (Wass & Stillion, 1988), if they have had experience with the death of an animal (Yalom, 1980) or if they have early experience with the death of a family member (Kane, 1979). For most children, the natural evolution of their ability to think rationally leads gradually to a mature understanding about death.

Cognitive Development: From Immaturity to Conceptual Understanding

Although Jean Piaget's work did not specifically address children's understanding about death, his theories concerning the development of children's thinking can be applied to this topic. I will focus on the three major developmental phases identified by Piaget and connect these with children's ideas about death in each phase.

The Young Child: Ages 2–7; Piaget's Preoperational Stage

According to Piaget, the preschooler tends toward magical thinking and egocentricity. He/she does not differentiate between thoughts and deeds, and therefore a young boy of this age may believe, when his sister dies suddenly in an accident, that his anger toward her caused her death (Kaplan & Joslin, 1993). The young child also cannot comprehend the irreversibility of death, and at this age may think that if he screams loudly enough he can awaken his deceased father, who he believes is sleeping (Saravay, 1991). Even when the young child has witnessed a burial he/she may not realize that the dead body in the casket no longer feels anything nor performs its usual activities. The child may wonder how the dead man can breathe with dirt on him and how he will go to the bathroom (Fox, 1985). A child in the movie *My Girl* insisted on putting eye glasses on her deceased friend in the casket so that he could see!

These vignettes all relate to Piaget's preoperational stage (ages 2–7), during which the child's thinking is concrete (literal) and may distort reality to conform to his/her idiosyncratic understanding, despite logical contradictions. Piaget refers to this type of thinking as "egocentric" since the child believes that everyone else sees the world as he/she sees it.

The work of Maria Nagy (1948) continues to be widely quoted with regard to her study and identification of three stages in children's perceptions of death. Nagy's first stage (ages 3–5) corresponds roughly to Piaget's preoperational phase. Nagy found that children at this age deny that death is a final event; they consider the state of death as temporary and reversible. Therefore, they wonder and may ask about when their dead father is coming home, even though they viewed his body in the casket at the wake. I will discuss the implications of these immature beliefs later in the chapter with respect to children's grieving. Before proceeding, however, I must caution against taking these age references too literally. Development is an individual process that proceeds generally as outlined, but—as with all matters human—individual variations are the rule. Furthermore, the lack of synchrony between ages in Nagy's and Piaget's stages should not cause serious concern. The main point is that development progresses gradually from immature to mature understanding about death.

The Latency-Age (Elementary-School-Age) Child: Ages 7–11; Piaget's Concrete Operational Stage

Reduced egocentricity and improved capacity for reasoning contribute to the progressive realization among children of elementary school age that death is irreversible. Fox states that "latency youngsters begin to know that dead is dead and that at some time each of us will die. However, their own increasing sense of power and control make it difficult for them to believe such a thing could happen to *them*" (1985, p. 11; emphasis in original). Solnit, referring to this realization, states that "the concept that inevitably each of us has to die becomes a threatening, unpleasant, ineffable quality of the *future*. Most children *are able to lay aside this oppressive sense of inevitability*, denying the feel of it because it is so far off. . . . [T]he juices of life and the joy of living help block out the fearful, painful conviction about death" (1983, p. 4; emphasis added). The elementary-school-age child's improved understanding of time permits this conceptualization about the "future" as a remote, distant expectation.

Piaget notes increased capacity for reasoning and the ability to organize sequentially and count backwards (subtract) during the period from
6 to 8 years (Piaget, 1955, 1972). The fact that children are learning to
read and use language further signals their developing cognitive abilities.

This development not only facilitates mastery of reading, writing,
and arithmetic, it also opens the child's thinking to more accurate compre-
hension of the mysteries of life and death. Whereas the concept of the
body and the spirit confuses the preschool child, who puzzles about how
the deceased can simultaneously be in heaven and in a grave at the
cemetery (Saravay, 1991), children of 9 or 10 can dramatize a puppet play
that expresses the wish to visit their parents in heaven, despite knowing
clearly that they are buried in a cemetery (Bluestone, 1999).

The elementary-school-age child knows that death is final and that
it will happen to everybody "sometime." However, children of this age
believe that death happens primarily to the elderly and weak who cannot
run fast enough to escape the pursuing "ghost, angel, or space creature"
who will cause their death (Fox, 1985; Nagy, 1948); 6- to 8-year-olds,
therefore, believe that young people their age usually do not die because
they can run fast! According to Lonetto, "death for the child from six to
eight years old is personified, externalized, and can be avoided if seen
in time. Death is not yet finalized; rather, it assumes various external
forms (skeletons, ghosts, the death-man)" (1980, p. 100). By 9 or 10 years
of age children develop a more realistic perception.

The Prepubertal Child: Ages 9–12;
Bordering on Piaget's Formal Operational Stage

"The mental development of the child appears as a succession of three
great periods. Each of these extends the preceding period, reconstructs it
on a new level, and later surpasses it to an ever greater degree" (Piaget &
Inhelder, 1969, p. 152). Thus, as we consider Piaget's third and "final"
stage of cognitive development, that of formal operations, we note the
building on preceding stages in addition to the ultimate spurt into the
complex arena of mature thought and understanding.

Piaget's stage of formal operations usually begins around age 11 or
12, when the youngster's thinking becomes truly logical, able to handle
many variables at once, and capable of dealing with abstractions and
hypotheses. Many authorities on the topic of children's understanding
about death (Anthony, 1971; Grollman, 1967; Kastenbaum, 1967; Lonetto,
1980; Nagy, 1948; Wolfelt, 1983) believe that children acquire a realistic
perception of the finality and irreversibility of death by age 9 or 10. Speece
and Brent (1996) in an examination of more than 100 studies of children's
understanding of death conclude that most studies have found that by 7

years of age most children have achieved a mature understanding. This is quite a bit earlier than Piaget's designation of the inception of formal thought "around the age of eleven or twelve" (1968, p. 63). Yet, perhaps it attests to the complexity of death itself—connecting both "concrete" elements, that is, a body that no longer functions (comprehensible to the 7- and 8-year-old), and the "abstract," that is, a notion of spirituality and life after death (understood by children older than 10). In Lonetto's (1980) study of children's drawings at different ages, an intriguing shift to the representation of death in abstract terms among 12-years-olds was found. They portrayed death with black crayon markings that they described as "darkness." Lonetto states that "children from nine to twelve years old seem capable not only of perceiving death as biological, universal, and inevitable, but of coming to an appreciation of the abstract nature of death, and of describing the feelings generated by this quality. This complex recognition pattern associated with death is joined by an emerging belief in the mortality of the self, but for these children death is far off in the future and remains in the domain of the aged" (1980, p. 157).

CHILDREN'S EMOTIONAL RESPONSES TO DEATH

What is the implication of children's cognitive development on their ability to mourn the death of a loved one? Can children grieve, and, if so, how do they grieve? Is children's grieving different from that of adults? What factors other than the child's age and level of cognitive development impact on the nature of the child's emotional response to death? This chapter (and others in this book) will explore these questions in detail, after first defining and distinguishing between the concepts of grief, mourning, and bereavement. Obviously, these terms all relate to loss following death, but they are not synonyms, even though the general public and some professionals use them interchangeably.

Bereavement

This term refers to the status of the individual who has suffered a loss and who may be experiencing psychological, social, and physical stress because a meaningful person has died; the term does not, however, spell out the precise nature of that stress (Kastenbaum, 1997). Corr, Nabe, and Corr (2000, p. 212) point out that three elements are essential in all bereavement: "1) a relationship with some person or thing that is valued; 2) the loss—ending, termination, separation—of that relationship; and 3) a survivor deprived by the loss."

Grief

Bowlby describes grief as "the sequence of subjective states that follow loss and accompany mourning" (1960, p. 11). Wolfelt points out that grief is a process, rather than a specific emotion like fear or sadness; it can be expressed by a variety of thoughts, emotions, and behaviors (1983, p. 26). A simple definition is that "grief is the reaction to loss" (Corr, Nabe, & Corr, 2000). These reactions can occur in feelings, in physical sensations, in cognitions, and in behaviors (Worden, 1991).

Mourning

The psychoanalytic definition of mourning describes it as "the mental work following the loss of a love object through death" (Furman, 1974, p. 34, quoting S. Freud, 1915/1954). This "mental work," often called "grief work," involves the "painful, gradual process of detaching libido from an internal image" (A. Freud, 1965, p. 67), thereby freeing libidinal energy for new relationships. This theoretical model of grief *requires disengagement from attachment to the deceased* in order for the grief to be resolved. The psychoanalytical definition of mourning, therefore, encompasses not only the initial grief reaction to the loss but also the future resolution of that grief (Grossberg & Crandall, 1978). In order for mourning to be resolved, according to Krueger, the bereaved person must comprehend the "significance, seriousness, permanence, and irreversibility" of his/her loss (1983, p. 590). In other words, in addition to feeling typical grief reactions such as sadness and anger, the individual must also come to understand that the deceased person will never return but that life can be meaningful nonetheless. This adaptation or acceptance to the irrevocable loss is referred to by Bowlby as "relinquishing the object" (1960, p. 11).

An alternative model of bereavement (Klass, Silvermen, & Nickman, 1996) that has received growing attention in the literature emphasizes the mourner's *continuing bonds* with the deceased. This approach differs drastically from models that posit disengagement and relinquishment as a goal of grief resolution. In contrast, in this view "it is normative for mourners to maintain a connection with the deceased" (p. 18) and this connection *continues throughout the life of the mourner.*

Can Children Mourn?

This question has been asked and debated in the literature, with responses depending on both the definition of mourning and on the specific theoretical framework of the respondent. If one's definition of mourning requires mature awareness regarding the finality of death, as stated above

by Krueger (1983), a positive response would not be possible until prepu-
berty. This is the position of Nagera (1970). At the other extreme, Bowlby
argues forcefully for the existence of grief and mourning in even very
young children when they are separated from their mothers. Quoting
Robertson's 10-year study of children ages 18–24 months who experienced
maternal separation, Bowlby presents the following position:

> If a child is taken from his mother's care at this age, when he is so
> possessively and passionately attached to her, it is indeed as if his world
> has been shattered. His intense need of her is unsatisfied, and the frustra-
> tion and longing may send him frantic with grief. It takes an exercise of
> imagination to sense the intensity of this distress. *He is overwhelmed as*
> *any adult who has lost a beloved person by death.* To the child of two with
> his lack of understanding and complete inability to tolerate frustration,
> it is really as if his mother had died. *He does not know death, but only*
> *absence;* and if the only person who can satisfy his imperative need is
> absent, *she might as well be dead.* (1960, p. 15, quoting Robertson, 1953;
> emphasis added)

Sigmund Freud, toward the end of his life, in discussing the responses
of young children to their mothers' absences, referred to their crying and
facial expressions as evidence of both anxiety and pain. Freud stated,
with regard to the distressed child, "it cannot as yet distinguish between
temporary absence and permanent loss. As soon as it loses sight of its
mother, it behaves as if it were never going to see her again" (1926/
1959, p. 169). These desperate reactions point to the child's total lack of
understanding that the mother continues to exist when she goes away
(object constancy). They also indicate the child's lack of a "mental representation" (memory) of the mother that can be evoked in her absence.
The beginning stage of object constancy usually occurs in the second half
of the first year of life, but the child's capacity to recall the mother's image
in her absence is ephemeral until completion of M. Mahler's rapproche-
ment stage at around 25 months of age (Furman, 1974; Masur, 1991).

It seems only logical that the child must have a clear idea about the
separate, independent existence of a person before the child can grieve
the loss of that person after his/her death. A. Freud (1960) maintains that
the child can mourn only when he/she has developed reality testing and
object constancy, and Furman (1974) agrees with this position.

While it is indisputable that even very young children react strongly
to the absence and loss of a meaningful person and that they show their
reactions in conformity with Bowlby's (1960) stages of protest, despair,
and detachment, it seems to me inaccurate to refer to these responses as
"mourning" when the young child understands neither the finality of the
loss not its significance in his/her life. Thus, feelings of sadness, rage,

and longing following the loss of a significant person may qualify as *grief reactions* but, without mature understanding of the finality and meaning of that loss, cannot accurately be termed as "mourning," in my view.

Although this may appear to be semantic hairsplitting, the implications for the grief counselor or therapist point to the necessity of respecting children's feelings without expecting more of the child than developmentally appropriate. Thus, the question "Can children mourn?" should ask instead, "Can children grieve?," to which an unqualified affirmative response can be given.

Does the Expression "Relinquishing the Object" Apply to Children—or Is the Concept of "Continuing Bonds" More Relevant?

The assumption that mourning can be "resolved" and that this resolution involves "decathecting" or "relinquishing" emotional investment in the deceased presents a challenge when applied to children's mourning. Some child therapists (Buchsbaum, 1987; Nagera, 1970; Wolfenstein, 1969) have pointed to children's ongoing psychological need to hold onto their relationship with their parents in order to successfully complete the tasks of development. Such a fantasized relationship with a deceased parent obviously hinders any "relinquishing" of libido from that fantasy until the adolescent stage has been completed. Nagera states that "the evidence seems to point to the fact that the latency child strongly cathects a fantasy life where the lost object may be seen as alive and at times as ideal" (1970, p. 381). This explains the position of Nagera and Wolfenstein that mourning is not possible until "detachment from parental figures has taken place in adolescence" (Nagera, 1970, p. 362).

A different view about childhood grief of Baker, Sedney, and Gross (1992) conceptualizes it as a series of psychological tasks that must be accomplished over time. In these authors' views, decathexis, or detachment, is not essential to the mourning process since they found that many children maintain an internal attachment to the mental image of the lost person that serves an important function in terms of the child's and later the adult's development. This is consistent with the views of Klass et al. (1996), as discussed previously.

Therefore, in my opinion, decathexis/detachment and "relinquishing the object" are not appropriate concepts to describe the mourning of children. While a child may certainly grieve the absence of the person who died and long to be with that person, these feelings need not interfere with the child's developmental course. In fact, my own experience as a bereavement counselor supports the convincing reports in the literature that an ongoing attachment relationship after the death of a loved person can help children withstand and overcome many stresses, as illustrated in the following examples.

CASE VIGNETTES

The Grief of a 6-Year-Old

This example comes from Krementz's *How It Feels When a Parent Dies* (1981/1991, pp. 107–110). A 7-year-old girl describes the events and her feelings around the sudden death of her father in a car accident 7 months prior to the interview. The child, Gail, discusses what she and her 3-year-old brother were told about the accident and about the family's funeral and memorial service. I will comment on aspects of the child's report that demonstrate both her developmental stage and that of her younger brother, especially with regard to their expressions of grief.

In describing the graveside service, Gail mentioned the number, color, type, and significance of flowers that the family put on the coffin. It was important to her that each family member place a rose on the coffin. Gail then spoke of "waving goodbye to Daddy," a concrete familiar activity that clearly symbolizes leave-taking. Later, when the family returned to their home and had another memorial service (since the funeral had occurred out of state), this confused Gail because she thought her father had "died again" and she did not like it. She also did not understand the explanation that crying would help people feel better. Crying made *her* feel very sad!

Gail reported that her brother (age 3) still believes that their father is "away" and that he is going to come back. When they returned home after a vacation, Gail's brother thought their father would be in the house waiting for them. Gail herself thinks her father is an angel in heaven, watching her from overhead.

Gail has many happy memories of times she shared with her father. She does not like to talk about him to other people, however, because she is afraid of being treated differently; and she thinks her friends might tease her.

Gail likes to sit in her father's chair on Saturday mornings. At these times she feels her father is out working and that he may come back. She does not like to have other people sit in his chair.

Comment

This child's reactions and those of her younger brother demonstrate the inability of the younger child to comprehend the finality of his father's death, and some evidence of more mature understanding on the part of the 7-year-old. The fact that Gail thinks of her father as an angel in heaven and yet at other times when sitting in his chair expects him to come home points to her *still* incomplete understanding about the irreversibility of his death. Also, she wants him to return. The fact that the interview occurred only 7 months after the death may account for some of Gail's denial. She is actively remembering her father and is very aware of missing him.

The Grief of a 9-Year-Old

Also from Krementz (1981/1991, pp. 29–35), this example involves another sudden death of a father in a car crash. Peggy, interviewed at age 11, was the eldest of three girls when her father died. She describes the physical sensations of her chest hurting as if someone had hit her when she learned of her father's death. She recalls screaming to "let all the anger out" and wanting to be left alone. Peggy went to the funeral but not to the burial. She says now that she is older she likes to visit the cemetery. She states, "I don't think I can grasp the fact that my father is really lying there underneath the ground. I think of him more as a ghost-like person floating around everywhere. *And I do keep thinking that maybe one day he'll come back*" (emphasis added).

Comment

Although 11 years of age when the interview was conducted, Peggy was still clinging to the possibility that her father's death was not final. This wish for reunion may be particularly strong among survivors of sudden death, who do not have the opportunities for anticipatory grieving as occurs in situations of terminal illness or disability preceding death. An element of this child's report that resembles the previous example and that may be especially vivid among latency-age children is the dislike of discussing the parent's death with peers because of the fear of being pitied.

The Grief of a 12-Year-Old

I selected another case example from Krementz (1981/1991, pp. 1–7) because it also involves a girl whose father died suddenly. Laurie, age 12, wrote about her father's death in a plane crash and about her reactions with regard to her peers, her mother, and her younger brother. Like the children in the previous examples, Laurie finds it hard to believe her father really died, and she would like to know all the details about why the plane crash occurred. She is quite protective of her mother, however, and hesitates to ask questions because of her fear of causing her mother any pain. Laurie has rationalized her father's sudden death as better than if he had to endure pain and suffering. She does not like to have people talk to her about her father, because it "makes her feel worse." She thinks about what should be done with her father's ashes and hopes that they will be scattered at her grandmother's farm, rather than in the church cemetery, because at the farm she would not have "to go visit him, so everything would be easier." Laurie is somewhat jealous of her younger brother, who has received special attention from his hockey coach since their father's death; however, she has been able to verbalize her feelings to her mother, who has been sensitive to her needs.

Comment

This example shares many similarities with the previous two and does not, in the brief vignette, reveal distinct progression toward mature understanding about death in the older child. Laurie exhibits a protective attitude toward her mother and seems to want her companionship. This may reflect either her age-appropriate preteen development or her concern about her mother's safety. Often children who have lost one parent worry about the possibility of losing the other.

Even 3 years later, Peggy wants to avoid reminders about her father's death. Although convinced of its reality, she still wishes that his ashes were not buried in the nearby cemetery, because she then has to visit it and, of necessity, think about her father's absence.

IS CHILDREN'S GRIEF DIFFERENT FROM THAT OF ADULTS?

The case vignettes, professional literature, and clinical experience with bereaved children all attest to some marked differences, as well as to some similarities, between the grief of children and that of adults. Wolfelt reminds us that "grief does not focus on one's ability to 'understand,' but instead upon one's ability to 'feel.' Therefore any child mature enough to love is mature enough to grieve" (1983, p. 20).

Denial, anger, guilt, sadness, and longing are felt by young and old alike in response to the loss of a loved person. Adults, who expect children to have many of the same feelings they themselves experience at a time of bereavement, may be able to help the children realize that these feelings are justified. It is even more important, however, for adults to recognize that most children have *limited ability to verbalize their feelings*, as well as very *limited capacity to tolerate the pain* generated by open recognition of their loss. Thus, in the vignettes, we note the children's various attempts to avoid talking about their losses.

We also note in the vignettes the children's *fear of being "different" from their peers with regard to having a deceased parent*. Unlike adults, who may obtain solace and comfort from the condolences of their friends, children *dread* this process, and frequently their peers feel equally uncomfortable at the prospect of having to speak to a bereaved friend. They don't know what to say, and they are afraid that their friend or they themselves will start crying. Children in latency and adolescence are trying hard to gain control over their feelings, so they resist and feel uncomfortable with an invitation to openly express their emotions. Furman (1974) comments that children consider crying babyish, so they may do their crying in private. The child's "short sadness span" (Wolfenstein, 1966) reflects the low capacity to tolerate acute pain for long periods, characteristic of childhood. Rando (1988/1991) explains that a child may manifest grief on an intermittent basis for many years in an approach–avoidance cycle with regard to painful feelings.

Children often use play as an escape from their pain and as a way to gain mastery over their complex and confused feelings about the death. Insofar as play is the language of childhood, children can deal with their feelings through play in a displaced, disguised manner. The trained play therapist understands and knows how to communicate in this symbolic language and, through the use of play therapy, can help the child work through his/her painful feelings. The purpose of this book is to demonstrate various techniques of play therapy that can help bereaved children with their grief.

In summary, the following considerations serve to differentiate the grief of children from that of adults:

1. Children's immature cognitive development interferes with their understanding about the irreversibility, universality, and inevitability of death.
2. Children have a limited capacity to tolerate emotional pain.
3. Children have limited ability to verbalize their feelings.
4. Children are sensitive about "being different" from their peers.
5. Children are able to express their feelings in play therapy.

RELIGIOUS/CULTURAL INFLUENCES ON CHILDREN'S CONCEPTIONS OF DEATH

Any analysis of a child's understanding about death must include not only the individual factors related to the child's cognitive and emotional development but also the influences impacting on the child that emanate from the cultural and religious beliefs in the child's home environment.

This will be discussed more fully in Chapter 2. A psychosocial assessment of the child examines both internal and external elements contributing to the child's understanding about death. McGoldrick et al. warn that "clinicians should be careful about definitions of 'normality' in assessing families' responses to death, [since] the manner of, as well as the length of time assumed normal for mourning differs greatly from culture to culture" (1991, pp. 176–177). They further point out that "cultures differ in major ways about public versus private expressions of grief" (1991, p. 178). Because of these differences, it behooves therapists to try to find out from a family member "what its members believe about the nature of death, the rituals that should surround it, and the expectations about afterlife" (p. 178). The child absorbs and interprets these beliefs and customs, questioning what is not clear, and supplying his/her own answers when the responses to his/her questions are vague and incomprehensible.

The Appendix to this book lists resources for information about the different religious practices and about mourning observances in different cultures. It is not practical to attempt a comprehensive overview of various religions and cultures here. However, grief counselors and therapists working with bereaved children must learn about the typical practices in the cultural and religious group of the bereaved child's family. It is especially important to know about whether the children are expected to participate in the formal and informal rituals of grieving or whether the children are excluded from these due to the belief that involving the children would be upsetting to them. Most thanatologists believe that it assists the child's grieving when he/she is included in the funeral and other rituals associated with the death of a loved one (Rando, 1988/1991; Wolfelt, 1983; Kastenbaum, 1997). When children are told in advance about what to expect and are given the opportunity to decide whether or not to participate, many elect to do so. Rando points out that rituals are well suited to children, since they are fascinated by these types of behaviors (1988/1991, p. 216). Of course, if there is an open casket at the funeral, the child must be prepared in advance for this and assured that the family will have some private time to say their farewells to the deceased. James Agee's Pulitzer Prize–winning novel *A Death in the Family* contains a moving, detailed account of a 5-year-old's viewing of his dead father at the wake, during which time the child came to synthesize his observations about his father's appearance in the casket with his first true understanding of the meaning of the word "dead" (1938/1969, pp. 288–298).

Children's accounts about attending wakes and funerals often project their ambivalence about the death. They prefer to remember their loved one when alive, but they also want to be included in the services. A

15-year-old boy in Krementz's book, whose mother died when he was 9, reflects as follows:

> The night before the funeral we all went to the funeral parlor, and I spent a lot of time right next to her coffin. She was wearing a white dress, but that's all I remember. I remember her more when she was alive because *I think my mind wants to remember her alive rather then dead.* I'm glad, though, that I got a chance to get a last look at her. I drew a picture for her and wrote a little note on it, asking her to wait in heaven for all of us. I gave it to daddy to put in her coffin with her, and even though she was dead, I like to think that she got that last message from me. (in Krementz, 1981/1991, p. 54; emphasis added)

Children differ in their feelings about how they want to remember their deceased relative, but the idea of avoidance of the cemetery is a theme that repeats in several children's accounts in Krementz's book. A 16-year-old Puerto Rican girl whose mother died when she was 11 states:

> I'm not sold on going to the cemetery. That's the worst place to remember her because I associate it with putting her into the ground. Why would I want to remember that part? My aunt is very religious and she's really into going to the cemetery and lighting candles in church and all that stuff. I don't think anybody should have to go the cemetery. I can't see it. I think the most vivid thing in a person's mind should be the happy moments, and when you visit the grave, you're left with the sad parts. ... I *cannot* relate to my mother by looking at her tombstone. It's hard to imagine there's a body underneath the ground even if I know it's there. The body's not that important to me. It's the soul that counts, and once that's gone, forget it. I wish my mother had been cremated. (in Krementz, 1981/1991, pp. 48–49; emphasis in original)

This child clearly has attained a mature understanding of death, and she appears to have accepted the finality of her loss while able to appreciate and remember "the happy moments" of her mother's life.

REFERENCES

Agee, J. (1969). *A death in the family.* New York: Bantam. (Original work published 1938)

Anthony, S. (1971). *The discovery of death in childhood and after.* London: Penguin.

Baker, J. E., Sedney, M. A., & Gross, E. (1992). Psychological tasks for bereaved children. *American Journal of Orthopsychiatry, 62*(1), 105–116.

Becker, E. (1973). *The denial of death.* New York: Free Press.

Bluestone, J. (1999). School-based peer therapy to facilitate mourning in latency-age children following sudden parental death: Cases of Joan, age 10½, and Roberta age 9½, with follow-up 8 years later. In N. B. Webb (Ed.), *Play therapy with children in crisis* (2nd ed.): *Individual, group, and family treatment* (pp. 225–251). New York: Guilford Press.

Bowlby, J. (1960). Grief and mourning in infancy and early childhood. *Psychoanalytic Study of the Child, 15,* 9–52.

Buchsbaum, B. C. (1987). Remembering a parent who has died: A developmental perspective. *Annual of Psychoanalysis, 15,* 99–112.

Corr, C. A., Nabe, C. M., & Corr, D. M. (2000). *Death and dying, life and living.* Belmont, CA: Wadsworth.

Fox, S. S. (1985). *Good grief: Helping groups of children when a friend dies.* Boston: New England Association for the Education of Young Children.

Freud, A. (1960). Discussion of Dr. John Bowlby's paper. *Psychoanalytic Study of the Child, 15,* 53–62.

Freud, A. (1965). *Normality and pathology in childhood.* New York: International Universities Press.

Freud, S. (1954). Mourning and melancholia. In *Standard Edition* (Vol. 14, pp. 237–258). London: Hogarth Press. (Original work published 1915)

Freud, S. (1959). Inhibitions, symptoms and anxiety. In *Standard Edition* (Vol. 20, pp. 77–175). London: Hogarth Press. (Original work published 1926)

Furman, E. (1974). *A child's parent dies.* New Haven, CT: Yale University Press.

Grollman, E. (Ed.). (1967). *Explaining death to children.* Boston: Beacon Press.

Grossberg, S. H., & Crandall, L. (1978). Father loss and father absence in preschool children. *Clinical Social Work Journal, 6*(2), 123–134.

Kane, B. (1979). Children's concepts of death. *Journal of Genetic Psychology, 134,* 141–153.

Kaplan, C. P., & Joslin, H. (1993). Accidental sibling death: Case of Peter, age 6. In N. B. Webb (Ed.), *Helping bereaved children: A handbook for practitioners* (pp. 118–136). New York: Guilford Press.

Kastenbaum, R. J. (1967). The child's understanding of death: How does it develop? In E. Grollman (Ed.), *Explaining death to children* (pp. 89–109). Boston: Beacon Press.

Kastenbaum, R. J. (1997). *Death, society, and human experience* (7th ed.). NewYork: Merrill.

Klass, D., Silverman, P. R., & Nickman, S. L. (1996). *Continuing bonds: New understandings of grief.* Washington, DC: Taylor & Francis.

Krementz, J. (1991). *How it feels when a parent dies.* New York: Knopf. (Original work published 1981)

Krueger, D. W. (1983). Childhood parent loss: Developmental impact and adult psychopathology. *American Journal of Psychotherapy, 37*(4), 582–592.

Lonetto, R. (1980). *Children's conceptions of death.* New York: Springer.

Masur, C. (1991). The crisis of early maternal loss: Unresolved grief of 6-year-old Chris in foster care. In N. B. Webb (Ed.), *Play therapy with children in crisis: A casebook for practitioners* (pp. 164–176). New York: Guilford Press.

McGoldrick, M., Almeida, R., Hines, P. M., Garcia-Preto, N., Rosen, E., & Lee, E. (1991). Mourning in different cultures. In F. Walsh & M. McGoldrick (Eds.), *Living beyond loss: Death in the family* (pp. 176–206). New York: Norton.

Millay, E. St. V. (1969). Childhood is the kingdom where nobody dies. In *Edna St. Vincent Millay collected lyrics* (p. 203). New York: Harper & Row. (Original work published 1934)

Nagera, H. (1970). Children's reactions to the death of important objects: A developmental approach. *Psychoanalytic Study of the Child, 25,* 360–400.

Nagy, M. (1948). The child's theories concerning death. *Journal of Genetic Psychology, 73,* 3–27.

Piaget, J. (1955). *The child's construction of reality.* New York: Basic Books.

Piaget, J. (1968). *Six psychological studies.* New York: Vintage Books.

Piaget, J. (1972). Intellectual evolution from adolescent to childhood. *Human Development, 15,* 1–12.

Piaget, J., & Inhelder, B. (1969). *The psychology of the child.* New York: Basic Books.

Rando, T. A. (1991). *How to go on living when someone you love dies.* New York: Bantam. (Original work published 1988)

Robertson, J. (1953). Some responses of young children to the loss of maternalcare. *Nursing Times, 49,* 382–389.

Saravay, B. (1991). Short-term play therapy with two preschool brothers following sudden paternal death. In N. B. Webb (Ed.), *Play therapy with children in crisis: A casebook for practitioners* (pp. 177–201). New York: Guilford Press.

Solnit, A. J. (1983). Changing perspectives: Preparing for life or death. In J. E. Schowalter, P. R. Patterson, M. Tallmer, A. H. Kutscher, S. V. Gullo, & D. Peretz (Eds.), *The child and death* (pp. 4–18). New York: Columbia University Press.

Speece, M. W., & Brent, S. B. (1996). The development of children's understanding of death. In C. A. Corr & D. M. Corr (Eds.), *Handbook of childhood death and bereavement* (pp. 29–49). New York: Springer.

Wass, H., & Stillion, J. (1988). Dying in the lives of children. In H. Wass, F. Berardo, & R. Neimeyer (Eds.), *Dying: Facing the facts* (pp. 201–228). Washington, DC: Hemisphere.

Wolfelt, A. (1983). *Helping children cope with grief.* Muncie, IN: Accelerated Development.

Wolfenstein, M. (1966). How is mourning possible? *Psychoanalytic Study of the Child, 21,* 93–126.

Wolfenstein, M. (1969). Loss, rage and repetition. *Psychoanalytic Study of the Child, 24,* 432–460.

Worden, J. W. (1991). *Grief counseling and grief therapy: A handbook for the mental health practitioner* (2nd ed.). New York: Springer.

Wordsworth, W. (1928). Now we are seven. In *The complete poetical works of William Wordsworth.* London: Macmillan. (Original work published 1798)

Yalom, I. D. (1980). *Existential psychotherapy.* New York: Basic Books.

2

✖

Assessment of the Bereaved Child

NANCY BOYD WEBB

Thanatologists agree that expressions of grief take many forms and that its duration varies (Wolfelt, 1983; Fox, 1985; Rando, 1988/1991) depending on individual, cultural/religious, and circumstantial factors. How, then, do we determine when a bereaved child's grief response is progressing on a "normal" course, and when does the child's reaction suggest the need for referral and assessment by a trained mental health professional? This question begs for a precise formula, yet its answer depends on the complex interplay among factors related to the child, the circumstances of the death, and the ability of the concerned adult to weigh these variables and arrive at a decision.

This chapter tackles the thorny question about "normal" and "pathological," or "disabling," grief as it applies to children, and offers some guidelines about when a professional assessment would be appropriate. Various therapeutic approaches helpful for bereaved children are outlined in Part IV of this book, as are the qualifications of the therapist or grief counselor who works with bereaved children.

DISTINGUISHING BETWEEN "NORMAL" AND "DISABLING" GRIEF

Granted the generous leeway for individual variability in both the nature and duration of grieving, how can we determine when the bounds of "normal" grief have trespassed into the dangerous territory of "disabling" grief? Furthermore, given the distinctions between adult and children's grief, as outlined in Chapter 1, how relevant is the literature on adult grieving to the normal and pathological assessment of children's grief? Is it helpful or pejorative to use the term "disabling" when referring to responses to a death that appear to greatly exceed the range, duration, or intensity of expression considered appropriate in a given situation? I will begin with the latter question.

Terminology

Lindemann's landmark article on the symptomatology and management of acute grief spelled out in great detail the "normal" grief reactions following traumatic experiences such as war or disastrous fire, and contrasted these with delayed or distorted responses, considered "morbid" or "pathological" (1944; reprinted in Parad, 1965, pp. 8–16). In studying 101 relatives and survivors of the Coconut Grove fire in Boston, and members of the armed forces, Lindemann concluded:

1. Acute grief is a definite syndrome with psychological and somatic symptomatology.
2. This syndrome may appear immediately after a crisis; it may be delayed; it may be exaggerated or apparently absent.
3. In place of the typical syndrome, there may appear distorted pictures, each of which represents one special aspect of the grief syndrome.
4. By use of appropriate techniques, these distorted pictures can be successfully transformed into a normal grief reaction with resolution. (1944; reprinted in Parad, 1965, p. 7)

I will not review Lindemann's work in detail here since it did not focus specifically on children's grief nor did it distinguish between various forms of "acute" grief. However, Lindemann's designation of delayed or distorted grief reactions does seem applicable to children's grief despite his unfortunate labeling of these responses as "morbid." Lindemann emphasized that "not only over-reactions, but under-reactions of the bereaved, must be given attention because delayed responses may occur at unpredictable moments and the dangerous distortions of the grief reaction, not conspicuous at first, may be quite destructive later" (1944; reprinted in Parad, 1965, p. 18). Rando refers to a category of grief she terms "unresolved grief," and within this group of responses she includes absent grief, inhibited grief, delayed grief, distorted grief, chronic grief, and unanticipated grief (1988/1991, pp. 81–84). Several cases in this book describe children who manifest various forms of unresolved grief. Indeed, one might propose that "absent," "inhibited," and "delayed" grief may be the *norm* for children because of their age-appropriate inability to bear the pain of extended grief.

Bowlby, in contrast to both Lindemann and Rando, focuses on the impact of loss in childhood. He believes that separation or death of a parent during the years of early childhood may predispose the individual to "unfavorable personality development" that leads to future psychiatric illness (1963, p. 500). Bowlby's views about the impact of loss on subsequent grief present a rationale about terminology that may be applicable here:

> If the experience of loss is likened to the experience of being wounded or being burned, the processes of mourning that follow loss can be likened to the processes of healing that follow a wound or burn. Such healing processes, we know, may take a course which in time leads to full, or nearly full, function being restored; or they may on the contrary, take one of many courses each of which has as its outcome an impairment of function of greater or less degree. In the same way, processes of mourning may take a favorable course that leads in time to restoration of function, namely to a renewal of the capacity to make and maintain love relationships, or they may take a course that leaves this function impaired in greater or less degree. *Just as the terms healthy and pathological are applicable to the different course taken by healing processes, so may they be applied to the different courses run by mourning processes.* (1963, p. 501; emphasis added)

With due respect to Bowlby's concern about the possible devastating effects of separation and loss in early childhood, it is reassuring to note his opinion that "not every child who experiences either permanent or temporary loss grows up to be a disturbed person" (1963, p. 527). This book is dedicated to the process of helping bereaved children so that their development can proceed despite their loss.

What, then, would be an accurate term to describe harmful grief when referring to a child? Any judgment about the appropriateness of a grief response always considers temporal factors related to the relative recency of the death. Since many, if not most, children avoid facing their upsetting feelings and can tolerate discomfort in only small doses, the terms "unresolved," "absent," or "delayed" grief do not seem apt for describing children's grief. One must expect children's grief to require the passage of time before expression and eventual resolution. Therefore, timeliness is not a useful consideration in evaluating children's grief.

Rather than the length of time of a child's grief reaction, it is the degree of intrusiveness into the child's life created by the grieving that must be evaluated. Specifically, we must determine the extent to which a child can carry out his/her usual activities and proceed with his/her developmental tasks despite the presence of grief reactions. When a child's social, emotional, or physical development shows signs of interference, his/her grief process can justifiably be considered "disabling," and our deliberate use of the term indicates that something is wrong. The grief has become all-encompassing and detrimental, instead of helping free the child to proceed with his/her life. The child is "stuck" and needs help which family members may be unable to provide. It is important to recognize and help such a struggling and blocked child so that, in Lindemann's words, "these distorted pictures *can be successfully transformed into a normal grief reaction with resolution*" (1944; reprinted in Parad, 1965, p. 7; emphasis added).

Although identifying a cluster of grief reactions as "disabling" may seem extreme and even pejorative, the result provides the avenue for professional intervention and avoids the unfortunate stance of joining the child's helplessness and hopelessness. Waiting for the child to "work it out" according to his/her individual timetable sounds respectful and logical, but such inaction also may fail the child who is floundering and even drowning in emotional crosscurrents. Use of the term "disabling grief" leads to preventative possibilities in the form of helping interventions. I prefer this term to others such as "unresolved" or "delayed" grief, which may inadvertently result in neglect of someone who truly needs and would benefit from timely professional intervention and assistance.

What, then, are the indicators that a child should be referred for an evaluation by a mental health professional, and what components will such an assessment include?

Indications for Professional Assessment

Grollman points out that the

> line of demarcation between "normal psychological aspects of bereavement" and "distorted mourning reactions" is thin indeed. The difference is not in symptom but in intensity. It is a *continued* denial of reality even many months after the funeral, or a *prolonged* bodily distress, or a *persistent* panic, or an *extended* guilt, or an *unceasing* idealization, or an *enduring* apathy and anxiety, or an *unceasing* hostile reaction to the deceased and to others. Each manifestation does not in itself determine a distorted grief reaction; it is only as it is viewed *by the professional* in the composition of the *total* formulation. (1967, p. 21; emphasis added)

Fox believes that "professional mental health services are indicated if there are questions about suicidal risk or if a child has been involved in some way in the death of another person" (1985, p. 17). Fox elaborates further regarding children who may require special assistance with the grieving. Referring to these as "vulnerable or troubled children," Fox identifies the following groups:

1. Children who themselves have a life-threatening or terminal illness.
2. Children who have already been identified as emotionally disturbed.
3. Children who are developmentally disabled and who may have difficulty understanding what has happened.
4. Children who remain "frozen" and in shock long after most grievers have returned to their usual daily activities. (1985, pp. 39–40)

In addition to identifying these groups of potentially vulnerable children, Fox enumerates some symptoms which she considers "red flags" suggesting the need for careful assessment of the grieving child. These "red flag" symptoms include the following:

- Suicidal hints
- Psychosomatic problems
- Difficulties with schoolwork
- Nightmares or sleep disorders
- Changes in eating patterns
- Temporary regressions

Fox clarifies that "none of these presentations suggests a formal diagnosis of emotional problems, but each is a possible indicator that the child's grief work may not be proceeding smoothly. Therefore, *each deserves the attention of someone who has been trained in the broad field of mental health so if intervention is indicated, it can begin promptly*" (1985, p. 42; emphasis added). Rando (1988/1991) wisely admonishes us that when there is a question, it is better to err on the side of going for professional help.

Symptoms of Depression

Many of the "red flag" behaviors noted by Fox and the distorted reactions listed by Grollman duplicate the clinical syndrome of depression as listed in the text revision of the fourth edition of the *Diagnostic and Statistical Manual of Mental Disorders* (DSM-IV-TR; American Psychiatric Association, 2000). See Table 2.1 for the precise diagnostic criteria for a major depressive episode, which Rapoport and Ismond (1990) state has been underdiagnosed in children. As indicated in the DSM-IV-TR criteria, there must be at least five of the symptoms present during the same 2-week period and this must represent a change from previous functioning. An important and possibly confusing consideration in identifying a child with "disabling" grief is the requirement in DSM-IV-TR that "the symptoms are

TABLE 2.1. DSM-IV-TR Criteria for Major Depressive Episode

A. Five or more of the following symptoms have been present during the same 2-week period and represent a change from previous functioning; at least one of the symptoms is either (1) depressed mood or (2) loss of interest or pleasure.

Note: Do not include symptoms that are clearly due to a general medical condition, or mood-incongruent delusions or hallucinations.
   (1) Depressed mood most of the day, nearly every day, as indicated by either subjective report (e.g., feels sad or empty) or observation by others (e.g., appears tearful). **Note:** In children and adolescents, can be irritable mood.
   (2) Markedly diminished interest or pleasure in all, or almost all, activities most of the day, nearly every day (as indicated by either subjective account or observation made by others).
   (3) Significant weight loss or weight gain when not dieting or weight gain (e.g., a change of more than 5% of body weight in a month), or decrease or increase in appetite nearly every day. **Note:** In children, consider failure to make expected weight gains.
   (4) Insomnia or hypersomnia nearly every day.
   (5) Psychomotor agitation or retardation nearly every day (observable by others, not merely subjective feelings of restlessness or being slowed down).
   (6) Fatigue or loss of energy nearly every day.
   (7) Feelings of worthlessness or excessive or inappropriate guilt (which may be delusional) nearly every day (not merely self-reproach or guilt about being sick).
   (8) Diminished ability to think or concentrate, or indecisiveness, nearly every day (either by subjective account or as observed by others).
   (9) Recurrent thoughts of death (not just fear of dying), recurrent suicidal ideation without a specific plan, or a suicide attempt or a specific plan for committing suicide.
B. The symptoms do not meet the criteria for a "Mixed Episode" (see DSM-IV-TR, p. 365).
C. The symptoms cause clinically significant distress or impairment in social, occupational, or other important areas of functioning.
D. The symptoms are not due to the direct pysiological effects of a substance (e.g., a drug of abuse, a medication) or a general medical condition (e.g., hypothyroidism).
E. The symptoms are not better accounted for by "Bereavement" (see DSM-IV-TR, p. 356), i.e., after the death a loved one the symptoms persist for longer than 2 months or are characterized by marked functional impairment, morbid preoccupation with worthlessness, suicidal ideation, psychotic symptoms, or psychomotor retardation.

Note. From American Psychiatric Association (2000, p. 356). Copyright 2000 by the American Psychiatric Association. Reprinted by permission.

not better accounted for by Bereavement, i.e., after the death of a loved one" (American Psychiatric Association, 2000, p. 356). The caveat implies that although some bereavement responses might duplicate many of the same symptoms as for a major depressive episode, if a loss has occurred, the symptoms are considered "secondary" to that; Rapoport and Ismond state that diagnostically "it is crucial . . . that the mood disturbance be primary and not secondary to some other disorder" (1990, p. 101). Although there is no diagnostic category for "complicated" or "disabling/ pathological" grief in DSM-IV-TR, it is clear that extensive overlapping exists between the term *depressed states* as used there and the term *disabling/pathological grief* as used by me. The designation of "Bereavement" in DSM-IV-TR clarifies that "some grieving individuals present with symptoms characteristic of a Major Depressive Episode (e.g., feelings of sadness and associated symptoms such as insomnia, poor appetite, and weight loss)" (American Psychiatric Association, 2000, p. 740).

As a child and family therapist, I am familiar with DSM and use it regularly in the assessment of clients who consult me with a variety of problems, some of which include bereavement. Several of my child clients have become bereaved unexpectedly during the course of my contact with them (see Chapters 3 and 4). I believe that all counselors who work with bereaved children would find it helpful to become knowledgeable about the DSM-IV-TR criteria for depression since they describe in detail many of the behaviors and responses that occur in grieving children, especially those whose grief has become "disabling." In my own practice, I have treated several children whose life experience combined depression and bereavement in different ways.

Preexisting Depression

Sometimes a child exhibits signs of depression prior to and independent of any experience with loss. Many of these children are "undiagnosed," since their form of depression permits minimal or passing school performance without extreme behaviors that draw attention to them. This category includes the quiet child who seems "withdrawn" but who "gets by." The child may have few or no friends, and sometimes he/she may be scapegoated because peers consider him/her "different."

These children are at extreme risk when they become bereaved, since their survival was precarious even before the loss. An example of such a child (Chapter 3) involves a boy with poor self-esteem (related to learning disabilities) who suffered the loss of two grandparents in 1 year. Without the loving familial support and the preexisting supportive relationship with his therapist, this child's grief might have become disabling.

Depressive Symptoms Following Loss

Sometimes symptoms of depression occur in a child with no previous psychiatric diagnosis. This speaks to the importance of the therapist obtaining a careful history to arrive at the correct diagnosis. Susan, in Chapter 8, illustrates an example of a child who was functioning normally until the sudden violent death of her friend precipitated a grief reaction with some accompanying symptoms of depression. When Susan's grief reaction was treated through play therapy, her depressive symptoms abated.

Suicidal Risk

Fox emphatically states that "each bereaved child must be considered potentially at risk for suicide" (1985, p. 16). While this advice may appear to be extreme, practice wisdom dictates caution. We know that many young children do not comprehend the irreversibility of death. Therefore, their wish to "go to heaven" to be with their deceased mother and father represents their literal interpretation of their experience and their remedy for their loss.

Even elementary-school-age children who understand the finality of death may express suicidal thoughts with reference to wanting a reunion with a deceased parent. Bluestone describes her skillful use of puppet play to assist two bereaved latency-age children who therapeutically "play out" their painful losses and longing for reunion with their deceased parents (1999, pp. 225–251). It is noteworthy that the therapist not only helped these children with their grief through play therapy but also conducted a suicide evaluation to determine the degree of suicidal risk of the girl who had been most upset during the play. When this case was presented at the annual meeting of the Association of Death Education and Counseling in 1992, one member of the audience was surprised that the therapist had taken the child's suicidal ideation "so seriously," since "it is common for bereaved children to fantasize about reunions with their parents."

I agree with Bluestone that we must take all such fantasies seriously, especially when they include the desire to escape the pain of the loss. We never know when a child might try to carry out his/her fantasy. Evaluation of degree of risk for suicide provides information about the individual's degree of intent and, in addition, provides the therapist the opportunity to discuss with the child his/her wish and longing for reunion while simultaneously emphasizing the vast difference between the wish and the irrevocable action that would implement it.

Counselors who are not familiar with the assessment of degree of suicide risk should consult Table 2.2 and the references at the end of this chapter (especially Pfeffer, 1986, and Peck, Farberow, & Litman, 1985). In situations where the counselor or therapist has any lingering doubts about the child's intent, it is wise to seek another opinion, and to tell the child and family that you are doing so because you are so concerned about him/her that you want to be certain that he/she will not do anything to

TABLE 2.2. Questions to Ask in the Evaluation of Suicidal Risk in Children

1. *Suicidal fantasies or actions:*
   Have you ever thought of hurting yourself?
   Have you ever threatened or attempted to hurt yourself?
   Have you ever wished or tried to kill yourself?
   Have you ever wanted to or threatened to commit suicide?

2. *Concepts of what would happen:*
   What did you think would happen if you tried to hurt or kill yourself?
   What did you want to have happen?
   Did you think you would die?
   Did you think you would have severe injuries?

3. *Circumstances at the time of the child's suicidal behavior:*
   What was happening at the time you thought about killing yourself or tried to kill yourself?
   What was happening before you thought about killing yourself?
   Was anyone else with you or near you when you thought about suicide or tried to kill yourself?

4. *Previous experiences with suicidal behavior:*
   Have you ever thought about killing yourself or tried to kill yourself before?
   Do you know of anyone who either thought about, attempted, or committed suicide?
   How did this person carry out his/her suicide ideas or action? When did this occur?
   Why do you think that this person wanted to kill him/herself?
   What was happening at the time this person thought about suicide or tried to kill him/herself?

5. *Motivations for suicidal behaviors:*
   Why do you want to kill yourself?
   Why did you try to kill yourself?
   Did you want to frighten someone?
   Did you want to get even with someone?
   Did you wish someone would rescue you before you tried to hurt yourself?
   Did you feel rejected by someone?
   Were you feeling hopeless?
   Did you hear voices telling you to kill yourself?
   Did you have very frightening thoughts?
   What else was a reason for your wish to kill yourself?

6. *Experiences and concepts of death:*
   What happens when people die?
   Can they come back again?
   Do they go to a better place?
   Do they go to a pleasant place?
   Do you often think about people dying?
   Do you often think about your own death?
   Do you often dream about people or yourself dying?
   Do you know anyone who has died?
   What was the cause of this person's death?
   When did this person die?
   When do you think you will die?
   What will happen when you die? *(continued)*

TABLE 2.2. (*continued*)

---

7. *Depression and other affects:*
   Do you ever feel sad, upset, angry, bad?
   Do you ever feel that no one cares about you?
   Do you ever feel that you are not a worthwhile person?
   Do you cry a lot?
   Do you get angry often?
   Do you often fight with other people?
   Do you have difficulty sleeping, eating, or concentrating on school work?
   Do you have trouble getting along with friends?
   Do you prefer to stay by yourself?
   Do you often feel tired?
   Do you blame yourself for things that happen?
   Do you often feel guilty?

8. *Family and environmental situations:*
   Do you have difficulty in school?
   Do you worry about doing well in school?
   Do you worry that your parents will punish you for doing poorly in school?
   Do you get teased by other children?
   Have you started a new school?
   Did you move to a new home?
   Did anyone leave home?
   Did anyone die?
   Was anyone sick in your family?
   Have you been separated from your parents?
   Are your parents separated or divorced?
   Do you think that your parents treat you harshly?
   Do your parents fight a lot?
   Does anyone get hurt?
   Is anyone in your family sad, depressed, or very upset? Who?
   Did anyone in your family talk about suicide or try to kill him/herself?

Note. From Pfeffer (1986, pp. 187–188). Copyright 1986 by The Guilford Press. Reprinted by permission of the publisher and author.

harm him/herself. It is better to overreact than to underreact in these circumstances.

When the Child's Bereavement Is Due to the Suicidal Death of a Family Member

Hurley (1991) points out that children bereaved by the suicide of a family member require urgent intervention, since there is evidence that such children are at greater risk for suicide and depression than are children in the general population. In particular, response to the grief of children bereaved by the suicide of a parent requires great professional skill and sensitivity, since the meaning of such a death "often becomes distorted in the mind of the child, who usually cannot face the 'voluntary' nature of the suicidal death" (Hurley, 1991, p. 238). Also, the family is usually emotionally devastated in this situation and may be incapable of offering the child essential information and support. When the family feels shame associated with the suicide, they may want to disguise or distort the truth about the death. This further confuses the child, who needs and wants accurate information about how his/her loved one died. The shame associated with stigmatized death such as suicide complicates the grief process for all involved and leaves the child bereft and angry. These children should be referred to a mental health professional for evaluation and treatment. (See Hurley, 1991, for an example of play therapy with a 4-year-old whose father committed suicide, and Elder & Knowles, Chapter 6 in this volume, for further discussion of suicide in the family.)

THE TRIPARTITE ASSESSMENT OF THE BEREAVED CHILD

Mental health practitioners, teachers, religious leaders, nurses, school-bus drivers, and scout leaders all may have had occasions to counsel a bereaved child. They may or may not have had training in grief counseling or in child development, but nonetheless most respond effectively out of their own compassion and instinctive respect for the child's feelings. Many bereaved children are not referred to mental health professionals, and many can go through their grieving without assistance from specialists.

Since the 1970s, however, there has been growing awareness in the general public about issues related to death and dying, sparked by the work of Kübler-Ross (1969) and reflected in the growth of the interdisciplinary field of death education. Interest in knowing more about how to help children has increased enormously.

Because of my firm belief in the necessity and value of a thorough assessment prior to counseling or treatment, I will now focus on the elements of such an assessment. I developed the tripartite assessment of the bereaved child as an adaptation of the tripartite crisis assessment that was originally designed to facilitate evaluation of the child in a variety of crisis situations (Webb, 1991, 1999).

Assessment of a bereaved child involves consideration of three groups of factors:

1. Individual factors
2. Factors related to the death
3. Family, social, religious/cultural factors

All of these interact and must be evaluated in order to appreciate fully the bereavement experience of a given individual. Figure 2.1 illustrates the components and interaction among the three sets of variables.

Individual Factors in Childhood Bereavement

The assessment of a bereaved child begins with studying the background and current status of the individual who has been bereaved. Many of the elements in the assessment of the individual focus on the reality of the

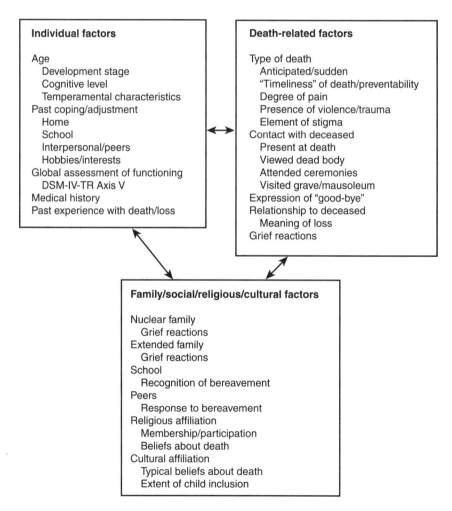

FIGURE 2.1. Tripartite assessment of the bereaved child: Webb.

child's life prior to the death, for example, his/her level of cognitive understanding and overall adjustment. I have developed a form (see Table 2.3) on which this information can be recorded to assist the bereavement counselor in organizing and summarizing the relevant personal information about the child. The five subcategories in this assessment consist of the following:

- Age/development/cognitive/temperamental factors
- Past coping/adjustment
- Global assessment of functioning: DSM-IV-TR, Axis V
- Medical history
- Past experience with death/loss

Age/Developmental/Cognitive/Temperamental Factors

Chapter 1 contains a detailed review of age/developmental/cognitive factors with reference to how these impact upon the child's understanding

TABLE 2.3. Individual Factors in Childhood Bereavement: Webb

1. Age ____ years ____ months   Date of birth _____
                                       Date of assessment _____
   a. Developmental stage   b. Cognitive level
      S. Freud _____   J. Piaget _____
      E. Erikson _____   c. Temperamental characteristics
                                 S. Chess and A. Thomas _____

2. Past coping/adjustment
   a. Home (as reported by parents) Good ____ Fair ____ Poor ____
   b. School (as reported by parents and teachers) Good ____ Fair ____ Poor ____
   c. Interpersonal/peers Good ____ Fair ____ Poor ____
   d. Hobbies/interests (list) _____

3. Global assessment of functioning: DSM-IV-TR, Axis V
   Current _____ Past year _____

4. Medical history (as reported by parents and pediatrician)—describe serious illnesses, operations, and injuries since birth, with dates and outcome. _____
_____
_____
_____

5. Past experience with death/loss—give details with dates and outcome *or* complete Wolfelt's Loss Inventory. _____
_____
_____
_____

Note. This form is one component of the three-part assessment of the bereaved child, which also includes an assessment of death-related factors (Table 2.4) and family/social/religious/cultural factors (Table 2.6).

of death. The temperamental components refer to Chess and Thomas's (1986) profiles of general temperamental style, which reflect a child's typical approach to routine and to stressful life experiences. Chess and Thomas identify three distinct profile categories differentiating children's levels of responsiveness, namely, the *difficult child*, the *easy child*, and the *slow-to-warm child*. Although these categories might seem overly simplistic, they are potentially useful to the bereavement counselor. It is valid to expect that a child who has always approached new situations with difficulty would have a harder time when faced with a death than would a youngster whose usual response to new and stressful experiences was generally adaptive.

Past Coping/Adjustment

While it may not be entirely true that the past determines the future (and most of us resist this idea strongly), it is only logical that someone who has been successful managing life stresses in the past will benefit from this track record and confront new challenges with a sense of confidence and resolve. Conversely, an individual who has barely managed to "get by" will probably have a more difficult time when he/she is confronted with a death experience. A rather harsh biblical teaching (Matthew 13:12, 25:29) maintains that the person who has much will be given more whereas the person with less becomes further deprived. The concept of ego strength explains why a child who is well adjusted will be more capable of dealing with the stress of a death than will a child who already is exhibiting difficulties in coping with routine daily stresses.

Global Assessment of Functioning: DSM-IV-TR, Axis V

This scale will be of use to mental health practitioners who wish to rate the child's overall psychological, social, and school functioning at the time of the evaluation and during the previous year. (See DSM-IV-TR [American Psychiatric Association, 2000, p. 34] for a description of the scale and how to use it.) A useful function of the scale is that it provides ratings for two time periods—the current and past year—so that the comparison may point to the need for treatment and the prognosis for future functioning, based on the scoring of the previous level of adjustment. The Global Assessment of Functioning constitutes a formalized, validated method of assessing past coping/adjustment.

Medical History

Sickness, injury, and hospitalization all constitute loss experiences in which the child has had to cope with his/her reality as an ill or injured person. None of us likes to be sick or hospitalized, least of all a child, who wants more than anything to view him/herself as strong and competent. The child who has had extensive past experience in which he/she has felt medically vulnerable or disabled may feel less than confident when confronting a death experience. Children who themselves are terminally or seriously ill may have very diminished reserves with which to undergo grieving for someone who has died.

Past Experience with Death/Loss

In addition to personal experiences of physical vulnerability, it is essential to obtain a history of the child's past experiences with death and loss, no matter how insignificant these may seem. Wolfelt (1983) has devised a detailed Loss Inventory that documents a whole range of losses from the death of a parent to a change in the child's living situation as minor as having to share a room. Wolfelt scores each loss in terms of degree of impact and also with regard to elapsed time since the loss, ranging from 0–6 months to 1–4 years. The Loss Inventory can help the grieving child understand that losses and attendant grief responses occur not only from death experiences but also from the myriad of seemingly petty problems of everyday life (Wolfelt, 1983, pp. 83–85). It also provides a literal summary of losses that contributes to documenting the possible effects of one individual's cumulative losses.

Death-Related Factors in Childhood Bereavement

Death is simple, and it is complex. A person stops breathing, and that single event can produce a sense of relief or of horror in the survivors. Family members who knew that their loved one was in a coma with no hope of recovery may have anticipated the death and feel relief when it occurs. In contrast, the cessation of breathing can create feelings of terror in a child who views his/her brother lying by the side of the road following a fatal car collision.

In evaluating the impact of a death on a child, we must consider the interaction of factors related to his/her personal background and experience, plus factors related to the death itself, and how these interact with influences of family/religion/culture and community to mediate the expression of grief. Death related factors include the following:

- Type of death
- Contact with deceased
- Expression of "good-bye"

- Relationship to deceased
- Grief reactions

Table 2.4 provides a form for recording these factors.

Type of Death

Children listen and try to understand the many comments made by family and friends about the circumstances associated with a death. Rando refers to "the death surround" to describe all the details of a death; these include the location, type of death, reason for the death, and the degree of preparation of the survivors (1988/1991, p. 52). Factors that I consider especially important with regard to children's understanding include whether the death was anticipated or sudden; whether family members consider it was "timely"; to what extent it might have been prevented; whether pain, violence, and trauma accompanied the death; and whether the death occurred due to circumstances associated with a sense of "stigma."

A sudden death contributes to a tendency toward denial among survivors. If a classmate who was not sick yesterday drowns today in his family pool, anxious feelings of personal vulnerability are stimulated among all his peers, who probably would not experience the same level of anxiety if the death had occurred to a different classmate who was known to be very sick with cancer. The degree of perceived preventability of the death is important both to adults and to children. Bugen (1983) discusses the interaction between the perception of preventability and the closeness of the relationship with the bereaved as predictors of the grief response. This is discussed more fully in Chapter 4 with reference to the death of a godfather who was terminally ill.

Children are very sensitive about pain. They fear it with reference to themselves, and if they hear details about a very painful death, this may arouse their anxiety, depending on the extent to which they can empathize. Elements of violence and trauma associated with a death also raise anxiety levels and may interfere with the grief process. Eth and Pynoos warn that "children are particularly vulnerable to the additive demands of trauma mastery and grief work. The obligatory efforts at relieving traumatic anxiety *can complicate the mourning process, and greatly increase the likelihood of a pathological grief response*" (1985, p. 179; emphasis added). Some children exposed to traumatic death may develop post-traumatic stress reactions that require special treatment (Pynoos & Nader, 1993; Nader, 1997). Cases involving treatment of traumatic grief are presented later in this volume in Chapters 7 (Bevin), 8 (Webb), and 10 (Nader).

Another important consideration with regard to the type of death is the degree to which the death may be associated with stigma. Some

TABLE 2.4. Death-Related Factors in Childhood Bereavement: Webb

1. Type of death
    Anticipated?   Yes _____ No _____ If yes, how long? _____ or sudden _____
    "Timeliness" of death   Age of the deceased _____
    Perception of preventability
    Definitely preventable _____ Maybe _____ Not _____
    Degree of pain associated with death
    None _____ Some _____ Much _____
    Presence of violence/trauma   Yes _____ No _____
    If yes, describe, indicating whether the child witnessed, heard about, or was
    present and experienced the trauma personally. _____

    _____

    Element of stigma   Yes _____ No _____
    If yes, describe, indicating nature of death, and degree of openness of family
    in discussing. _____

    _____

    _____

2. Contact with deceased
    Present at moment of death?   Yes _____ No _____
    If yes, describe circumstances, including who else was present and whether the
    deceased said anything specifically to the child. _____

    _____

    Did the child view the dead body?   Yes _____ No _____
    If yes, describe circumstances, including reactions of the child and others who
    were present. _____

    _____

    Did the child attend funeral/memorial service/graveside service?   Yes _____
    No _____ Which? _____
    Child's reactions _____

    _____

    Has the child visited grave/mausoleum since the death?   Yes _____ No _____
    If yes, describe circumstances. _____

    _____

3. Did the child make any expression of "good-bye" to the deceased, either spontaneous
    or suggested?   Yes _____ No _____
    If yes, describe. _____

    _____

    _____

Note. This form is one component of the three-part assessment of the bereaved child, which also
includes an assessment of individual factors (Table 2.3) and family/social/religious/cultural
factors (Table 2.6).

examples of stigmatized deaths are those occurring because of suicide, AIDS, drug overdose, or murder/homicides. Doka (1989) uses the term "disenfranchised grief" to refer to losses that cannot be openly acknowledged, socially sanctioned, or publically mourned. The concomitant feelings of shame complicate the grief process and compound reactions of guilt and anger in all of the survivors.

Contact with Deceased

As I have previously indicated, children are very literal and they are also curious. Family members may argue about the degree to which they believe that children should be included with the family in their various rituals associated with a death. I will consider four pivotal points in time at which the child may be permitted to have personal contact with the deceased. These include the following:

- Being present at the death
- Viewing the body
- Attending ceremonies
- Visiting the grave or mausoleum

Rando (1988/1991) is adamant about the appropriateness of including children with the family in all rituals and observances surrounding a death. According to Rando, when children are separated from the family and not given accurate information, they will have more difficulty resolving their loss (1988/1991, p. 215). However, some children may prefer not to attend a funeral when they understand that many people will be crying. Most mental health professionals and thanatologists believe that the child should be given the choice after having been told about the circumstances that will occur at each event.

Expression of "Good-Bye"

Some form of farewell to the deceased can help a child comprehend the reality of the death. The wake and/or funeral ritual may serve this purpose for adults, who "pay their last respects" as a final good-bye. Situations of sudden death, in which the body may be lost (as in a drowning at sea) or when families do not engage in any formalized funeral or memorial, deprive all family members of personal contact with their loved one's body which can help them confirm the reality and finality of the death.

Children, who may be unable to comprehend the abstraction "death," may benefit from doing something tangible for the dead person. Some of the children described by Krementz (1981/1991) expressed their satisfaction about placing a rose on the casket or putting a note with a poem inside the casket. Bowen (1976) relates a moving example of his work with a family in which a young mother died very suddenly of a heart attack, leaving her husband and three young children. Each of the children benefited from the private viewing of his/her mother's body, during which time each child spontaneously said or did something special or meaningful in the spirit of good-bye. Perhaps the value of these gestures is that they give some measure of personal control in a situation that is beyond everyone's control.

Relationship to Deceased

The closer the relationship, the more profound will be the impact on the survivor. Wolfelt's Loss Inventory (1983) ranks the death of a parent or sibling as having the highest impact, the death of a close relative next, and the death of a friend several points lower in terms of impact on the child. Unfortunately, there is no ranking for the death of a pet, which constitutes the first experience of death for many children and which can be quite devastating to a child.

It is very important to consider the personal meaning of each loss in terms of the unique aspects of that relationship to the surviving child. The grief counselor can obtain details about this by asking the child to talk about the dead person and, especially, about what they used to enjoy doing together.

Grief Reactions

In the assessment of the bereaved child, the therapist will note the grief reactions that the child currently demonstrates, including in this review both the child's feelings and behaviors as self-reported and as observed by the family and by the counselor. Table 2.5 provides a means of recording the details about the nature of the child's grief.

Family/Social/Religious/Cultural Factors in Childhood Bereavement

The growing child becomes socialized into the belief systems of the adults in his/her family, school, and community. Those adults, in turn, maintain beliefs about life and death based in large part on their own childhood experiences. A book about childhood bereavement would have to be enormous in size to include the practices and beliefs of all cultures and religions. This is not my intent here, as I indicated in Chapter 1. I believe, however, that the therapist or counselor must take into account the partic-

TABLE 2.5. Recording Form for Childhood Grief Reactions: Webb

Age of child _____ years _____ months   Date of birth _____
                                        Date of assessment _____

See the form "Individual Factors in Childhood Bereavement" (Table 2.3) for recording of personal history factors.

Date of death _____
Relationship to deceased _____
  Favorite activities shared with deceased _____
  What the child will miss the most _____
  If the child could see the deceased again for 1 hour, what would he/she like to do
  or say? _____

Nature of grief reactions (describe) _____

  Signs of the following feelings? Y = Yes; N = No
  Sadness _____ Anger _____ Confusion _____ Guilt _____ Relief _____
  Other _____
Source of information on which this form has been completed:
  _____ Parent _____ Observation _____ Other

Note. This form is an extension of "Death-Related Factors in Childhood Bereavement" (Table 2.4), focusing specifically on the nature of the child's grief.

ular belief system (cultural/religious) of any bereaved child with whom he/she is working.

The significance of the following general spheres of influence on the bereaved child are included as part of the assessment, and may be recorded on Table 2.6:

- Family influences (nuclear and extended)
- School/peer influences
- Religious/cultural influences

Family Influences

Bowen points out that "family systems theory provides a broader perspective of death than is possible with conventional psychiatric theory, which focuses on death as a process within the individual" (1976, quoted in Walsh & McGoldrick, 1991, p. 92). My position is that *both* individual and family systems factors must be assessed. Certainly it is essential to know how the family perceives the death and to what extent the child is included in the mourning rituals of the family. A family that believes it is appropriately shielding a young child from pain by arranging an outing with a favorite baby-sitter at the time of a grandmother's funeral cannot be

TABLE 2.6. Family/Social/Religious/Cultural Factors in Childhood Bereavement: Webb

1. Family influences
    Nuclear family: How responding to death? Describe in terms of relative degree of openness of response.
        Very expressive ____ Moderately expressive ____ Very guarded ____

        To what extent is the child included in family discussions/rituals related to the deceased?
        Some ____ A great deal ____ Not at all ____
    Extended family: How responding to death? Describe, as above, in terms of relative degree of openness of response.
        Very expressive ____ Moderately expressive ____ Very guarded ____

        To what extent do the views of the extended family differ or agree with those of the nuclear family with regard to the planning of rituals and inclusions of the child?
        Very different ____ Very similar ____
        If different, describe the nature of the disagreement

2. School/peer influences
    The child's grade in school ____
    Did any of the child's friends/peers attend the funeral/memorial services?
        Yes ____ No ____
    Was the teacher informed of death?   Yes ____ No ____
    Did the child receive condolence messages from friends/peers?
        Yes ____ No ____
    Does the child know anyone his/her age who has been bereaved?
        Yes ____ No ____
        If yes, has the child spoken to this person since the death?   Yes ____ No ____
    Does the child express feelings about wanting or not wanting peers/friends to know about the death?   Yes ____ No ____
        If yes, what has the child said?

3. Religious/cultural influences
    What is the child's religion? _____
    Has he/she been observant?   Yes ____ No ____
    What are the beliefs of the child's religion regarding death? _____

    What about life after death? _____
    Has the child expressed any thoughts/feelings about this? _____
    _____

Note. This form is one component of the three-part assessment of the bereaved child, which also includes an assessment of individual factors (Table 2.3) and death-related factors (Table 2.4).

criticized for being cruel. Families differ greatly in their degree of comfort about open expression of feelings, and the child might indeed become upset upon witnessing adults in the throes of grief.

Family members may hold differing views about the rightful role of children as participants in significant life passages such as death, and their beliefs will be determined by their cultural backgrounds. Some parents, at a time of diminished emotional reserves, do not have the resolve to argue their position with a member of the older generation who may appear weak and vulnerable but who may hold more "traditional" views about "protecting innocent children" from exposure to the pain of death. In the ideal situation, young and old family members cry together and obtain strength and comfort from the unity of their mutual support. Thus, in the years to come, it is to be hoped that there will be increasing inclusion of children in all of the family's rituals and personal expressions following death.

School/Peer Influences

The preschool child who attends day care may have growing awareness of the wider world outside the family. Nonetheless, young children continue to be influenced mainly by the attachment figures in their close family network. Once a child enters school, however, he/she is much more alert to the opinions of teachers and classmates. When a child experiences a death of a loved one, the reactions of friends and school personnel are important to him/her. As I have already discussed, children have a strong need to "fit in" and feel accepted by their peers. Frequently they interpret this to mean conformity. When someone close to them dies, this event makes them "different" from their peers, and many children feel uncomfortable about the difference. They may need reassurance that they will still be respected and admired for their own qualities, even though they may no longer have a father or mother. Similar to the need to reassure the young child that he/she will still be taken care of after a death, the friends and teachers of the school-age child may need to remind him/her of their continuing esteem and friendship. A child grieving the loss of a family member or friend is in a very vulnerable state and will appreciate genuine communications that recognize his/her value and importance as a person and the intent of peers to maintain their friendship.

Religious/Cultural Influences

In counseling a bereaved child, it is helpful to know not only what the child has been taught but also what he/she has "caught" with regard to the religious/cultural practices of the child's family. When children are confused, they combat their confusion with their own idiosyncratic logic. Thus, the child in the movie *My Girl* whose friend died of an allergic reaction to numerous bee stings began to feel better when she reasoned that her own mother, who had died in childbirth and who now "lived" in heaven, could take care of her recently deceased young friend.

We have learned more about the views of children following parental death from the work of Silverman and Worden (1992) and Klass, Silverman, and Nickman (1996), whose findings suggest that many bereaved children think about their deceased parent as "watching over" them from heaven. This view incorporates not only the concept of the parent as "superego" but also the feeling of parent as loving protector.

SUMMARY

The complete assessment of the bereaved child weighs the interactions between the various components of the individual factors in childhood bereavement, the death-related factors, and the family social/religious/cultural factors. While few therapists or counselors have all this information at their fingertips, nonetheless they must appreciate the power of both what they know and what they do not know as potentially influential on children's grief responses.

REFERENCES

American Psychiatric Association. (2000). *Diagnostic and statistical manual of mental disorders* (4th ed., text rev.). Washington, DC: Author.

Bluestone, J. (1999). School-based peer therapy to facilitate mourning in latency-age children following sudden parental death: Cases of Joan, age 10½, and Roberta age 9½, with follow-up 8 years later. In N. B. Webb (Ed.), *Play therapy with children in crisis* (2nd ed.): *Individual, group, and family treatment* (pp. 225–251). New York: Guilford Press.

Bowen, M. (1976). Family reaction to death. In P. Guerin (Ed.), *Family therapy* (pp. 335–348). New York: Gardner Press.

Bowlby, J. (1963). Pathological mourning and childhood mourning. *Journal of the American Psychoanalytic Association, 11,* 500–541.

Bugen, L. A. (1983). Childhood bereavement: Preventability and the coping process. In J. E. Schowalter, P. R. Patterson, M. Tallmer, A. H. Kutscher, S. V. Gullo, & D. Peretz (Eds.), *The child and death* (pp. 358–365). New York: Columbia University Press.

Chess, S., & Thomas, A. (1986). *Temperament in clinical practice.* New York: Guilford Press.

Doka, K. (Ed.). (1989). *Disenfranchised grief: Recognizing hidden sorrow.* New York: Free Press.

Eth, S., & Pynoos, R. (1985). Interaction of trauma and grief in childhood. In S. Eth & R. S. Pynoos (Eds.), *Post-traumatic stress disorder in children* (pp. 171–183). Washington, DC: American Psychiatric Press.

Fox, S. (1985). *Good grief: Helping groups of children when a friend dies.* Boston: New England Association for the Education of Young Children.

Grollman, E. A. (Ed.). (1967). *Explaining death to children* (pp. 3–27). Boston: Beacon Press.

Hurley, D. J. (1991). The crisis of paternal suicide: Case of Cathy, age 4½. In N. B. Webb (Ed.), *Play therapy with children in crisis: A casebook for practitioners* (pp. 237–253). New York: Guilford Press.

Klass, D., Silverman, P. R., & Nickman, S. L. (1996). *Continuing bonds: New understandings of grief.* Washington, DC: Taylor & Francis.

Krementz, J. (1991). *How it feels when a parent dies.* New York: Knopf. (Original work published 1981)

Kübler-Ross, E. (1969). *On death and dying.* New York: Macmillan.

Lindemann, E. (1944). Symptomatology and management of acute grief. *American Journal of Psychiatry, 101,* 141–148. (Reprinted in Parad, 1965, pp. 7–21; see below.)

Nader, K. O. (1997). Childhood traumatic loss: The interaction of trauma and grief. In C. R. Figley, B. E. Bride, & N. Mazza (Eds.), *Death and trauma: The traumatology of grieving* (pp. 17–41). Washington, DC: Taylor & Francis.

Parad, H. (Ed.). (1965). *Crisis intervention: Selected readings.* New York: Family Service America.

Peck, M. L., Farberow, N. L., & Litman, R. E. (1985). *Youth suicide.* NewYork: Springer.

Pfeffer, C. R. (1986). *The suicidal child.* New York: Guilford Press.

Pynoos, R. S., & Nader, K. O. (1993). Issues in the treatment of posttraumatic stress in children and adolescents. In J. P. Wilson & B. Raphael (Eds.), *International handbook of traumatic stress syndromes* (pp. 535–559). New York: Plenum Press.

Rando, T. A. (1991). *How to go on living when someone you love dies.* New York: Bantam. (Original work published 1988)

Rapoport, J. L., & Ismond, D. R. (1990). *DSM-III-R training guide for diagnosis of childhood disorders.* New York: Brunner/Mazel.

Silverman, P., & Worden, J. W. (1992). Children's reactions in the early months after the death of a parent. *American Journal of Orthopsychiatry, 62*(1), 93–104.

Walsh, F., & McGoldrick, M. (Eds.). (1991). *Living beyond loss: Death in the family.* New York: Norton.

Webb, N. B. (1991). Assessment of the child in crisis. In N. B. Webb (Ed.), *Play therapy with children in crisis: A casebook for practitioners* (pp. 3–25). New York: Guilford Press.

Webb, N. B. (Ed.). (1999). *Play therapy with children in crisis* (2nd ed.): *Individual, group, and family treatment.* New York: Guilford Press.

Wolfelt, A. (1983). *Helping children cope with grief.* Muncie, IN: Accelerated Development.

PART II

*

Death in the Family

3

🐟

Deaths of Grandparents and Parents

NANCY BOYD WEBB

Death is a part of life and can occur without warning to young and old alike. The dream of most parents and grandparents is to live to see their children and grandchildren grow into adulthood and have children of their own. However, about 5% of children lose a parent to death before they reach the age of 18 (Wessel, 1983, p. 125), and certainly a much higher percentage experience the death of a grandparent. This chapter deals with the impact of the deaths of parents and grandparents on their children and grandchildren and on the role of professional counselors in assisting the children's bereavement process.

Use of the tripartite assessment (Chapter 2) helps practitioners evaluate each death according to the unique factors of the individual child and family's history and current circumstances, together with the specific nature of the death, and the level of support in the school, religious, and secular community environment.

THE DEATH OF GRANDPARENTS

Children who were blessed with grandparents have gained much to sustain and enrich their lives. They have learned that death can be regarded as a peaceful completion of life, rather than something to be feared. . . . Children of any age in grieving

are unconsciously expressing gratitude for the gifts from the
past given to them.
—PATTERSON (1983, p. 77)

A child's first experience with death may be the death of a grandparent,
and the child's reaction to the death varies depending on the quality of the
attachment relationship (Raphael, 1983; Crenshaw, 1991). The closeness of
the relationship and the warmth and frequency of the interaction will
determine the nature of the child's response. Sometimes grandparents
are very important figures in the child's life as sources of unconditional
love and caregiving (Hatter, 1996). However, in other situations, "the
death of their grandparents is a nonevent. The [children] know that
the death has occurred but cannot really feel much about it because of
the lack of relationship with their grandparent. While they may be quite
affected by their own parent's distress at the loss, they may have little to
grieve for themselves " (Rando, 1988/1991, p. 150). The child, therefore,
responds to the grandparent's death in both *personal terms*, based on the
quality of the lost relationship, and in *family systems terms*, based on the
reactions of other family members to the death. Walsh and McGoldrick
point out that in cases where the grandparent has suffered a prolonged
illness, the parent will be "stressed by pulls in two directions: toward
the heavy responsibilities of caring for young children and toward filial
obligations for the dying and surviving parent" (1991, p. 40).

In the following case example a 9-year-old boy who was in therapy
for difficulties related to problems at school and problematic family relationships experienced the terminal illness and death of his grandmother,
followed after a few months by his grandfather's death. The case illustrates
the interaction of both individual and family factors as the boy and his
family dealt with these stressful experiences of loss.

Family Life Cycle Considerations

It is understandable that the serious illness and death of any family
member will "lead to disruption in the family equilibrium" (Brown, 1989,
p. 458). In determining the degree of disruption Brown weighs the following factors:

1. The social and ethnic context of death
2. The history of previous losses
3. The timing of the death in the life cycle
4. The nature of the death or serious illness
5. The position and function of the person in the family system, and
6. The openness of the family system. (1989, p. 458)

These factors will be discussed with regard to the Silver family.

Case of the Silver Family—
Siblings, Ages 11, 9, and 5

Family Information

Father, Edward, age 42, insurance business
Mother, Joan, age 39, high school teacher/substitute
Children: Victoria, age 11, sixth grade
           Todd, age 9, fourth grade
           Flora, age 5, kindergarten

Extended family
Mr. Silver, Sr., "Grampa," age 81, retired lawyer; blind; diabetic
Mrs. Silver, "Grammy," age 79, cancer—2 years; recent terminal diagnosis

The diagnosis of terminal cancer in Mr. Silver's mother was an implicit warning of her imminent death in "several months' time." "Grammy" lived a few blocks from the Silvers in a home she shared with her husband, 81, who was almost blind and suffered from a variety of physical ailments. The grandchildren visited their grandparents several times a week for short visits. The severity of Grammy's condition meant that she would no longer be able to cook and perform routine chores, especially the physical care of her husband. Fortunately, the elderly couple had resources to pay for home nursing and housekeeping care.

Edward Silver has two older siblings: an unmarried sister, 9 years his senior, and a married brother, 4 years older; both live out of state.

Joan Silver's parents are in their late 60s; they are retired and live nearby. Joan has one married sister, 9 years her junior, who lives out of state.

Background on Referral

The family was referred by the hospital social worker who had been involved with Grammy's medical treatment. The parents had expressed their concerns to her about Victoria's "impossible" behavior which led to daily screaming fights between Joan and her eldest daughter. The hospital social worker, who had met all family members, described them as "a family of screamers." The parents had welcomed her suggestion that they seek therapy to try to reduce the tension and stress.

Summary of Initial Contacts with the Parents and Victoria

Many of the issues presented by the parents as disturbing to them reflected rather typical preadolescent behaviors, such as Victoria's messy room, the timing of her homework completion, her refusal to wear her night brace, and her frequent arguments with her brother, Todd. After meeting with the parents and Victoria several times I concluded that their conflict was "the last straw" that added stress to everyone at a time they all were concerned about Grammy's serious illness. They all nodded solemnly as I predicted that the months ahead might be even *more* stressful and that especially during this difficult time they needed to be supportive rather than hostile toward one another. I offered to work with them around the agreed-upon goal of "fight reduction" so that the tension in their family could be reduced. I also mentioned that as Grammy's death became imminent, they might benefit from some anticipatory bereavement counseling.

Comments

With reference to the life cycle considerations enumerated by Brown (1989) I noted that the Silver family was Jewish, white, and middle class, with no experience of deaths among their immediate or next generation of relatives in either the mother's or father's family. They were sad but resigned to the certainty of Grammy's death, and they agreed that her death was "timely." She had lived a long, healthy life, and their concerns were to make her last months as comfortable as possible while the family provided emotional support to her and to "Grampa." Brown states that "generally the farther along in the life cycle, the less is the degree of family stress associated with death and serious illness. *Death at an older age is viewed as a natural process*" (1989, p. 463; emphasis added).

The death in this family actually proved to be less significant than were the unresolved old sibling conflicts that the anticipatory bereavement stirred up among Edward Silver's siblings. Matters of necessary decision making such as arranging health care, planning for Grampa's care after Grammy's death, and selling their home and disposing of its contents all provoked discord between Mr. Silver and his middle-aged brother and sister. The deaths of the first generation provided me with an intergenerational perspective of the sibling rivalry I had been witnessing firsthand between Victoria, age 11, and Todd, age 9. Mr. and Mrs. Silver were very open with me regarding their difficulties with Mr. Silver's siblings, and this information deepened my diagnostic understanding and led to some strategies intended to release Mr. Silver from his unconscious need to replay his own sibling battles through his children.

Of Brown's (1989) aforementioned six factors affecting the impact of death and serious illness on the family system, the fifth, "the position and function of the person in the family system," seemed to be the most relevant in this case. The prospective deaths of the family patriarch and matriarch led to great instability and jockeying for control among their adult second-generation offspring. Viewing this case in a family systems context increased my appreciation of intergenerational family issues that were precipitated by the anticipated and subsequent deaths of the first-generation "heads of the family."

Scapegoating following a Death

Although increased solidarity in a family is a frequent reaction to death, according to Goldberg, "scapegoating may also occur in a family as a way of re-achieving homeostasis when the previous family balance included a scapegoat" (1973, p. 402). This proved to be an operative factor in this case situation with regard to the criticism and disdain expressed by Edward Silver's siblings toward him. Their attitudes seemed exaggerated and unwarranted in view of Mr. Silver's essential and valuable role in supporting his parents. In time, I came to learn that Mr. Silver's father, Grampa, was considered by the family as a demanding tyrant who was very inconsiderate of his wife's feelings. This, evidently, was one of the few areas of agreement between Mr. Silver and his siblings; they had all relied on Edward and Joan Silver to hire and orient health aides and intervene in his mother's behalf. Grammy was to be "protected" from the insensitivity and lack of consideration of her tyrannical/scapegoat husband. Once Grammy died, the family institutionalized Grampa, and, in the process, they began to criticize Edward Silver's financial management over the past few years. In a family accustomed to a scapegoat as the brunt of their own hostilities, the death of the beloved matriarch led to the "punishment" of her partner through nursing home placement; then, the resultant vacuum sucked Edward into the scapegoat role. This is also the position of Todd within his nuclear family, a matter I understand better now than I did while working with the family.

Ethnic/Religious Considerations

According to Brown, "Jews are well prepared to deal with life's tragedies and life's suffering. . . . They are a very expressive ethnic group with a tradition of shared suffering. . . . These values and characteristics assist the Jews in dealing with death openly and directly. If they need assistance in this regard, it is to get in touch with the personal aspect of the death" (1989, pp. 460–461). I knew that the Silver family was accustomed to open expression of their feelings and that Edward and Joan were appropriately preparing their children for the probability of Grammy's death by following some suggestions I had given them.

However, the reason they had contacted me originally was for help in dealing with Victoria's obstinate personality, not about Grammy's impending death. After several months of parent counseling and individual play therapy sessions with Victoria, the parents asked me to evaluate Todd. Their conflict with Victoria had subsided significantly. Todd, however, presented unique problems that subsequently proved to be due to attention-deficit disorder. He had many fears and was highly anxious. At the time of Grammy's death I was seeing Todd individually, alternating every other week with parent counseling sessions. His problems, although certainly magnified by the family stress regarding his grandmother's impending death, were separate and idiosyncratic.

A question for me was how to recognize the death when it occurred and whether or not to attend the services or visit the home. I expected that Todd would be quite upset about his grandmother's death, and I wanted to be available to offer support to him and other family members. I knew that this family would follow traditional Jewish practices following the death, including immediate burial and subsequent observation of the mourning period (shivah). Mr. Silver had described the practices to me, indicating that there would be elderly relatives from out of town spending time with them, talking about his mother's life as part of the expected mourning process. I decided that it would not be appropriate for me to intrude on this intimate family gathering. I asked Mr. Silver to notify me when the death occurred, and I suggested that it might be helpful to all of them to meet together with me in my office soon after all the relatives had returned home. I also made it clear that I would be available by telephone if any of the family wanted to talk with me after the death. (The details of the family bereavement session are given in a later section.)

Preliminary Assessment and Treatment Plan

An overview of the presenting problem suggested several sources of strain for this family: first, Victoria's preadolescent development, especially her push toward autonomy and challenge to parental authority; second, Todd's emotional and learning problems; and, third, the serious illness and impending death of Mr. Silver's mother. These family life cycle transitions could be viewed as "normal" developmental passages, capable of arousing anxiety and requiring adjustment. This family, which had been functioning reasonably well up to the time of referral, seemed to lack the psychological reserves to cope with the combined stress of the losses of the prospective death of a member of the older generation and the difficulties of their two elder children. On a symbolic level the parents may have felt an increasing sense of loss of control.

My initial assessment, thus, was that this was a family struggling to cope with the stresses of normal developmental transitions, characterized by losses associated with growth and with death. I believed that a short-term behaviorally focused intervention would help them to relieve the tension generated by the parent–child conflict. Meanwhile, I hoped that my work with them around this would help build a relationship that would increase my ability to assist them with bereavement issues at the time of Mr. Silver's mother's death.

Treatment Summary. Using a psychoeducational approach I helped the family implement the contract to which they all had agreed, namely, that all would consciously try to avoid fighting with one another. Some techniques they learned to use successfully were "time-out" hand signals, refraining from arguing when a disagreement was brewing by leaving the scene, saving the disagreement for discussion in family sessions with the therapist, and planning special pleasurable times together. I encouraged mutual expressions of praise and genuine positive regard, which had been absent in the negative spiral of anger and recrimination.

After several months Mr. Silver's mother continued to weaken, and the parents and Victoria spoke of Grammy "gradually fading away." I had become more aware of the intense sibling conflict between Victoria and Todd and suggested that he join some of the sessions. The parents were open to this and said that they hoped I would see Todd separately as well, since at times he seemed to them as "totally out of it," in a world of his own.

The next phase of treatment, therefore, included some sessions with the parents, joint sessions with Victoria and Todd, some with Victoria alone, and some with Todd alone. After a few months, the focus shifted more to Todd, since he appeared to be a very needy 9-year-old boy whose frustration tolerance and ego development seemed very immature.

Preliminary Assessment of Todd

Todd presented as a tall, lanky youngster with a variety of somatic complaints and many anxieties and fears. He was not doing well in school and required intensive parental involvement to complete his homework. He resented being reminded to do his schoolwork and would frequently whine, complain, and provoke very negative responses from his parents.

These difficulties did not, however, seriously interfere with Todd's social adjustment: He was perceived as a "nice kid" who had friends, and who was quite proficient in gymnastics and baseball.

The parents wanted Todd to be tested for possible learning disabilities since he seemed frequently to "forget" his school assignments and appeared unable to follow directions or to prioritize. The subsequent psychological evaluation confirmed their impressions.

My own assessment of Todd was that he was struggling to find his acceptance in this family as the only boy and middle child, between a very bright older sister and a younger sister who was "spoiled rotten," according to the mother. Todd was not comfortable with the idea of growing up. Because of his height people often mistook him as being older, yet his response to my question about what age he would like to be was "In my mommy. Then I'd be safe from everything except a nuclear bomb!"

Because Father more typically brought Todd to sessions with me whereas Mother brought Victoria, I tuned in to the issues of male identification. Father evidently also had been learning disabled, although undiagnosed; he had also gone through several years of psychotherapy when he was Todd's age. Father's affect in conveying this to me in a resigned manner was that of "history repeating itself."

The Grandmother's Death

In the midst of Todd's evaluation, Edward Silver's mother died. Mr. Silver telephoned me, stating that her death had been peaceful and that, although he had not been with her at the exact moment of death, he had been with her for several hours earlier that same day.

I asked about the children's reactions, and Mr. Silver said that Victoria had cried, that Flora was very excited about going to the funeral, and that Todd had been "distraught." He moaned and became very clingy, to the point that Mr. Silver asked the rabbi to speak to him. On the evening after the death (the night before the funeral) Todd had gone to his best friend's house to sleep. The family evidently felt that they could not console him and that his agitation would subside in the company of his friend.

Mr. Silver mentioned that Todd's class was anticipating a special holiday outing to see a ballet, *The Nutcracker*, on the day of the funeral. Mr. Silver said that his instinct was to permit Todd to go with his class, since Todd indicated that he wanted to go. Mrs. Silver's sister was coming to be available to the children after the service. Mr. Silver felt that it might not be appropriate for the children to witness the burial service during which, as part of the tradition, the mourning family shovel dirt onto the lowered casket.

I expressed my condolences, and Mr. Silver said that "even when you expect it, the feeling of loss is very real." I indicated my concern for his feelings and then asked to speak to Victoria and Todd. Each of them came to the phone, and we spoke briefly. I set the appointment with Mrs. Silver for a family bereavement session 5 days later. The family planned to sit shivah for 3 days following the funeral and burial. I suggested that Mrs. Silver bring to the session pictures of the children with their grandparents. Mrs. Silver said that she would do this and asked if she could also bring Flora to this meeting.

The Bereavement Counseling Session

My goal in suggesting this session was to provide a setting and a method (the photos) whereby the children could tune in to their memories about their grandparents and recognize that the grandparents had a life with their parents even before their own births. Todd and Flora were at the age in which "concrete thinking" still prevailed to some extent. I reasoned, therefore, that seeing pictures of their grandparents with their parents (when their parents were young) might convey to them the message of their family's history in a way that merely talking about memories would not. Even though I realized that the appreciation of a sense of "family history" could be an unreasonable goal for 5-year-old Flora, I believed that it was possible for both Todd and Victoria and that it would help them grieve the loss of their grandmother.

I had received some recent training in phototherapy and was eager to use "people's personal photos and their interactions with these images as powerful adjunctive tools to move beyond the constraints of traditional verbal-only therapy" (Weiser, 1988, p. 339). My own feelings in anticipating this session were a mixture of apprehension about whether it would accomplish a meaningful purpose and whether Flora would be able to participate appropriately.

Summary of Session.[1] The family meeting, using the photographs as a way to reminisce and talk about the grandparents, was partly successful, and especially meaningful to Mr. Silver. However, the session was a rude reminder to me that the death of a grandparent does not change family relationships. Todd became whiny and irritable as he noted that there were more pictures of the grandparents with Victoria than with him. His strong feelings of sibling rivalry surfaced as he viewed the old photos. Weiser comments that when we look at photos we interact with them and project onto them the meanings we need unconsciously at that time (1988, p. 353). I had intended the photos to help the mourning for the grandparents, but Todd was not ready for that process and needed to project onto them his own feelings of rivalry and disappointments. Nonetheless, the family session served a purpose that the photos facilitated. The parents clearly experienced the review of the photos as meaningful to them. In addition, the photos helped the parents affirm the grandpar-

---

[1]A detailed script of this session appears in the first edition of this book.

ents' love for all their grandchildren. This was an important message for the children to hear.

Session with Todd and Father

A few months later, Todd came for an individual session accompanied by his father. His psychological evaluation had been completed and he was taking Ritalin on a daily basis to counteract the effects of attention-deficit disorder. The parents had commented on the calming effect of the medication and on the concomitant improvement in Todd's ability to concentrate.

I noticed a positive change in Todd's ability to carry on a conversation without fidgeting. There was also a dramatic decrease in his whining and regressive squirming. Typically, Mr. Silver came into the session at the beginning with Todd, and then Todd and I would spend the remainder of the time together. This time, Todd asked his father to remain while we played a game together.

I mentioned that I had a new game they were welcome to play with me for the first time. It was Gardner's (1988) *Storytelling Card Game*, a therapeutic board game based on the creation of stories, using cardboard cutout figures and an array of story card settings. These backgrounds include different household rooms (such as the kitchen, bathroom, or bedroom), community scenes (such as the supermarket parking lot, the doctor's office, the school, or a cemetery), and several blank cards with which the child can create his/her own scene and story (Gardner, 1988). The players have a choice about the backgrounds they use for the creation of their stories, since the spinner permits a choice among four different background cards each time.

Because of this range of choices, I was very surprised when in the middle of the game Todd selected card 7, the cemetery scene (see Figure 3.1); he had three other choices and looked at all the backgrounds carefully before opting for the cemetery.

I knew that Todd had not participated in his grandmother's burial ritual, but I was certain that he knew about it and that he had probably overheard conversations about the event. I was curious about what kind of a story Todd would create. His manner in the telling of his story was very matter of fact. Mr. Silver was playing the game with us, and I could sense his tension at Todd's selection of the cemetery scene. My best recollection of Todd's story follows:

> Todd: *(Placing a family group of the cardboard figures in the cemetery, around a monument in the center)* Somebody has just died, and the family is here to throw dirt on the casket. The rabbi says

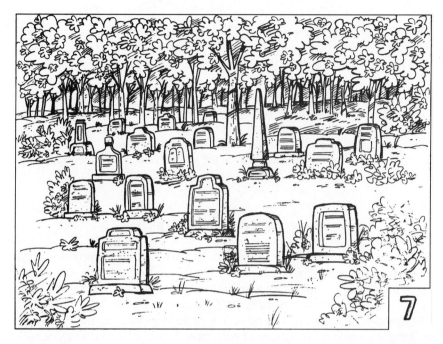

FIGURE 3.1. Card 7, the cemetery scene, from Gardner's (1988) *The Storytelling Card Game* (Creskill, NJ: Creative Therapeutics). Reprinted by permission of the author.

prayers. The family all say things about the person. They feel very sad, and some of them are crying.

THERAPIST: What happens next?

T: They go home, because they are still a family.

(Mr. Silver and I exchange a meaningful glance, and I repeat Todd's last phrase, "They are still a family.")

Comments

This is a family with both strengths and vulnerabilities. I have no doubt that they could have "made it" without professional intervention. However, I have frequently thought about the hospital social worker who referred them at the time of Mr. Silver's mother's terminal diagnosis. She gave the family the means to free themselves from the chains of the past and to work on current sibling conflicts. The parents became aware of the ghosts from the past, which made them far more able to respond to their own children in terms of current realities rather than old scripts. I am optimistic that Victoria's and Todd's children in years to come will not need to repeat the same pattern of sibling hostility.

The death of a family member is a crisis which, like all crises, offers both dangers and opportunities. In this case the grandmother's death was anticipated and the children could witness her decline with their own eyes. They also were able to say their "good-byes" to their grandmother and to experience a sense of closure because of this. The following section includes two cases of parental death, one of which involves the terminal illness and death of a mother, and the other, the sudden death of a father.

THE DEATH OF PARENTS

Because of the implicit role of parents as nurturers and caretakers, their loss stirs up distressing feelings of anxiety based on the ongoing attachment relationship and the dependency needs of the survivors, regardless of their age (Ainsworth & Bell, 1971; Mahler, Pine, & Bergman, 1975). The impact of a parent's death on a child depends on many factors, and the unique circumstances of each case require that we analyze each situation in order to assess how to respond and whether help is needed, and if so, what kind. As discussed in Chapter 2, the tripartite assessment of the bereaved child was developed to assist in this process.

A parent's death can have a catastrophic impact on their children because young children invest almost all of their feelings in their parents (in comparison with adults who divide their love among several meaningful relationships): "Only in childhood can death deprive an individual of so much opportunity to love and be loved and face him with such a difficult task of adaptation" (Masur, 1991, p. 164, referring to Furman, 1974).

This section discusses some typical responses of children to the death of a parent, utilizing two case examples to illustrate (1) the terminal illness and death of a mother, and (2) the sudden death of a father. These will be presented following a discussion of risk and protective factors that can help or hinder a child's adjustment to parental death.

Risk Factors for Children Related to a Parent's Death

Most studies of parental bereavement have focused on the death of the *father*. Consistent differences have been found, as reported by Kastenbaum (1998, p. 291), between children whose father died and children who have both parents alive; children whose father died tend to exhibit the following characteristics: [They]

- Are more submissive, dependent, and introverted
- Show a higher frequency of maladjustment and emotional disturbance, including suicidality
- Show a higher frequency of delinquent and criminal behavior
- Perform less adequately in school and on tests of cognitive functioning

[In summary] parental [especially paternal] bereavement must be regarded as a *potential problem* in many areas of a child's life. (pp. 291–292; emphasis added)

We must not be deterministic, however, since many children who lose their parents in childhood grow into achieving and well-adjusted adults. Whereas the death of a parent in the life of a child does seem to create a risk, many other factors (discussed below) can intervene to help and support the child with his/her ongoing growth and development.

Resilience and Protective Factors for Children Related to a Parent's Death

Resilience refers to both internal capacities of the individual and to the transactional process between the individual and the supportive factors in the environment (Davies, 1999). Protective factors include positive influences from the wider social environment (school, religious community, peers), and risk factors may include individual vulnerabilities of the child, impaired parenting, and socioeconomic or institutional factors such as poverty and social disadvantage (Davies, 1999, pp. 48–49).

The importance of protective factors to balance risk factors is demonstrated in the case of Sabrina, a 7-year-old child whose mother died of cancer following several months of steady decline (Webb, 1996). The child's reactions must be evaluated in the context of the responses of her father and the extended family. The fact that Sabrina's half-brother had died of a drug overdose 1 year prior to her mother's death certainly was a complicating factor and an added risk in this child's bereavement experience.

Sudden Death of a Sibling and Terminal Illness and Death of a Mother: Case of Sabrina, Age 7[2]

Family Information

Child, Sabrina, age 7, first grade
Mother, Lida Rossi, age 47, psychologist (currently unemployed);

---

[2]A full discussion of this case with detailed scripts of treatment sessions appears in Webb (1996).

history of cancer; operations for a colostomy and a vaginectomy 18 months ago
Father, Dan Rossi, age 40, editor at publishing house
Half brother, John Sand, died of heroin overdose, age 19 (1 year ago)

Extended family
Paternal grandparents, in their 70s, live nearby
Paternal aunt, Carol, age 44, lives nearby
Cousins (Carol's children) Katie, age 10, and Gregg, age 4
Maternal grandmother, age 70, lives out of state
Maternal aunt, Ann, age 45, lives out of state
Cousin, Ann's son, Steve, age 7
Maternal aunt, Jean, age 43, lives out of state

Mrs. Rossi had been married previously; her first husband died of a heart attack at age 45 when John was 4. Dan and Lida Rossi have been married 9 years.

Summary of Contacts with Family (Prior to Mother's Death)

The initial contact with this family occurred prior to Mrs. Rossi's surgery. It included sessions with Mr. Rossi and John, as well as separate sessions with Sabrina and with her mother. The early focus was on planning for family tasks during the time when Mrs. Rossi was in the hospital, and on preparing Sabrina for her mother's absence and subsequent period of convalescence. After the operation I continued to see various members of the family at 2-week intervals. John had begun individual therapy with another therapist. The family mood was optimistic despite the ongoing concerns about John, who drank excessively, was unemployed, stayed out late, and spent many hours drawing graffiti on walls. Mrs. Rossi was hoping to return to work, and Sabrina was doing well at school and at home.

Eight months after Mrs. Rossi's operation John was found dead of a heroin overdose in a friend's apartment. The family's state of disbelief, anger, and sadness was compounded by their shame at the manner in which John had died. Although Sabrina was too young to comprehend the full implications of her half brother's death, she felt his absence as a profound loss that meant that now she was an "only child." I spent many sessions with Sabrina in which she expressed her grief through drawings, recalled memories of her brother, and played the board game *Clue*. I believe that the game provided her with a way to repeat and attempt to work through her own (and the family's) struggle to understand

John's death and their ongoing questions about how and why John had died.

Her son's death took a terrible toll on Mrs. Rossi, whose medical condition steadily deteriorated in the following months. The physicians recommended that the family engage Hospice to provide nursing and home health care services. After several weeks of being bedridden and approximately a year after John's death, Sabrina's mother died. Three days before Lida had told her daughter that "God wanted her" and that "God would take care" of Sabrina and her father. She also told Sabrina that she would be watching over her.

Comment

The responses of the extended family and school helped to mitigate the impact of these two tragic and untimely deaths in Sabrina's life. She had previously been doing well socially and academically, and fortunately the paternal grandparents were able and willing to help with Sabrina's care before and after school. Furthermore, the school social worker coordinated with Sabrina's teacher and therapist in order to closely monitor her school adjustment.

Sabrina was a very resilient child. Even the dual losses of her half brother and her mother did not seriously interfere with her ongoing development. The fact that her paternal grandparents lived near, as did many aunts, uncles, and cousins kept this child from feeling isolated and abandoned. The extended family system served as essential "protectors" for a child whose adjustment might otherwise have been seriously compromised after the deaths of her half brother and her mother. Christ (2000) points out that the events that follow parental death may be of equal or more importance in determining the child's adjustment than that of the death itself.

Accidental Death of a Father: Case of the Turner Family[3]

When a father dies leaving four children ranging in age from 4 to 12 years old we can see differences in the children's responses based on their ages and on their different levels of adjustment prior to the death. The following case illustrates some important factors that must be considered when a parent dies: First, children comprehend and interpret the death

---

[3]An earlier version of this case discussion appears in Webb (2001). Copyright 2001 by Columbia University Press. Adapted by permission.

according to their ability, based on their age and developmental stage. Second, the anxiety and stress associated with a death can magnify preexisting conditions, or lead to acting out behaviors that require a therapeutic response which recognizes the underlying meaning of the behavior. Third, the ability of the surviving parent to focus on the children's needs and to maintain structure and routine in the home impacts strongly on the children's adjustment. Fourth, a parent's ability to interact appropriately with the children depends on the support that the parent receives from the extended family, friends, and the community. In this case, like that of Sabrina's, there was a large extended family who rallied around and offered help. In addition, the community and the father's work associates also provided exceptional and ongoing support. This family appeared to have been functioning well prior to the crisis of the death. They were already resilient, and although the sudden death certainly was a terrible loss, the support they received contributed to their ongoing growth and development.

Family Information

> Mother, Betty, age 34, part-time cashier
> Father, Greg, age 35, policeman and volunteer fireman; killed in
>   house fire
> Children: Mary, age 12, seventh grade
>   Greg Jr., age 9, fourth grade
>   Brian, age 6, first grade
>   Lisa, age 4, nursery school

Referral

Three months following the death, the policeman/MSW social worker who was on the "crisis debriefing team" that visited the family immediately after the death suggested to Betty that it would be a good idea for her to consult a play therapist for the children because of the traumatic nature of their father's death. The policeman/social worker telephoned me to provide information and to alert me to expect a call from Betty. Mrs. Turner agreed to bring all the children for a family session. I mentioned that following this initial meeting I would like to see each family member, including her, individually. I said that depending on my assessment of their individual needs, we would agree on a plan of how to proceed. Mrs. Turner mentioned that her husband's and Mary's birthdays were coming up soon, and she thought that this was going to be "hard" on all of them. The birthdays also coincided with an upcoming ceremony planned by the fire department and the town to name a street after her husband. I indicated my understanding of the combined honor and pain of this event, and mentioned my wish to do whatever I could to help her and the children get through this difficult period.

Family Counseling/Therapy Following the Death of a Parent

Whenever possible, it is important to see the family together for at least one session following the death of a parent. This is to acknowledge that they have all experienced the same loss, and also to point out that different people in the family will respond differently to this loss. The social work counselor models a tolerance for differences, which can be particularly important for the children, who may feel guilty because they still want to go out and play and have fun with their friends while their surviving parent may be sitting sadly in the house.

During the family session it is also helpful for the worker to indicate that most people's feelings change over time and that their preference for counseling at one point may change later. The worker also should state that sometimes it will be helpful to see different family members alone or together in sibling groups. A model of flexibility respects everybody's changing needs.

First Family Session. This consisted of an opportunity for me to meet all the family, to acknowledge the terrible loss they have each experienced, and to explain some of the ways I might be helpful to them. I described my role as someone who "helps children and families with their troubles and worries, and that sometimes we talk and sometimes we play" (Webb, 1996, p. 68). I suggested that we begin by everyone making a drawing of a happy memory of their family. The boys each drew a picture of an outing in the park, the mother helped Lisa draw a snowman, and Mary drew some flowers. The purpose of this warm-up exercise was to help the children begin to feel comfortable with me. I also used the drawings to refer to their father, asking his whereabouts in the scene each drew. I had suggested that Mrs. Turner bring some pictures of her husband with her to this session, and she shared them at this time, pointing out the individual children with their father when they were much younger. I was impressed by Mrs. Turner's ability to focus on her children when I knew that she had suffered a great loss herself.

The pictures also showed some older family members and other relatives. I learned that Mrs. Turner's parents had both died during the past year, as had her mother-in-law. I said with great feeling, "This family has lost a lot of important people in a very short time!" Mary said that she believed in reincarnation and that she thought that life continues in other forms. She elaborated that several of her aunts had had babies this year, and she thinks that her grandparents' spirits will be felt in these new lives. I said that I was very impressed by her spiritual beliefs. Addressing the younger members of the family particularly, I mentioned that no matter what happens after death, we still miss the person and wish he was still with us. There was some discussion among the boys about who would own their father's fire helmet and jacket.

Four-year-old Lisa was getting quite squirmy, and I suggested that we all play a board game called *The Goodbye Game*. This is a therapeutic game that incorporates the stages of grief (denial, anger, bargaining, acceptance) by permitting the players to respond to questions (printed on different-colored cards) about death when they land on corresponding color sections of the board. Because Lisa couldn't read (and it turned out that 6-year-old Brian couldn't either), Mary read their cards for them. One of Greg's cards requested, "Draw a picture of death." He drew a picture of a narrow casket with a thin figure in it (see Figure 3.2).

As Greg drew, Brian asked if he could draw also, and of course I agreed. Brian drew a burning house (see Figure 3.3).

When we were looking at the drawings, I commented that they were both probably thinking about their father. I noticed that Mary's eyes filled with tears several times while playing the game.

At the end of the session I set up appointments to see Mrs. Turner and each child separately. I said that I know that it is hard to think and talk about someone you loved who died but that I thought it would be helpful to them. I also mentioned again that we could play as well as talk.

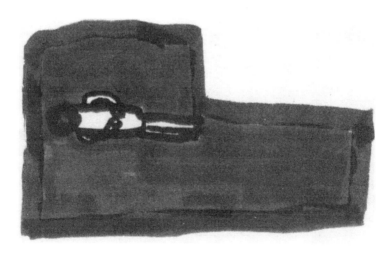

FIGURE 3.2. Greg's drawing, "Picture of Death."

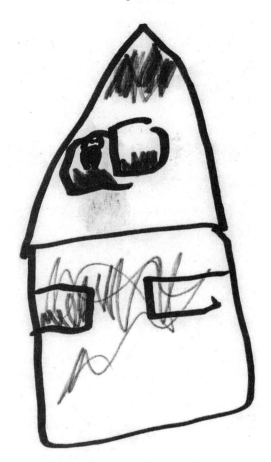

FIGURE 3.3. Brian's drawing, "Picture of Death."

Comment. This family was fairly easy to engage; the challenge was the wide age range of the children, between 4 and 12 years. Because of this I knew that there was a vast difference in Lisa's and Mary's understanding of death. I realized that in a family session such as this it is difficult to meet the individual needs of different family members. Nonetheless, the family session served the purpose of engagement and beginning the therapeutic relationship with each individual. I knew that in future sessions with the individual children I would use play therapy techniques with the two younger children, mostly talk with Mary, and a combination of talking and playing with Greg.

Individual Therapy/Counseling Following the Death of a Parent

"Some of the distinct advantages of individual therapy over group or family therapy are that it permits maximum attention to the particular needs of the child, and allows the therapist to move at the child's pace in a careful in-depth exploration of the child's underlying feelings about the death" (Webb, 1993, p. 51). Individual counseling is *always* recommended in situations of traumatic bereavement or following a suicidal death. This is because the individual (child or adult) must deal with their frightening ideas/images about the gruesome nature of the death before they can engage in the normal mourning process. Mourning, by definition, requires remembering the person who died. When the death has been traumatic, very frightening elements become superimposed upon these memories and interfere with peaceful and healing recollections (see Chapters 8 and 10). Counseling the traumatically bereaved is a stressful process for both the individual and the social work counselor/therapist. Before undertaking this anxiety-producing work, the worker should have received specialized training in counseling traumatized individuals (see the Appendix to this book for lists of training programs).

Individual Session with Mrs. Turner. I used this meeting to build my relationship with the mother and to strengthen her resolve to help her children. I made a referral to a bereavement group for Mrs. Turner, but she said she didn't feel ready yet but that she might want to go "later." We also discussed the status of each child individually. Mrs. Turner stated that Mary told her after the family session that she didn't want to come back for individual sessions. The mother felt that Mary was "doing very well" and that she didn't really need help, in contrast to the other children. She was concerned about Greg, who had started to be aggressive with other children in school and whose schoolwork was deteriorating. Brian had always been disorganized, according to Mrs. Turner, and she felt that now he was "in a daze." Lisa simply did not comprehend what had happened, according to Mrs. Turner. She would say, "My Daddy died in a house fire," but then hearing someone enter the house the very next moment she would say, "That's Daddy!"

I reviewed some of children's expectable responses to a parent's death and helped Mrs. Turner understand that many of their reactions were normative. At the same time, I asked for permission to contact the boys' schools and to confer with the school social worker about their academic and behavioral status. Mrs. Turner was glad to have me do this and signed the necessary release forms.

Summary of Individual Sessions with the Children. As planned, I saw each child individually for several play therapy sessions. Greg was able to admit that he was losing his temper "a lot lately." We spoke together about how much stress he was under because of his father's death, and I referred to the fact that many people, adults and kids, feel angry when someone they love dies suddenly. He made a picture of a volcano, at my suggestion, and we talked about how, when feelings are held in, they can "explode like a volcano." I also gave him clay to mold and twist as we talked about what it's like now that his father isn't home, and he reminisced about some of the things he used to enjoy doing with his dad.

Within 3 weeks I noticed a visible relaxation of Greg's tension. His mother said that there had been no more negative reports from school, and the school social worker reported that he was spending time with Greg every week talking about their shared interest in basketball.

Brian's reactions and behavior in therapy were quite different. He typically brought an assortment of toys with him from home and dumped them in the middle of the office floor, creating a very chaotic scene. He would then add my firemen dolls, trucks, and the whole array of police and medical dolls in my collection, together with an assortment of family dolls of all sizes, ethnicity's, and ages. Brian re-created on the playroom floor the chaos he was feeling internally. I understood the symbolic meaning of his play and verbalized to him that "everything seemed all mixed up and confused." His play came to no resolution or conclusion, and he would not permit me to "play out" any rescue efforts. About 3 months after I began seeing him and on the last day before I was to go away on an extended leave, he played out a house fire, the deaths of many people, and the inability of the hospital to save the people. This was a very sad scene, and I verbalized feelings of sadness and helplessness for Brian. He permitted me to cover up the "dead bodies" (with Kleenex), and he joined me in doing this. After a quiet and intense interval I said something about missing those people very much and trying to remember how much they loved us. This very active child became quite focused and serious during this play, which I believe had deep meaning to him.

When I first began seeing Brian I was concerned about his poor speech and encouraged his mother to request an evaluation at school. In the midst of the period of therapy, she reported to me that the school was arranging special help for him. I felt quite certain that these difficulties were independent of his father's death. But it also seemed likely that his problems with speech and learning were increased by the death.

Lisa also had a speech impairment, but it was not serious, considering her young age. However, because I had some difficulty understanding her, I subsequently suggested that her mother have her evaluated. In the play sessions with me Lisa turned all the adults in the dollhouse family into females, even those who were clearly male. When I asked her to tell me who was in the family, she did not name a father. I asked her, "What happened to the daddy in this family?" and she responded, "We can't find him." This response is understandable in view of Lisa's young age. She has heard people say that her father is dead, but she doesn't understand that death is irreversible. That is why she can switch from saying that her father died in a house fire to announcing his arrival at the front door. My response (and one I later suggested that mother repeat to Lisa) was that "maybe the daddy is dead, and when people are dead, we don't see them anymore and they don't come back." It was not necessary to continue play therapy sessions with Lisa, because I believed that her mother would respond patiently and appropriately to the child whenever necessary.

CONCLUSION

Death is a part of life, and neither grandparents or parents can guarantee their ongoing survival throughout the lifespan of their children/grandchildren. Social workers, therefore, must be prepared to provide services to families following deaths and to assist schools and community agencies with the creation and provision of programs for bereavement counseling. Depending on the nature of the death and the age of the surviving relatives, services may be offered through Hospice programs, through schools, through mental health clinics, through religious organizations, through funeral homes, or by private practitioners. Regardless of the locale of the services, the bereavement counselor should make an assessment of the individuals, taking into account the various components of potential risk and resilience factors as enumerated in the tripartite assessment (Chapter 2). Special attention should be given to the age and level of cognitive understanding of the children, as well as to the nature of the death and the quality of existing support. The outcome of this assessment will point to the type of intervention that is appropriate.

A variety of treatment options should be considered, depending on the circumstances of each case. Among these are bereavement support groups, individual and family therapy, or a combination of various treatments. The social work value of client self-determination argues for participation of the client in the choice of the particular treatment modality. Certain methods may be more acceptable to different individuals at different stages of their bereavement process. It is important to move at the clients' pace and to be respectful of their wishes. Children usually do not have the autonomy or sufficient awareness to participate fully in selecting a treatment method that appeals to them. However, we must try whenever possible to include the children in this decision since this will enhance their subsequent motivation to participate. The child, obviously, had no control over the death, but many children can voice their preference about whether to see a counselor by themselves, with their family, or in a group with other bereaved children if the choice is presented to them. For example, Sabrina declined my suggestion that she attend a weekend "summer bereavement camp" which would have necessitated her being away from her father for 2 nights. At the time, her mother had been dead for approximately 7 months and I had been seeing her with her father in bimonthly counseling sessions. I thought that she might be ready to deal with her grief issues in the company of other bereaved children. However, as an only child (now that her brother had also died), Sabrina was not comfortable with the prospect of being separated from her one surviving parent even for a weekend. I respected the child's wishes and continued to see Sabrina with her father in cojoint sessions, helping each of them express their anxieties about safety and separation issues.

In contrast, 12-year-old Mary in the fireman's family did not want to commit to either family or individual therapy after one family session 4 months following her father's sudden death. However, this girl did agree to attend a school-based bereavement group and, according to her mother, benefited greatly from the experience. Her three younger siblings participated regularly and enthusiastically in one-to-one individual play therapy over a period of 5 months following the death. The widowed mother attended a bereavement group during this period.

In summary, choices about different treatment options should be offered in the spirit of respecting the clients' preferences. Whereas a death is the end of a life, it must not result in despair and depression for the families of the survivors. Social work can perform a vital service by setting up appropriate programs, referring bereaved clients to them, and providing bereavement counseling on an age-appropriate level.

DISCUSSION QUESTIONS

1. Comment on the family bereavement counseling sessions in the Silver and Turner families. Do you think that this was helpful to each family? If so, how? How could it have been more beneficial to them?

2. What is the appropriate role for the counselor/therapist at the time of the death of a family member? Do you agree with this therapist's decision *not* to make a condolence visit in the Silver case? On what basis should this decision be made?

3. Do you agree with the therapist's assessment about the sibling hostility reenactment across generations in the Silver family? How else might the therapist have intervened with regard to this source of family conflict?

4. Compare and contrast the use of individual, family, and group approaches in situations of bereavement. Compare Sabrina's unwillingness to accept a referral to a bereavement group with Mary's ability to participate in a school-based group. Can you think of any way to help Sabrina accept the referral? Role-play how you might approach Sabrina and deal with her anxiety about attending the group.

5. What play therapy methods are especially helpful to use with bereaved children?

REFERENCES

Ainsworth, M. D. S., & Bell, S. M. (1971). Attachment, exploration, and separation: Illustrated by the behavior of one-year-olds in strange situation. In S. Chess & A. Thomas (Eds.), *Annual progress in child psychiatry and child development* (pp. 41–60). New York: Brunner/Mazel.

Brown, F. (1989). The impact of death and serious illness on the family life cycle. In B. Carter & M. McGoldrick (Eds.), *The changing family life cycle: A framework for family therapy* (2nd ed., pp. 457–482). Boston: Allyn & Bacon.

Christ, G. H. (2000). *Healing children's grief: Surviving a parent's death from cancer.* New York: Oxford University Press.

Crenshaw, D. (1991). *Bereavement: Counseling the grieving throughout the life cycle.* New York: Continuum.

Davies, D. (1999). *Child development: A practitioner's guide.* New York: Guilford Press.

Furman, E. (1974). *A child's parent dies.* New Haven, CT: Yale University Press.

Gardner, R. A. (1988). *The Storytelling card game.* Creskill, NJ: Creative Therapeutics.

Goldberg, S. B. (1973). Family tasks and reactions in the crisis of death. *Social Casework, 54*(7), 398–405.

Hatter, B. S. (1996). Children and the death of a parent or grandparent. In C. A. Corr & D. M. Corr (Eds.). *Handbook of childhood death and bereavement.* New York: Springer.

Kastenbaum, R. J. (1998). *Death, society, and human experience* (6th ed.). New York: Macmillan.

Mahler, M., Pine, F., & Bergman, A. (1975). *The psychological birth of the human infant: Symbiosis and individuation.* New York: Basic Books.

Masur, C. (1991). The crisis of early maternal loss: Unresolved grief of 6-year-old Chris in foster care. In N. B. Webb (Ed.), *Play therapy with children in crisis: A casebook for practitioners* (pp. 164–176). New York: Guilford Press.

Patterson, P. R. (1983). The grandparent teaches the child about living and dying. In J. E. Schowalter, P. R. Patterson, M. Tallmer, A. H. Kutscher, S. V. Gullo, & D. Peretz (Eds.), *The child and death* (pp. 75–78). New York: Columbia University Press.

Rando, T. (1991). *How to go on living when someone you love dies.* New York: Bantam. (Original work published 1988)

Raphael, B. (1983). *The anatomy of bereavement.* New York: Basic Books.

Walsh, F., & McGoldrick, M. (Eds.). (1991). *Living beyond loss: Death in the family.* New York: Norton.

Webb, N. B. (1993). *Helping bereaved children: A handbook for practitioners.* New York: Guilford Press.

Webb, N. B. (1996). *Social work practice with children.* New York: Guilford Press.

Webb, N. B. (2001). Death of a parent. In A. Gitterman (Ed.), *Handbook of social work practice with vulnerable and resilient populations* (2nd ed., pp. 481–499). New York: Columbia University Press.

Weiser, J. (1988). Phototherapy: Using snapshot and photo-interactions in therapy with youth. In C. E. Shaefer (Ed.), *Innovative interventions in child and adolescent therapy* (pp. 339–376). New York: Wiley.

Wessel, M. A. (1983). Children, when parents die. In J. E. Showalter, P. R. Patterson, M. Tallmer, A. H. Kutscher, S. V. Gallo, & D. Peretz (Eds.), *The child and death* (pp. 125–133). New York: Columbia University Press.

4

🍃

Complicated Grief—
Dual Losses of Godfather's
Death and Parents' Separation

Case of the Martini Family—
Sisters, Ages 8 and 10

NANCY BOYD WEBB

This chapter discusses the therapy with a family in which the parents were initiating a marital separation at the same time that a close family friend and the godfather of Linda, age 10, was terminally ill with cancer. Ironically, the family was drawn together to support one another during the 3-month period of the godfather's illness and ultimate death at the same time they were facing the dissolution of their intact family as they had known it.

The literature on grief reactions following death or divorce points out many similarities, as well as distinctions, between the two forms of loss. In the Martini family, because of the juxtaposition of the "loss" of the father (due to marital separation) and the anticipated and subsequent death of the godfather, the grief reactions of the girls were complicated.

The term "complicated grief" refers to mourning in which the mourner attempts to "deny, repress, or avoid aspects of the loss" and also wants to hold on and "avoid relinquishing the lost loved one" (Rando, 1993, p. 149). Complicated grief may occur following multiple losses and after sudden or traumatic death (Goldman, 1996). In this chapter, the term refers to the responses of the Martini girls as they faced two simultaneous losses of important paternal figures in their lives.

GRIEF FOLLOWING DEATH

Furman (1974) refers to numerous clinical studies of normal mourning following death; these specify affects of pain, sadness, grief, anger, and guilt among mourners. Bowlby (1960, 1961, 1963) considers anger as a critical component of grief, related to yearning for the lost object. Bowlby (1980) also believes that discharge of anger serves a constructive role in the mourning process. Furman (1974) comments that "children, more easily than adults, acknowledge anger at the dead, both for having died and for their shortcomings when still alive" (p. 258). Anger is quite pronounced in the case of these bereaved girls. However, rather than directing their anger toward either of their "lost" paternal objects, they turned it toward one another in the form of intense sibling conflict.

Bowlby (1980) identifies four phases of mourning, following the loss of a close relative:

1. Numbing (duration of a few hours to a week)
2. Yearning and searching (duration from months to years)
3. Disorganization and despair
4. Reorganization

While many of these reactions have been observed in child as well as adult mourners, we do not know about the likelihood of their occurrence following the death of a nonblood relative such as a godfather. Burgen (1983) offers a conceptualization of childhood bereavement that seems applicable to this situation. Burgen proposes that the intensity and duration of bereavement are related to two dimensions: *the closeness of the relationship* and the mourner's *perception of preventability* of the death. In Burgen's model, "a griever who considered the deceased to be a central person in his life, and does not consider the death preventable in any way, is likely to experience an intense, but brief grief reaction" (1983, p. 359). This would seem to apply to the Martini girls' reaction to the death of Linda's godfather from a fatal disease; he was a beloved person, helpless in the grip of a terminal illness.

GRIEF FOLLOWING DIVORCE

The professional literature indicates that the mourning of losses associated with divorce parallels in many ways that of grief following death. Doka (1986, p. 442) refers to the intense grief reactions associated with divorce which can include "high levels of anger, guilt and ambivalence." Viorst (1986) enumerates sorrow, pining, yearning, denial, despair, guilt, and feelings of abandonment as similar grief reactions in both types of losses. A major difference between the two is the intensity of the anger response following divorce. This is often more pronounced because of the conflicts that precipitated the breakup and the underlying sense of blame and guilt about the failed marriage. Raphael (1983) notes that in divorce "the bereaved must mourn someone who has not died" (p. 228), and Weiss (1975) refers to the necessity in families of divorce for the couple to relinquish their attachment to one another.

In the Martini family, the parents were at the very beginning stage of initiating a marital separation. The girls did not have a clear idea of how their future might change, and this was frightening to them. In fact, both parents in this family were determined to retain their own special relationship with their daughters. They each tried to clarify that the divorce was between the adults, promising that it would not change their relationship with them. However, despite these reassurances, fear, anxiety, and anger inevitably surfaced and was expressed by the girls toward each other and, in a more guarded way, to each of their parents.

In separation and divorce situations children must mourn the loss of their intact family. Their mourning is especially complicated because of the possible reversibility of the decision which plays into their wish and fantasy about parental reunion (Wallerstein & Kelly, 1980; Wallerstein & Blakeslee, 1989; Wallerstein, Lewis, & Blakeslee, 2000; Jewett, 1982). According to Burgen's conceptualization of childhood bereavement, the most intense and prolonged grief response occurs when the griever "considers the deceased to be a central person in his life and also believes that the death was preventable" (1983, p. 357)

If we extend this concept to the loss and grief of divorce and apply it to Linda, age 10, and Amanda, age 8, it is clear that the prospect of having their parents separate and their father move out qualifies as a situation in which intense and prolonged grief might be expected. Certainly their father was very important to each of them, and—although they knew that their parents were in conflict—they probably believed that this could have been resolved if the parents made more of an effort to preserve their family.

ROLE AND SIGNIFICANCE OF GODPARENTS

In Catholic families the function of godparents includes the responsibilities of accompanying the godchild through important milestones, religious ceremonies such as baptism and confirmation, as well as providing security for the godchild. Falicov comments that "godparents are equivalent to an additional set of parents who act as guardians or sponsors of the godchild and care for him or her in emergencies" (1982, p. 143). If we consider Moitoza's (1982) statement that godparentage reflects the belief that survival is ensured with a second set of parents (p. 420), the impact on Linda of her godfather's imminent death at the same time she and Amanda learned of their father's plans to move out of their home certainly has great significance. It must have seemed to these girls that they were losing *two* primary male sources of affection and protection at the same time.

IMPACT OF MULTIPLE STRESSORS

The text revision of the fourth edition of the *Diagnostic and Statistical Manual of Mental Disorders* (DSM-IV-TR; American Psychiatric Association, 2000) provides for a listing of psychosocial and environmental problems that may affect diagnosis and treatment. These are to be listed on Axis IV. Problems related to the individual's primary support group are listed together, and included among these are the death of a family member, health problems in a family, and disruption of the family by separation, divorce, or estrangement. Clearly Linda and Amanda are suffering several problems at once. The impact of multiple crises can lead to disorganization and fragmentation of coping abilities (Webb, 1999). Furthermore, Bowlby states that "persons subjected to multiple stressors are more likely to develop a disorder than are those not so subjected" (1980, p. 187). Certainly either the departure of the father from the home or the terminal illness of the godfather qualifies as a stressful event for Linda and Amanda, and their combined impact puts the girls at considerable risk.

INDIVIDUAL FACTORS IN ASSESSING THE IMPACT OF LOSS

I have identified five factors in making an assessment of the child in crisis (Webb, 1999). Since terminal illness, death, and parental separation obviously are crises, it is appropriate to consider the interactive influences of these factors in the case under consideration. A form for recording the specific elements of these factors is available in a previous publication (Webb, 1999). The factors included in assessing a child in crisis are as follows:

- Age/development
- Precrisis adjustment
- Coping style/ego assessment

- Global assessment of functioning: DSM-IV-TR, Axis V
- Specific meaning of the crisis to the child

These factors will be considered with regard to Linda and Amanda following the presentation of family and referral information.

CASE OF THE MARTINI FAMILY

Family Information

Mother, Ann, age 34, buyer for department store
Father, Jim, age 35, architect in building firm, recovering alcoholic
(12 years)
Linda, age 10, fifth grade, on gymnastics team
Amanda age 8, third grade, very artistic
Linda's godfather, Robert, age 35, former restaurant manager, recovering alcoholic (12 years)
Linda's godmother, Terry, age 34, secretary
Note: The godparents have two children, ages 6 and 4.

Amanda and Linda refer to Robert and Terry as "Aunt" and "Uncle." Robert was Jim's Alcoholics Anonymous (AA) sponsor; they generally attend meetings together three times per week. Ann has attended Alanon in the past (sometimes with Terry), and the girls attended a group for children of alcoholics several years ago. At the time of intake, both Ann and Jim were in therapy separately.

Religious/Cultural Heritage

This is a Catholic family that observes major milestones such as baptisms and first communions according to the expected practice in their religion. Their participation in church services tends to be sporadic; Ann says, "We believe, but we are not really strict." The parents are of European cultural background; both are third-generation Americans. Ann is Polish and Jim is Italian.

Past History

Linda

The initial referral occurred about 9 months prior to the events that constitute the focus of this chapter. The parents originally consulted their pediatrician because of their concern about a sleep disturbance Linda had been experiencing for approximately 2 months; she would wake in the middle of the night, turn on many lights, enter the parents' bedroom, and quietly stand by their bed until one of them awoke and took her back to her own room.

A very frightening incident had initiated this sleep disturbance while the family had been vacationing with Linda's godparents, Robert and Terry, and their children. Linda awakened in the middle of the night, convinced that a robber/kidnapper was in the vacation cabin. Actually in her disoriented state in a strange location Linda had witnessed her godfather carrying his child in the dark to the bathroom. Her panic over this case of confused identity seemed excessive, but her parents were sympathetic initially, trying to comfort her, and convinced that the nightly waking would improve once the family returned home. When it continued unabated for a 2-month period, the parents appropriately sought a consultation from me, a child and family therapist.

Linda's therapy consisted of 11 sessions over the course of a 3-month period. Using a combination of art therapy, behavior modification, and parent counseling, complete symptom alleviation occurred after approximately 6 weeks. Termination followed gradually lengthening intervals between sessions. In the course of work with this family I was impressed with their ability to follow through with the treatment plan we established together. Once or twice during this time I had met Amanda briefly, as she accompanied her sister and mother and waited in the room adjacent to the office (see Webb, 1996, for a full account of this treatment).

Amanda

Approximately 6 weeks after termination of my sessions with Linda, Ann called with the request that I evaluate Amanda. The reason for the referral was not precise but alluded to Amanda's not being happy about the way she looked and about her tendency to cry and overreact when things did not "go her way." I saw Amanda several times in play therapy sessions, where she became very involved in doll play, drawing, and using clay. I was still in the process of evaluating Amanda when Ann requested a family session to discuss with both girls the parents' decision to initiate a marital separation.

Presenting Problem

The parents had decided to separate, and realizing that this would have serious consequences for their daughters they sought support and help from me, the child and family therapist who knew them and with whom they already had had a positive therapeutic experience. I suggested that all family members attend the session, with the understanding that I might see the girls individually after first meeting with the family as a group. In actuality, Jim did not come to the family session since Robert had been hospitalized on that day with pancreatic cancer and Jim felt obliged to remain with him in the hospital during visiting hours, which coincided with the appointment for the family session. Ann and the girls planned to go to the hospital after the session to see Jim briefly, since the hospital was located midway between their home and my office.

Although the family was not focused on their concerns about Robert's illness at this time, it was evident to me that the impact of the two major stressors needed to be considered in evaluating the girls' responses to their parents' imminent separation.

First Family Session

This meeting began with Ann, Linda, and Amanda together. They all sat together on the couch, with Ann, the mother, in the middle; Linda sat closest to me and appeared to be the most comfortable of the three, in that she showed no apparent anxiety; Amanda, by contrast, sat very close to her mother and appeared to lean on her. Ann had lost quite a bit of weight and looked very pale, fragile, and somewhat anxious during this meeting. Excerpts from the session follow.

Content of Session	Analysis and Feelings
THERAPIST: Hello! It's unusual to see *all* of you together! Even though I know each of you and you each know me, we haven't all met together as a group before. I'm sorry your dad couldn't be here also, but I know he must be *very* worried about Uncle Robert.	Want to recognize that this session is different, while pointing out that they have some past experience with me and with therapy.
AMANDA: Do you know that he has *cancer?*	Wondering what this means to an 8-year-old.
T: Yes. I knew he was being treated for cancer before he went to the hospital.	
AM: We're going to see him after we leave here.	
T: Have you ever visited anyone in the hospital before? What do you think it will be like?	

AM: *(Eagerly) I want* to see him. I want him to know that we love him!

How touching! I worry that the oncology floor might frighten her.

T: I'm sure that will mean *a lot* to him, I know that your families are very close. You may be able to help in other ways also, as time goes on. (*to Ann and Linda, trying to include them while opening up the discussion for other possible topics*) There certainly is a lot going on right now in your family!

Responding in concrete terms that might help Amanda.

Also wondering how Ann and Linda are feeling.

ANN: The girls know about Jim and me. We talked about it on the way here.

T: That's really why you're here tonight. So we can talk about it all together. It's a *big* step! (*to Linda and Amanda*) How do you feel about your parents separating?

Want to clarify the purpose of session and give everyone permission to express their feelings.

LINDA: *(Shrugging her shoulders and looking down)* It's okay I guess. They fight a lot and maybe it'll be better for them.

Has beginning understanding but looks upset.

T: But what about *you?* What do you think it will be like for *you?*

L: I don't know. I never lived with separated parents before. (*Ann laughs nervously.*)

Sounds sarcastic.

AM: Dad says we'll still see him every Wednesday and every other weekend, and we're *not* going to sell the house. I *love* my room and he put in bookshelves and my bed just where I wanted them.

Denying that things will be different.

T: Many kids do worry that their lives will be different after their parents split up.

Giving permission to express fears.

L: (*to Ann*) Are you and Dad going to get a *divorce? (Says the word with great distaste.)*

Groping with future possibilities.

ANN: We don't know yet. This is a trial separation. We're both in therapy, and we're going to see how it goes. We may end up getting a divorce and we may not.

T: (*to Linda and Amanda, but also to sensitize Ann about the girls' feelings*) It's going to be hard not knowing what's going to happen, but you're just going to have to "hang in" and wait. It's really up to your mom and dad to make this very important decision, and because it is so important, they need time to be sure. I'm sure they'll tell you as soon as they decide.

Important for the girls to realize that this is an *adult* decision and that they need to trust their parents.

At this point I offered to see each girl separately because I wanted to explore their individual reactions. Since Linda is 2½ years older than Amanda, the younger girl tends to defer to her older sister. In the separate interviews, Linda expressed her thoughts that maybe in the future she would choose to live with her father, but she did not know how she could tell her mom this without hurting her. I offered to help, if and when the time came.

In the separate session with Amanda she admitted that she felt very "scared." She could not identify what precisely frightened her the most but agreed that not knowing about what was going to happen was hard. I reassured her of her parents' deep love for both her and Linda, and also that I would try to be helpful to everyone in the family as time went on.

Preliminary Assessment and Treatment Plan

This is a family in crisis, with the prospect of the marital separation creating considerable anxiety for both children. In addition, the terminal illness of Robert, Jim's close friend and Linda's godfather, posed the possibility that the father's involvement with his friend might interfere with his ability to support and reassure the girls at the time they truly needed reassurance that they would not be "losing" him when he moved out of the home.

On the positive side, I knew of both parents' genuine concern for the well-being of their daughters. Because of my past positive relationship with them, I felt optimistic about their openness to parent counseling in matters relevant to the girls. I also felt relieved to know that each parent was engaged in individual therapy and hoped that this might reduce the acting out that sometimes occurs between couples in situations of marital conflict. I wanted to recommend marital counseling, but Ann made it clear that they were "not ready yet."

The *treatment plan* was for biweekly play therapy sessions with Linda and Amanda, and parent counseling with the parent who brought them to sessions. The parents were to alternate bringing their daughters, so that I could remain in contact with each of them on a monthly basis.

My *goals* with the girls were to provide support at a time of destabilization and crisis in their lives. I wanted to give them a place where they could safely express their fears and anxieties, and to offer clarification and intervention with their parents, when appropriate. I also wanted to prepare the girls for their godfather/uncle's future death and help them get ready to say good-bye to him in a manner that would be developmentally appropriate and meaningful to them.

With regard to the *individual assessment* of each girl, I noted that they both were doing well in school and each was involved in an activity outside of school. Furthermore, each had friends in her own peer group and appeared to be developing normally. At ages 8 and 10 they had a fairly realistic idea about the finality of death, and because of the nature of their godfather's terminal illness and the family's plan for frequent contact with him, I believed that they would naturally enter a phase of anticipatory grieving. The only area of concern about the girls was that each had some previous difficulty that had required therapeutic involvement. Given that this was a family in which therapy was the "norm," nonetheless I made a mental note to watch for signs of excessive lability and possible depression in Amanda, and for indications of phobic fears and possible regression in Linda. On DSM-IV-TR, Axis V, Global Assessment of Functioning (American Psychiatric Association, 2000), I ranked the girls as follows: Linda—past year, 50; current, 90; Amanda—past year, 70; current, 80.

Play Therapy Sessions

The usual pattern of these meetings consisted of a 20-minute family session with the girls and whichever parent brought them, followed by 20 minutes with the girls together. Sometimes, depending on issues raised in the individual session, I would see the parent alone for 10 minutes at the end (always related to something specific, and always with the child's permission to discuss the matter with their parent).

It was notable from the beginning that Linda and Amanda were involved in intense sibling conflict. This often began in the car with a battle over which one would sit in the front seat with the parent, and it continued in therapy around which one would come in to see me first. We resolved this initially with a toss of a coin and a plan to rotate each time, but since we all tended to forget whose turn it was from session to session, the argument persisted. During the occasional times I consulted with a parent following the individual sessions, the girls would resume their battle in the waiting room, fighting about a desired magazine or what station to listen to on the radio. The fighting sometimes was physical and included hair-pulling, screaming, and punching, often requiring my setting very firm rules with them, since they seemed to ignore their parents' attempts to intervene. I believe that this fighting clearly represented regressed behavior, and also served to show both me and their parents how angry and "out of control" they felt in view of their present life circumstances. Selected segments from the family therapy and individual play therapy sessions follow.

Two Weeks after Initial Family Session

Content of Session

This session begins with Father and the girls together. Seating is similar to that of the initial session with Mother, except this time Amanda sits with her arm locked with Father's. Linda sits at the side, appearing more independent.

THERAPIST: Hello, Jim. It's been a while since I've seen you. I'm so *sorry* to hear about Robert!

JIM: He's in pretty bad shape. I'm sorry I couldn't get here for the family meeting last time. Robert doesn't have much time left, and I'm trying to be with him as much as possible.

T: This must be incredibly *hard* for you!!

J: He's such a young guy, he's the same age as me—35. He was always so strong and healthy. Now he's just skin and bones. I can't believe it.

T: (*to Amanda and Linda*) Have you been visiting Uncle Robert?

AMANDA: Yeah. He's got all tubes and stuff connected to him. The first time he was sitting in a chair, but the next time he was lying in his bed and I thought he was *dead*. I ran out of the room crying!!

T: That must have been very scary! Were you with your mom?

Analysis and Feelings

This man is really in the throes of grieving. How hard to have to watch a close friend die!

Vulnerability factor: "If it happened to him, it could happen to me." Wonder if the girls are thinking this also.

Amanda expresses all the details and her fears while Linda watches and listens.

AM: Yeah, but I ran ahead into his room alone. He's so *skinny* now.

T: It's hard to see someone change like that. But he's still the same person inside that skinny body. Did you tell him that you love him like you wanted to?

AM: Yes, and I gave him a big kiss.

I am moved by her openness and affection.

T: What about you, Linda? What is it like for you, seeing your Uncle Robert now?

LINDA: We know he's going to die. I hate to see him suffer.

J: *(Strongly)* We're not going to let him suffer. The doctor may start giving him very strong medication so he won't feel the pain.

Jim is trying to be reassuring.

T: That could mean that Uncle Robert won't be able to talk with you. *(to Jim)* Do you think it's important for the girls to keep on visiting?

Wanting Jim to consider that it is okay for the girls *not* to visit.

J: That's up to them.

T: *(to Linda and Amanda)* How do you feel about it?

L: There usually are a lot of people there—all his friends from AA and his family. Sometimes I take care of John and Susi [Robert's kids] so they won't make too much noise and bother the other patients.

She has found a way to be helpful, despite the sad situation.

T: That's really helpful. I'm sure Aunt Terry is pretty upset, and she must really appreciate your playing with John and Susi.

AM: Mom says she is going to sleep over at their house sometimes

There has been some advance planning for the last stages of Robert's illness.

T: You're *all* doing your part to help, and I'm impressed. *(to Linda and Amanda)* Is there anything else you want to tell or do for Uncle Robert while he can still hear you?

Crediting their caring, and helping them plan for this death.

L: Just that we're praying for him and
we love him. *(Amanda nods.)*

T: That may sound like a little, but it re-   Sad reality.
ally is a lot. And it's really all you
can do for him.

J: I want him to know that his kids will   How touching that he thinks
always have a father as long as I am   to reassure Robert about his
alive.   children.

T: I hope you each will spend a special   Does this sound preachy? I re-
moment with Robert and whisper in   ally feel moved and saddened
his ear just what you have said here.   by what this family has to ex-
Then you can feel that you have   perience.
done all you can for him. It's very
sad, but there's nothing more anyone
can do except help his family and let
him die in peace.

At this point I saw each of the girls separately. They made drawings,
and played board games with me (Linda: *Connect Four*; Amanda: *Candyland*). I learned that Jim planned to move out this coming weekend, and
that he had given each girl his new phone number and they had set up
a visitation plan in which they would spend weekends with him in the
family's vacation home. This weekend visiting would not start right away,
however, because of Robert's illness and Jim's decision to spend as much
time as possible with him in the hospital.

Summary. Sessions took place, as planned, at biweekly intervals during the next month. Robert's condition continued its inevitable decline.
Jim reported that Amanda was "all over me" (needing a lot of physical
contact) and that Linda was "angry, but keeping it all in, like me." During
the session before the Thanksgiving holiday Amanda asked her father
why he would not be with them for Thanksgiving dinner at Gramma's
house, as usual, this year. Jim tried to explain that it would not be "comfortable" for Ann and him to be together; he told the girls that they would
have "their own" Thanksgiving together with him that weekend.

This change in traditional plans around a major holiday seemed to
mark the girls' first *true* realization that their parents had separated. In fact,
all of the hospital visiting and collaboration to help Robert's family had,
understandably, masked the reality of their own changed family situation.

Session Following Death

The week after Thanksgiving Ann telephoned to say that Robert had died
the night before and that a memorial service would be held at his home

the coming Saturday. We scheduled a family session to which Ann and the girls came. In retrospect, I cannot recall why Jim did not come with them. I am certain that I would have invited him. I suspect the reason was that because the couple was in conflict they avoided situations where they would have to talk with one another.

Content of Session	*Analysis and Feelings*
THERAPIST: Well, your uncle has died. Even though we all knew it was coming, it must be hard to believe.	I wonder how the girls are feeling and how much they will be able to verbalize their feelings. I want to be helpful and wonder just how far words can go at a time like this in view of the girls' ages.
LINDA: We were all sleeping at Terry's so she could be at the hospital. Uncle Robert's friends and Dad were there with him. Someone called Mom in the middle of the night to tell her.	
T: So it's all over now.	Stressing the finality.
AMANDA: There's going to be a memorial service at their house on Saturday.	
T: Do you know what that will be like?	Wanting to anticipate the situation and help prepare the girls.
L: The priest will be there to say prayers, and someone is going to play a guitar and sing.	
ANN: And different people will get up and talk about Robert and his life. I asked Linda if she wanted to write something.	
T: *(to Linda)* Is that something you want to do?	Wondering if Linda feels pressure to produce something.
L: I might. Last year in school when a teacher's wife died we all wrote notes, and he told us later that they helped him feel better.	The idea of doing something "concrete" is certainly age-appropriate.
T: *(to Amanda)* Are you wondering what you might be able to do?	
AM: I could draw a picture for Terry and make her a card.	
T: That's a good idea. We could all work here on a big, joint "card picture" like a collage. *(The girls seem interested, and I proceed to get out the construction paper, scissors, glue, markers,*	Are we moving away from expression of feelings here, or will the feelings come in conjunction with the activity?

and some magazines.) Sometimes you can find pictures in magazines that remind you of something about a person. You can either draw on the paper, or cut something out and paste it on.

I want to offer possibilities for evoking memories that do not depend on drawing abilities.

The girls and Ann became very involved in looking through magazines, cutting out pictures, and reminiscing about Robert. It proved to be a meaningful activity that encouraged sharing of significant memories. Each of them recalled different aspects of their relationship with Robert. They planned to give the collage to Terry, and I learned later that she not only thanked them warmly for it but displayed it prominently at the memorial service. Linda wrote a poem for her "uncle" which Ann read at the service. It is printed here with her permission.

My Uncle Robert

My Uncle Robert was brave and strong
There was no test, I wasn't wrong
He loved us so very much
I know we will miss him much
And I couldn't help crying when my Uncle was dieing [sic]
But now he is dead and we bow our heads
So god up there take good care of my Uncle Robert

Two Weeks Later: Summary of Session with Father and Girls

We discussed Robert's death, the memorial service, and what "an ordeal" (Jim's words) they had all been through. The upcoming Christmas holidays were a concern as related to Terry and her children, but Jim made it clear that both he and Ann would see to it that they were not alone. It seemed to me that the focus remained on Robert and his family, rather than on their *own* situation. When I expressed this, Jim mentioned his concern because the girls fought so fiercely at times when they stayed overnight with him. He attributed this to their reaction, both to Robert's death and to the separation. While I agreed with him, I emphasized the necessity of his intervening firmly to keep them from hurting one another. I told him that he must convey to them a sense that he will protect them and that he will not allow them to hurt each other.

Two Months after Death: Summary of Family Session with Mother and Girls

Conflict between Ann and Linda seemed to be escalating. Some of this might have been preadolescent turmoil, but some also seemed related to tension around the separation. Ann believed that Linda was similar to Jim insofar as she held things in and then exploded. When this happened Ann overreacted, treating Linda as if she represented her father rather than as an anxious 10-year-old. Linda may have believed that the separation was Ann's fault since Jim told the girls that he still loved their mother and always would. Linda probably felt a sense of divided loyalty.

Linda and Amanda continued to argue and tussle with one another. When I saw them jointly to discuss this, Linda said perceptively, "I guess *we* should get a divorce!!" When I suggested that Linda draw her feelings (on a paper plate "mask") while I was speaking individually to Amanda, she drew a fearsome "Mr. Warewolf" with sharp teeth, which clearly depicted her anger (Figure 4.1).

Linda later gave me this drawing, and I said that it certainly looked angry and scary; I offered to keep it for her in my office, where it would not get "on the loose" and hurt anybody. Linda smiled and accepted

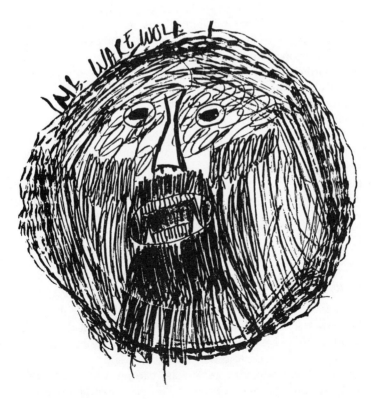

FIGURE 4.1. Linda's drawing of "Mr. Warewolf."

my offer without hesitation, seeming to welcome this view of the safety function of the therapist's role.

A separate session with Amanda included extensive doll play in which she played the nurturing caretaker to twin infant dolls. I did not interpret any of this play but emphasized wherever possible "how lucky those babies were to be so well cared for." One time, in playing a card game, *The Game of Feelings*, with Amanda, she responded to an Angry card: "I felt angry when my parents split up." I agreed that this was understandable, but she declined my offer to talk and so we went on with the game.

Five Months after Death: Summary of Family Session with Mother and Girls

Tension and arguments continued between Ann and Linda as Linda persisted in finding issues to present to Ann that suggested that her mother was treating her unfairly. For example, as a means of saving money and respecting Linda's growing "maturity," Ann had dismissed the regular after-school baby-sitter (Linda was now almost 11, and Amanda 9). This caused inevitable problems between the girls, who complained to Ann about each other. Linda wanted the privilege of being left without supervision, while she thought that her sister should be expected to go to the sitter's house, as previously. Linda whined to her mother, "I went to the sitter when I was 9!"

My role in this was to point out that in view of the girls' difficulty getting along, it was *not* a good idea to leave them alone together. I also reinforced the idea that it was, indeed, appropriate to treat them differently, respecting the age difference and giving Linda some added privilege due to her age.

I noted that at this time there was an absence of dissension about who would go first for therapy, and I complimented the girls about their improved "maturity" with me. I said that I hoped they were getting along better at home as well.

Nine Months after Death: Summary of Telephone Sessions with Amanda

When I went away for my usual 2-month summer vacation, I left my telephone number with Ann, clarifying with her that it was perfectly all right to call me if the need arose. I received two phone calls from Amanda during this time. Amanda told her mother that she wanted to talk to me because she got worried when she was reading a book and the words "seemed to jump out at her." When I talked to Amanda she seemed very puzzled about this and denied any event that might have been upsetting to her. I suggested that sometimes when we are reading our minds wander and maybe that was what happened. I said to Amanda that she should not be overly concerned about what happened but that I wanted her to call me again in a week. A week later when Amanda called she told me that she had had a dream about her mother dying. I said that must have been very frightening, even though it was only a dream. We had an upcoming appointment at the end of my vacation, and I made it clear to Amanda that we would try to understand more clearly these upsetting experiences when we met in person.

One Week Later: Session with Amanda

This was a very interesting session insofar as this 9-year-old came in to therapy having already figured out the source of her own symptoms, which she then refused to explore any further with me.

Content of Session	Analysis and Feelings
THERAPIST: It's good to see you in person, after those phone calls. I'm glad you called, but we need to take some time to try to understand what all of your concerns mean.	Wondering if some events in Amanda's life have changed, or whether she has experienced a delayed reaction to her difficult year.
AMANDA: I think I know what happened. Those words on the page had "angry" voices. That must mean that I am angry inside of me.	Wow! This girl is really making some connections! Or has she discussed this with her mother?
T: It sounds like you've been thinking a lot about this. Were you really worried about what happened?	Trying to figure out the meaning of this experience to Amanda.
AM: It's been a very *rough* year!	Sounds like what she may have heard Mom or Dad say. True!
T: Yes. I know you've been through a lot, and I wouldn't be surprised if you were angry. You certainly have a *right* to be angry.	
AM: I'm not mad at anyone *right now*.	Back off. Even though she made her own interpretation, she does not want to see herself as an angry person.
T: It sounds like you don't want to think of yourself as having angry feelings, even though part of you thinks that might be the reason you had the experience with the words in the book and the dream.	

AM: It's okay now. I haven't had
    any trouble for a long time
    now.

T: I'm glad you're feeling better. I do
   agree with what you said before,
   that some anger inside may be slip-
   ping out. That's okay. Anger can't
   hurt you, and if it happens again,
   we'll talk about it.

She wants to drop it. Shall I
go along with her, or pursue
it?

One Year after Death: Summary of Session with Mother and Girls

Father had let me know that he no longer wanted to bring the girls for therapy and he had conveyed to them his doubts about whether they still needed to come. Mother believed they did and was willing to bring them. In discussion with the girls, they seemed ready to terminate, and we discussed this in the process of reviewing the past year. Parents had now decided to proceed with getting a divorce. The girls said they felt okay about this, because it was now much better than before when the parents were fighting all the time. Father had moved out, and everyone agreed that there was less fighting both between Linda and Amanda and between Ann and Linda (and, of course, between Ann and Jim!). The girls were doing well in their new school classes, and they all seemed happy. The visitation plan had worked well; they saw their father twice a week.

In my individual session with Linda, she asked to play with the wooden blocks (she had never used these before). She built an elaborate house constructed on stilts, using all the blocks in my set. When I asked her if she wanted to put some people in the house she used a male and female doll, referring to them as "the girlfriend" and "the boyfriend." She declined my offer to make up a story about the house and the people, but wanted to invite her mother and sister in to see it before she packed it up, prior to leaving. In Amanda's separate session, she again played with the baby doll, having the mother doll give birth.

Approximately Two-and-a-Half Years after Godfather's Death

I contacted Amanda and Ann by mail, asking whether Amanda (now age 12) would be willing to appear in a videotape in which she and I would discuss her therapy while we demonstrated some of the games and activities that had been helpful to her. They readily agreed, and Amanda came for a follow-up therapy session in which we talked about why she had come originally for therapy, and about how she was doing currently (Webb, 1994). I did not invite Linda to participate since she was then 14 years old, which was beyond the age range of focus on the video-tape.

The taped session with Amanda portrayed her as a poised and sensitive preadolescent who spoke openly about the "rough year" when her "uncle" died and her parents got divorced. She mentioned on the tape that she and her sister had had only one fight in the previous year and that it had occurred at the time their mother was in the hospital for minor surgery. They resolved their differences by telephoning their mother in the hospital to mediate their conflict. On the tape Amanda participated in working with clay, which had been one of her favorite activities in therapy, and we also played the *Deck of Feelings* card game, a "therapeutic" card game that elicits comments from the players about a range of different feelings. I felt very good about this follow-up session in which Amanda reflected her developing maturity.

Three Years after the Death: Summary

Ann was planning to remarry, and Jim, who had kept the family home up to now, planned to sell it. Ann and the girls had moved out to live with the maternal grandmother the previous year. Amanda asked her mother to let her see me to discuss some of her conflicts with her father and her anxieties about her new school. Both girls continued to do well in school and reported feeling very positive about their future stepfather.

RETROSPECTIVE COMMENTS AND CRITIQUE

The first edition of this book was published almost 4 years after the original referral, and approaching 3 years after the marital separation and death of the godfather. At that time I identified and tracked various stages of mourning and its resolution as expressed by these latency-age girls. Insofar as they experienced two very stressful losses almost simultaneously, it was impossible to know how much of their anger was related to the parents' separation and how much was related to bereavement associated with the godfather's death. My own belief is that since the death was unavoidable, and thus "unpreventable" in Burgen's (1983) terms, the mourning associated with this resolved more completely and that "acceptance of the inevitable" death became the operable family dynamic to which the girls also subscribed.

However, the separation and ultimate decision to divorce presented greater challenges to these child grievers. The separation created the possibility of blaming someone, and it also permitted the girls (and sometimes the father also) to hope that the marriage could be saved. Even I shared this wish. I believe strongly in the value of marriage counseling, and I had recommended it to each parent. However, they were not open to this and I had to abide by their decision. In retrospect, my own self-critique makes me wonder if I was as effective as I might have been with regard to the conflict between Linda and her mother. Part of me was also angry with Ann. Although I liked her very much, I realized that the separation had been initiated by her, and I worried about the future impact on the girls of growing up in a divorced family. This points to the challenge in family therapy when the therapist may be pulled to take sides with one or more members, despite conscious efforts to maintain therapeutic neutrality. Fortunately, I had the opportunity to see Ann for one separate session at her request when her therapist was away. This meeting was tremendously beneficial to my understanding of the reasons for the marital breakup. It taught me about the potential value in the therapist's conducting individual sessions with *all* family members from time to time, to promote professional objectivity based on an understanding of each family member's position.

At the time of termination, Linda and Amanda were proceeding with their development and I was optimistic about their future. Linda had expressed her anger openly following the death and separation, and then seemed to have moved beyond it. Amanda, who was younger, benefited from symbolic expression through play therapy. Whenever she experienced some tension related to changes in her life, her positive past experience in therapy prompted her appropriately to seek assistance. I was confident that these girls would continue to develop normally. Although the mourning of the loss of an intact family may never be complete (this may be an unrealistic goal), they had come to an acceptance of their lives and were enjoying their teenage years.

UPDATE

I continued to have intermittent contact with the family, primarily at the time of the remarriages of both Ann and Jim. Prior to Ann's remarriage I had a family session (at her request) to discuss the potential stresses associated with the girls' acceptance of their new stepfather. This actually proceeded quite smoothly, with little conflict. A new baby sister was born within a year, and the girls appeared to dote on her.

In contrast to the ease with which the girls accepted their stepfather and half sister, their relationship with their new stepmother was very strained at first. I had several sessions with the girls alone, with Jim and his new wife, and finally with the girls and their father and stepmother. To everyone's credit, they were eventually able to work out an amicable relationship, but this was complicated because Jim and his new family were living in the home in which the girls had grown up. (He had decided not to sell it once he planned to remarry.) Wallerstein et al. (2000) conclude that children whose parents are able to rebuild happy lives after divorce and include the children in these lives have an easier adjustment as adults. Fortunately, this appears to be true for Amanda and Linda.

When Linda graduated she received a scholarship to attend a college out of state. About the same time, Jim's wife became pregnant and Amanda came to see me about all the changes in her families and her anxiety about having Linda leave home. To Amanda's credit, she always sought and benefited from short-term treatment when she was anxious.

I contacted the girls, now 19 and 21, respectively, in anticipation of writing this update for the second edition of this book. Both were willing and signed permission for me to discuss their current status. Amanda is now a senior in college and is involved in a meaningful relationship. She continues to live at home during school vacations. She looks forward to becoming an early childhood teacher and to getting married after graduation.

Linda shared less of her life. She had left college prior to completion of her degree and was living out of state. Her mother was not pleased about this, and I believe some tension in their relationship may still exist.

The fact that both young women immediately gave me permission to write about them and each wrote personal notes to me verified my own belief that they recognized the significance of their therapy over the course of various life crises during their school-age and adolescent years. For them there is reason to hope that the legacy of their parents' divorce may not continue to haunt them into adulthood.

DISCUSSION QUESTIONS

1. Discuss the early treatment plan with regard to the focus on the girls, rather than on the family as a unit. Consider the advantages and disadvantages of other possible treatment modalities.

2. Discuss the issue of multiple therapists in a family where marital separation is occurring. Do you think it would have been helpful for the therapist treating the children to have been in touch with each of the parents' therapists? Explain your reasons.

3. Comment on the issue of sibling therapy. Evaluate how the therapist dealt with the sibling rivalry and conflict, and suggest how this might have been managed differently.

4. How do you evaluate the girls' respective play themes in the termination session? Do you agree with the therapist's decision about terminating at that time?

6. How successfully did these girls mourn (a) the death of their godfather and (b) their parents' separation? Do you agree with the therapist's optimism about their future?

REFERENCES

American Psychiatric Association. (2000). *Diagnostic and statistical manual of mental disorders* (4th ed., text rev.). Washington, DC: Author.

Bowlby, J. (1960). Grief and mourning in infancy and early childhood. *Psychoanalytic Study of the Child, 15*, 9–52.

Bowlby, J. (1961). Process of mourning. *International Journal of Psycho-Analysis, 42*, 317–340.

Bowlby, J. (1963). Pathological mourning and childhood mourning. *Journal of the American Psychoanalytic Association, 11*, 500–541.

Bowlby, J. (1980). *Attachment and loss: Vol. III. Loss.* New York: Basic Books.

Burgen, L. A. (1983). Childhood bereavement: Preventability and the coping process. In J. E. Schowalter, P. R. Patterson, M. Tallmer, A. H. Kutscher, S. V. Gullo, & D. Peretz (Eds.), *The child and death* (pp. 357–365). New York: Columbia University Press.

Doka, K. J. (1986). Loss upon loss. The impact of death after divorce. *Death Studies, 10*, 441–449.

Falicov, C. J. (1982). Mexican families. In M. McGoldrick, J. K. Pearce, & J. Giordano (Eds.), *Ethnicity and family therapy* (pp. 134–163). New York: Guilford Press.

Furman, E. (1974). *A child's parent dies.* New Haven, CT: Yale University Press.

Goldman, L. (1996). *Breaking the silence: A guide to help children with complicated grief.* Washington, DC: Accelerated Development.

Jewett, C. L. (1982). *Helping children cope with separation and loss.* Cambridge, MA: Harvard Common Press.

Moitoza, E. (1982). Portuguese families. In M. McGoldrick, J. K. Pearce, & J. Giordano (Eds.), *Ethnicity and family therapy* (pp. 412–437). New York: Guilford Press.

Rando, T. (1993). *Treatment of complicated mourning.* Champaign, IL: Research Press.

Raphael, B. (1983). *The anatomy of bereavement.* New York: Basic Books.

Viorst, J. (1986). *Necessary losses.* New York: Baltimore Books.

Wallerstein, J. S., & Blakeslee, S. (1989). *Second chances.* New York: Ticknor & Fields.

Wallerstein, J. S., & Kelly, L. (1980). *Surviving the break-up: How children and parents cope with divorce.* New York: Basic Books.

Wallerstein, J. S., Lewis, J. M., & Blakeslee, S. (2000). *The unexpected legacy of divorce: A 25 year landmark study.* New York: Hyperion.

Webb. N. B. (1994). *Techniques of play therapy: A clinical demonstration* [Videotape]. New York: Guilford Press.

Webb, N. B. (1996). *Social work practice with children.* New York: Guilford Press.

Webb, N. B. (Ed.). (1999). *Play therapy with children in crisis* (2nd ed.): *Individual, group, and family treatment.* New York: Guilford Press.

Weiss, R. (1975). *Marital separation.* New York: Basic Books.

5

❧

The Grief of Siblings

BETTY DAVIES

When asked what they like about their brothers or sisters, young children will often groan, "Like?? I don't like anything about them!" But, when questioned further, many describe positive attributes of their relationship: "He helps me with my homework," "She let's me play with her toys," or " She talks to me about things no one else will talk about." Adolescent siblings sometimes express gratitude for the watchful eye of their older brother or sister: "He always looked out for me—made sure that I didn't get into trouble." Ambivalence often characterizes relationships between siblings. Furthermore, sibling research characterizes siblings as attachment figures, antagonists, playmates, protectors, and socializers (B. Davies, 1999). Through a shared history and common bonds, siblings have the potential for providing one another with intense emotional experience, support, guidance, information, and companionship. Consequently, the significance of the sibling relationship portends the profound effect that the death of one child can have upon brothers and sisters.

Despite the potentially traumatic effect of sibling bereavement, little attention has been directed to children's reactions to the death of a brother or sister. The earliest publication to address sibling bereavement appeared in 1943 (Rosenzweig) and discussed the relationship between sibling death and schizophrenia. This paper stood alone on the topic for two decades. Four articles appeared in the 1960s (Cain, Fast, & Erickson, 1964; Hilgard, 1969; Pollack, 1962; Rosenblatt, 1969); all focused on the effect of childhood bereavement on adults under treatment for psychiatric disorders. Authors writing on the topic in the next decade continued to be mostly psychiatrists and psychologists, who expanded beyond pathology to include the potential growth among bereaved siblings and a family perspective (Blinder, 1972; Binger, 1973; Tooley, 1973; Pollock, 1978; Nixon & Pearn, 1977; Krell & Rabkin, 1979). During the 1980s, authors represented additional health care disciplines, and a dramatic increase in the number of papers was evident. The concern shifted from considering sibling bereavement as a psychiatric problem to a concern for promoting children's health (Balk, 1983b; Martinson, Davies, & McClowry, 1987). As well, attention was directed toward siblings of various ages, including adolescents (Balk, 1983a, 1983b, 1996; Mufson, 1985; Hogan, 1988, Hogan & DeSantis, 1992, 1996), and toward the various factors, particularly the family, that may influence siblings' experience (Lauer, Mulhern, Bohne, & Camitta, 1985; McCown, 1984; Davies, 1988a, 1988b). During these years, the setting shifted from psychiatry to oncology. More recently, interest has turned to developing and testing intervention programs for bereaved siblings (Gibbons, 1992). Much still remains to be done to assess the complex interactions of multiple factors affecting sibling bereavement, to assess bereavement interventions for siblings and their families, and to continue the exploration of long-term effects of sibling bereavement.

SIBLING RESPONSES

Early reports in the literature provide contradictory findings with regard to children's reactions to a sibling's death. Some investigators reported disturbed reactions in the form of significant behavior problems (Cobb, 1956; Cain et al., 1964; Binger et al., 1969; Binger, 1973). In contrast, others reported no significant problems (Futterman & Hoffman, 1973; Stehbens & Lascari, 1974). The variability in findings raises questions about whether the behavior evidenced by grieving siblings represents pathology or a range of bereavement responses.

Range of Behaviors

Bereavement literature indicates that sadness, irritability, feelings of being alone, complaints of bodily discomforts, sleep disorders, and loss of appetite are common to both children and adults who are grieving. These are manifestations of normal grief, and unless they occur with severe intensity or for long periods of time, they are not necessarily indicators of maladjustment (Webb, 1993, and Chapter 2, in this volume). Rather than assessing children's response to a death by identifying the presence or absence of any of these behaviors, it is more important to consider the intrusiveness created by the grieving in the child's life (Webb, 1993). Moreover, the absence of typical grieving behaviors is not necessarily cause for alarm; not all children are affected in the same way or to the same degree by a sibling's death. Parents, in fact, need to be advised that each child in the family will react differently and that, for some children, their reactions may not become evident until later.

Absence of behavioral changes should not negate the significance of the event for siblings since responses may be internal and not readily apparent. However, some siblings have obvious difficulty, and it is important for adults to be alert to the needs of these children. In some studies, about 25% of bereaved siblings demonstrated behavioral problems at levels comparable to those of children referred to mental health clinics; in the general population, behavior problems of only 10% of children reach this level. Unfortunately, there is no certain way to identify those children whose behavior is a sign that they are in trouble, but a number of behaviors may signal those children who might require further attention. Watch for children who persistently show the following signs of problematic sibling bereavement:

- Persistent sadness, unhappiness, or depression
- Persistent aggressiveness or irritability
- Loneliness and social withdrawal
- Worrying
- Persistent anxiety or nervousness
- Ongoing eating difficulties or recurrent nightmares
- Low self-esteem
- Poor school performance

It is important to remember to look for *persistent changes* in the child's behavior and for a *pattern* of problems. No one problem by itself is necessarily an indication of trouble. Though not requiring formal intervention, most bereaved siblings can benefit from opportunities to talk about their responses not only at the time of the death but for many years following. If they are denied opportunities to talk about the death and their reactions, children will suffer needlessly.

Duration of Bereavement

The impact of sibling bereavement lasts for a lifetime. Years following the death, many bereaved siblings report that they still think about, talk to, and miss their deceased brother or sister. They often experience renewed and intense grief on occasions that would have been significant in their lives together, such as graduations, weddings, the birth of babies, career challenges, and even retirement in their later years. It is helpful to warn parents and older siblings about the recurring grief they may experience, and to reassure them that such reactions are common and are not signs of emotional disturbance.

Growth Potential

A child's death not only has the potential of negative effects on surviving siblings; psychological growth often results as well. In one study, bereaved siblings scored higher than the standardized norms on a measure of self-concept (McClowry, Davies, May, Kulenkamp, & Martinson, 1987). Many siblings felt they had matured as a result of their experience, and they felt good about their abilities to handle adversity. As one teenage boy commented, "I have a better outlook on life now; I mean, I realize how important life is as a result of my sister's death." Interviews with parents also indicated that they perceived their children as more sensitive, caring individuals who had matured as a result of their experience with death. Many parents described their children as more compassionate and aware of other people's problems. In the words of one mother about her 15-year-old daughter, "She has learned a lot from her brother's death. It hasn't been easy, but she has gained such insight about life and death. She has been exposed to things that most kids of her age are not. She had to grow up faster, and she is very sensitive and patient. She is so much more tolerant of others as well."

As indicated earlier, there has been an ever-expanding effort in recent decades to learn more about sibling bereavement. Researchers and clinicians share the common goal of wanting to reduce as much as possible the untoward effects of sibling bereavement on children and adolescents. To this end, studies have focused on one or more influencing factors, such as age, gender, suddenness of death, self-esteem, family environment, and their effect on behavior and emotional outcomes. Though contributing to our knowledge about sibling bereavement, such studies do not provide sufficient guidance for intervention since a combination of factors influence how siblings respond to the death of a brother or sister.

Looking more closely at the conceptual relationships among the variables and siblings' responses provides a comprehensive description that provides direction for assisting grieving children (B. Davies, 1999). The impact of a child's death on siblings results in four general responses:

- "I hurt inside."
- "I do not understand."
- "I do not belong."
- "I am not enough."

"I Hurt Inside"

This first response focuses on the emotional and psychophysiological responses normally associated with grief. These include sadness, anger, frustration, loneliness, fear, anxiety, irritability, and guilt. These responses are common to all who grieve, including children—it hurts to grieve. However, unlike adults who more readily describe their emotions, children manifest their hurt in other ways. They may cry, withdraw, seek attention, misbehave, complain of aches and pains, pick fights easily, argue, have nightmares, fear the dark, lose their appetites or overeat.

"I Do Not Understand"

How children begin to make sense of death depends in large part on their level of cognitive development. As children mature, they move from concrete operational ways of thinking toward more abstract or conceptual ways of thinking (see Chapter 2). If children are not assisted to understand and in their own way make sense of death and related events, they become very confused. Their confusion only compounds the anxiety they feel, and in turn their anxiety adds to their confusion.

"I Do Not Belong"

A death in the family disrupts the usual day-to-day activity of family life. Parents are distressed, and familiar and unfamiliar visitors invade the home. Children feel overwhelmed with the flurry of activity and with the outpouring of emotions. They often feel as if they do not know what to do; they may want to help but do not know how. They may begin to feel as if they are not a part of the activity, that they don't belong. Sometimes, children's unique ways of responding are not tolerated by the adults. For example, a teenager who prefers to go out with friends rather than stay at home with other family members may be harshly criticized by adults who think that the family should be together during the crisis. Bereaved children frequently feel different from their peers; again, this may contribute to their feelings of not belonging.

"I Am Not Enough"

This response may result when children feel as if the child who died was a favored child. They feel that the dead child was special in some way, or in many ways, and that they themselves are not at all special. Such children may conclude that *they* should have been the one to die. No matter what they do, they are "not enough" to make their parents happy ever again.

Sibling Responses in Context

Siblings' reactions to the death of a brother or sister do not occur in isolation. Characteristics of the children themselves, the circumstances surrounding the death, and environmental factors play a role. These various factors, characterized as individual, situational, and environmental characteristics, interact with one another, coming together to impact on siblings' responses to the death of a brother or sister (E. Davies, 1983; B. Davies, 1995, 1999; see Figure 5.1).

Aside from emphasizing children's level of cognitive development and their associated understanding of death, there is very little in the literature relating individual characteristics to bereavement outcome in siblings. Paying attention to individual characteristics, however, is basic to perceiving each child as his/her own person. It requires knowing about what makes each sibling unique; it requires knowing about the factors that influence the child's vulnerabilities to loss. Individual characteristics include physical characteristics (such as gender and age, dependence,

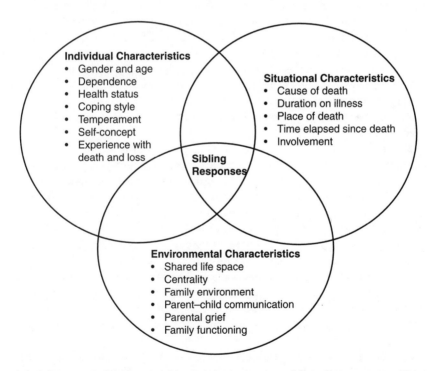

FIGURE 5.1. Mediating variables impacting upon sibling bereavement. From Davies (1999). Copyright 1999 by Taylor & Francis, Inc. Reprinted by permission of Taylor & Francis, Inc., http://www.routledge-ny.com.

and health status), coping style, social-emotional characteristics (such as temperament and self-concept), and experience with death and loss. The circumstances surrounding the death also contribute to how siblings respond. These variables include the cause of death, the duration of illness preceding the death, the place of death, the time elapsed since the death, and the extent of involvement in the death and death-related events.

Environmental variables constitute the third category of factors that influence siblings' bereavement response. These are factors that contribute to the social-emotional atmosphere of the child's context. The nature of the predeath relationship between siblings is of significance. The closer the relationship between two siblings, the more difficulty the surviving child will have after the other's death. Closeness may override age and gender differences. Family environment, particularly family social climate, level of functioning within the family, and parental grief responses, also are instrumental in sibling bereavement response. Children react strongly to these factors since they are dependent on their families for the information and the support they receive. Families characterized by open communication about the death and about feelings tend to provide environments supportive of grieving children. Children learn from their parents and from other adults about death and grief, and how to deal with them. If children see their parents openly sharing their own sorrow, if children hear conversations in which their parents talk about their sadness and confusion and how to deal with these reactions, then children are more likely to learn effective ways of expressing and managing their own sadness.

The cause of death, that is, whether the death is sudden and unexpected or whether it follows a downhill illness trajectory, is one situational factor that is commonly viewed as significant to bereavement outcome. It has been widely documented in the literature on adult bereavement that sudden death results in more intense grief of longer duration (Ball, 1976/1977; Carey, 1977; Fulton & Fulton, 1971; Parkes, 1975; Vachon, 1976). This seems to be the case for sibling bereavement as well. Regardless of the cause of death, all siblings require a clear understanding of what happened. In cases of accidental or violent death, however, issues of fault or preventability come into play, often resulting in feelings of responsibility for family members, including siblings (Kaplan & Joslin, 1993). In addition, elements of trauma and violence raise anxiety levels among children since they may fear a similar fate. When the death is suicidal, surviving children are at risk for disturbed grief reactions (Stephenson, 1986; Brent et al., 1993). Not only are the surviving children left to cope with their grief as well as their possible feelings of rejection by the deceased child, but they also bear the burden of coping with the negative and social stigma that accompanies suicide (Doka, 1989).

The death of a child from a long-term illness implies that the surviving children have had the opportunity to learn about the disease and to prepare for the ill child's eventual death. It is often assumed that anticipatory grief somehow makes it easier for the families of these children. However, this is not the case. All parents hope that their child will be the miracle child who will recover at the last moment. They struggle to put aside their fears of death. Siblings also tend to appraise the situation in positive ways (Brett & Davies, 1988). As a result, there is always an element of the unexpected in a child's death. Moreover, the stress of a long-term illness on families is profound. As a result, siblings may come to the death with a "backlog" of unmet needs and feelings of resentment because their parents have had little time to spend with them. Each family's situation and the experience of each surviving sibling must be assessed individually.

Sibling responses occur within a larger familial and social context as well. Cultural and community values and priorities also contribute to the experiences of bereaved siblings. Within their immediate family, or within their extended families and communities, the interactions that siblings have with the significant adults in their lives are integral to how siblings manage and adapt to the death of a brother or sister.

ADULT INTERACTIONS WITH BEREAVED SIBLINGS

The four major sibling responses listed earlier can serve as a guide to adults who are striving to help grieving children (B. Davies, 1999). For children who are "hurting inside," the goal for parents and other adults is to comfort and console. Adults must accept the child's feelings and behaviors as normal manifestations of grief. They must be patient in allowing children to express their own thoughts and feelings in their own time and in their own ways. Adults who endeavor to share their own thoughts and feelings with children instill a sense of being together with them and offer hope for feeling better in the future. On the other hand, when adults limit expression of feelings, children may conclude that there is something wrong with their feelings. In such situations, children frequently learn to stifle their feelings.

Parents and other adults play a major role in helping children who "don't understand." Adults must explain and interpret all that is happening. Adults need to remember that confusion and ignorance contribute to additional hurt. Therefore, adults must provide honest information in ways that children can understand. They must provide explanations and offer information ahead of time so that children know what to expect. Children learn that it's okay to ask questions if they have adults in their lives who offer explanations of feelings and not just events and who help the young to interpret their own feelings and reactions. They also learn that not all questions have answers; in the company of understanding parents, they learn to accept the uncertainties of life.

Adults can do much to prevent bereaved siblings from feeling as though they "don't belong" if they include and validate the children. When children are included in what is happening, when they have an active role to play in plans and activities, when they are prepared in advance for what is happening, children can manage very well. They feel as if they are part of the family, as if they have valuable contributions to make. On the other hand, when children are excluded from the plans and activities, when they are not given a choice about the nature of their involvement, or when they are not adequately prepared for what to expect, they feel as if they don't belong; their presence and contributions are invalidated. Such children often seek a place of attention through acting out, risk taking, avoiding home, or withdrawing into themselves or their schoolwork.

When children hurt inside, feel as if they are stupid because they don't or can't understand what has happened, or perceive they don't belong, feelings of "I am not enough" are enhanced. This response can be lessened by adults reassuring and confirming through both word and deed that the children are, indeed, special. Through both verbal and nonverbal messages from adults, children must be made to feel that they are loved, appreciated, and valued. Children who feel as if they are not enough may deal with their feelings of inadequacy and inferiority by overachieving, taking on the identity or characteristics of their deceased sibling, excelling at meeting the needs of others, or becoming unrealistically good.

A child's death has lifelong implications for that child's brothers and sisters. However, siblings who are comforted, taught, included, and validated feel they learn from their experience. They feel as if they have become better people, are better able to help others who are grieving, and are better prepared to handle death in the future. Siblings who are belittled, disregarded, left out, or shamed live with feelings of regret and remorse where they feel that nothing good came of their experience. Of course, the experience of any sibling is not entirely one way or the other, but the goal of helping bereaved siblings is to assist them integrate their losses in ways that are regenerative rather than degenerative in the continual unfolding of their lives.

CASE OF JAN, AGE 18, WHOSE BROTHER
DIED WHEN SHE WAS AGE 5

Family Information

Jan Thomas, 18 years of age, just completed her first year of study at the local university, majoring in philosophy. She lives at home with her parents. Jan is the youngest of three siblings. Her older sister, Julia, is 23 years old; she too is attending college but in another state. Her brother, Mark, died at age 11, when Jan was 5 years old.

Presenting Problem/Circumstances

Jan was recruited by a classmate to talk with me about her reaction to Mark's death. She had learned that I was conducting research about sibling bereavement, and she sought the opportunity to share her own experience and, as she said, to "reflect on what I have learned and where I am going with it." The interview was tape recorded and transcribed. Names and identifying information have been altered to protect the anonymity of this individual and her family.

Jan's story clearly demonstrates the long-term effects of a sibling's death with the impact sometimes not fully realized until later in the child's life. It also illustrates the significance of parents' interactions for how children cope with the death.

Content of Session	Analysis and Feelings
INTERVIEWER: Tell me about what happened.	
JAN: My brother, his name was Mark and he died when I was really young, when I was 5 years old. He would have been 11 or 12. He died of a brain tumor in children. At the time the doctors didn't know what it was, what caused it or how to cure it. He woke up Thanksgiving morning and he couldn't walk. It came on really suddenly. There was no warning sign; he just woke up in the morning and he couldn't walk. And then that went on for about a year. Then, on my aunt's birthday, he died in the hospital. I guess my first childhood memory, the first thing I can remember, as far back as I go without peo-	What a frightening and worrisome situation for everyone in the whole family. The brother perhaps died of a brain tumor, although the exact cause of his death is not certain. Without adequate explana-

ple actually telling me what happened, is the viewing of the body at my brother's funeral. It's probably one of the worst memories I have too, because I can remember standing there and looking at my brother and I can remember feeling no remorse, nothing. I think its because I was so young, I didn't even know what was going on.

tions, young children do not understand what has happened nor how to behave. They are confused by their own reactions.

I: You didn't know what was going on.

J: No. I can remember looking and seeing my dad, and it looked like my dad had just no expression on his face. He didn't show any reaction on his face, and I thought that's the way it was for a long time.

Parents' lack of expressing and talking about their own grief not only deprives the child of learning about grief but also may result in the child's drawing inaccurate conclusions about parents' responses. Jan perhaps thought that this is how she should respond.

I: But at the time what you remember is that you didn't think your dad showed any expression of grief or sadness or remorse?

J: Right.

I: So as a little kid, you assumed that your brother's death didn't affect your dad.

J: Right. And I didn't exactly remember that until I was somewhere in the sixth or seventh grade—I would have been 12 or 13. That was the first, the first time that I actually started to realize that I had had a brother that had died on me.

The impact of a sibling's death on children may surface years after the death.

I: What happened to make you realize this?

She says "died on me"—note the personalization of his death.

J: I remember . . . in sixth grade at my school there was an award at the end of the year that was given out to the kid that was the most exceptional student and it was called the Mark Thomas Award [named for her brother]. Mark was your model A student, your model A person, and so when he died the school started to give an annual award to the person graduating from sixth grade who was also a model student, like Mark. When I was in the seventh grade—they usually had the person that won the award give it away the next year—but that year the person moved away so they asked me to give it. That was really . . . it wasn't an eerie feeling but it was a different feeling, giving away an award named for my brother and I had no idea really who he was.

I: And that's what got you thinking about this brother who died.

J: Yeah, that's that's what got me started thinking about it, and I could never talk to anybody in my family about it. We never talked about it as a family, so I went on just trying to, trying to figure out what it all meant. It was the first time I started to deal with my brother's death. That really sparked the interest that I had growing up, a big interest in death. I wanted to know what it was and why my brother died.

When siblings receive no explanation about the death and related events, and when there is no opportunity to discuss the death openly in the family, children will search for answers on their own. She also is close to the age when he became ill; this is often a trigger for thoughts about a deceased sibling.

I: How did you know or find out how he died?

J: This I didn't find out until when I was enrolled in college, the death and dying class. Through that class—it was the first time that I started to discuss it with my family, and not until then did I know a lot of things.

I wonder why it was that she never felt that she could ask even a factual question about her brother's death. The power of a "no talk" rule in families can be profound.

I: So it was kind of like a mystery until then?

J: Right, because growing up right through junior high and high school, I would never bring it up to my parents.

I: Why was that, do you think?

J: Well, my father is the type of person that doesn't let his emotions show.

A climate closed to the discussion of death and to the ex-

He had a lot of deaths in his family that affected him, and he doesn't let his emotions out. And we never talked about it. I can never remember talking about it as a family. They told me that we never did even when I was little.

I: Like his name wasn't mentioned?

J: Well, I mean it would be mentioned here and there, but you would never sit down and talk about it, about his death. Occasionally you might talk about something he did, but you never talked, you never mentioned that he died. When I was starting to deal with it, I could remember some of the times when my mother had broken down with grief because of certain things happening. Like something Mark made had broken and Mom would break down. I must have been about 7. And I knew the way my dad was—where he would never show his emotions—so it was just a natural thing to not talk about it. I was just scared to talk to them about it.

I: You were scared to talk about it because if you talk, your mom's going to break down and you don't know what your dad will do?

J: Right. Because he doesn't let you know. So I just felt like I couldn't talk to them and there wasn't really anyone to talk to. Not when I was a little kid, and not growing up when I was really thinking about it. There wasn't anybody else outside of the family to talk to. I wasn't thinking that I could go talk to some of my friends or something like that.

I: You felt as if there was no one to talk to, no adults. Not even aunts, uncles?

J: Right. It just didn't feel to me that that's something that should be done. I was also brought up in a fam-

pression of emotions inhibits children from talking about death or asking questions.

Children are aware of their parents' distress. It's often frightening for young children (and even older ones) to see their mother cry. Children will often resolve to do nothing (like asking questions) that they believe will cause their parents further distress.

When a young child cannot talk freely with his parents, it is difficult to talk to others and it compounds the child's loneliness and sadness.

When families function by keeping "secrets" within the family, children perceive it is ily where problems within the family stay in the family, and that's how things are dealt with.

I: In the family?

J: Right. In the family. So even going outside our immediate family would have, you know, felt uncomfortable. It was just never brought up so we never talked about it. And then I started to get interested in it and I started to read some stuff on that and that led to other interests.

I: So this interest started when you were in the sixth or seventh grade with the award, and you had no one to talk to, and so you started to read about death and dying?

J: Yeah, and I wanted to know *why* my brother died at such a young age. It's probably a good thing I didn't start thinking much about it earlier, like before I could find stuff to read on my own. I wasn't Catholic, I was Protestant, but you still go through some classes to be in the church.

I: Classes to prepare you to belong to the church?

J: To belong to the church, right. I can't remember what it was called. So I was starting to go to those, and I was learning some things through religion. I started to read stuff on death. There are a lot of inner connections between death and religion. When I was in high school, reading so much religion and trying to find the answers, that's what got me interested in philosophy.

I: So your studying philosophy now stemmed from your interest in death?

J: Right. I think that's an effect my brother's death had on me. It just affected how I looked at religion. Anytime I

"wrong" to talk with anyone outside the family.

Now that she has started to talk about her brother's death, she is even willing to participate in this project!

She seemed to be looking for a religious explanation.

Sounds as if she is/was going through a spiritual struggle.

A sibling's death has long-term and sometimes profound effects on brothers and sisters.

look at a religion, I base my
thoughts on my brother's death to
see if that religion can justify it. I
stopped being active in the Christian
religion, I stopped believing in a
Christian God because I felt that it
couldn't justify my brother's death.
And I held that against Christianity,
and I still do. So his death has led
me to the way I live now.

> This is almost like an existen-
> tial problem for her. What is
> the *meaning* of this death?

I: Being unable to find a reason for his
death took you away from the Christian religion.

J: Yeah, exactly.

I: Have you found that other religions answer some questions for you?

J: I've found different religions that answered different things. Like the
Quaker religion is really misunderstood but it answers certain things.
And I have some Native American
in me, so I've gone back to their religions and they have things in them
that help a bit. But there isn't one religion that I can say I went to and it
answered my questions and now I
can follow that religion. It's like an
ongoing search. I would like to have
a religion, but it's something I cannot do right now.

I: There's nothing that really seems to fit
what you're looking for.

> She is looking for answers.

J: Right. It's really difficult to justify that
to other people. You can try to explain why you're that way, but other
people still don't accept that.

I: You can try to explain that you are
looking for answers?

J: Yeah . . . I am trying to find out *why*
my brother had to die. They don't
know what to do with that.

I: People don't know what to do with
you if you don't have answers?

J: Yeah, mostly because you don't know what to do with yourself.

I: Let me see if I have this right. You are searching for answers about your brother's death. You haven't found answers in any one religion, and you are still trying to understand why it is your brother died. And other people don't seem to understand your need to find this out.

J: Yeah. They don't understand why I have to find out and settle this for myself.

Making sense of finding meaning in a sibling's death is a personal journey that can be lonely and isolating.

I: That sounds like a lonely task.

J: You bet it is. But it's getting better.

I: And so taking this course [on Death and Dying] was another way to find some answers?

J: Exactly. This course has made it possible to do lots of things that I couldn't do before.

As siblings get older, they often find creative ways to explore their experiences with death.

I: So what was it like for you to take this course?

J: For the first time, I talked to my mom and dad.

What a breakthrough!

I: And what was that like?

J: It was a lot easier to talk to my mom. In fact, I didn't talk to my dad through the whole course. I would write the papers and I'd take them home, and my mom kept wanting to read them. She didn't even know what the class was.

I: She didn't know it was a class on Death and Dying?

J: She knew I was taking the class, but she didn't know what it was or what we were doing. I was reluctant to let her read my papers, but then I decided to let her read the first group of papers and then I got to talking with my mom about it. We talked

Jan's mother was open to learning and sharing with her daughter.

and she said that she would have liked for me to talk to her about it earlier on. But I was just a little kid when it happened, so I couldn't really be the one to set the stage. It was really hard for her, to lose a child. She had some mental problems as a result. That was at the same time as I was doing all my reading in high school. There were times I started to feel sort of suicidal, and my mother said she could tell that, but that was never brought up either. She said she had always prayed that when she came home I'd be there.

I: She was worried about you.

J: Right. Because she knew that these things were going through my head. I didn't know this at the time. But she never brought them up and she never talked about them. So, finally we talked during this course. I talked to my mom about my papers, and that's when I started to get answers. Before the class—when I knew I was going to take the class—I wanted to settle some things with myself. I went to the graveyard. I couldn't ask my parents where Mark's grave was, so my friend asked them. Then, I went and saw the grave for the first time, and that was just last summer. I still couldn't talk to my parents about it. Then, after the class, with the discussions with my mom, I started to get some answers. I had all these questions for so long, but no relief. I had no way to get the answers before.

I: The class gave you a way of beginning to talk to your parents.

J: Right. I finally got some of the answers that I wanted. Like I said, I hadn't talked to my father through the

Individual grief is always distressing, but lack of open expression in families compounds the individual distress.

The fear of talking openly about sensitive topics results in greater isolation. The silence has taken a toll on Jan's mother also.

Seeing the gravesite of a deceased sibling offers more information about the death and her brother.

whole ordeal. That really bugged me. So for my final paper, I wrote about how I wanted to talk to my dad, that I wanted to bring these things up and speak to him. I took it home and I left it somewhere, and he found it and read it. He didn't say anything for a while. He started to write something back to me, and then one day he let me read what he wrote. It was about four or five pages of what happened when he grew up, about how his mother died during the Vietnam War. He didn't really know her before he went off to war, and then she died before he had a chance to get to know her. He explained to me how all of these things affected him and that's why he is the way he is now. So I was finally able to talk to my dad—it was the first time that I ever saw him emotional. He doesn't want to show emotion, and this was the first time he did. That was really hard for me to take because I'd never seen it before.

Now this clarifies the father's inability to deal with his son's death. When a father is not usually expressive, seeing a father's distress is often difficult for children even though they value such expression.

I: And it was so different from what you expected.

J: Right, right. So since then we talk about it in spurts. I kept wanting to talk about it more, but he wasn't ready. Then he started to read certain books on things that happen in your childhood and how they affect you. He's given me some of the books to read, and he wants to talk about those in the hope that we can start a real conversation. We still haven't actually talked about my brother's death, not specifically.

Open discussion about death develops slowly in families where expression has been minimal.

I: But it sounds as if the door has opened.

Trying to be helpful.

J: Right. It's been opened. I know what he's doing—hoping that these books

Talking about related topics first can lay the groundwork

can start us talking on these terms
and then have that lead into talking
about my brother's death.

I: Sounds as if he's using a similar strategy
to what you used when you left the
papers you had written so that your
mom and dad would find them and
read them, and begin to talk to you.

J: Yeah, I think so. He thinks he's the
kind of father who was always open
with his kids and always able to talk
to them. So it really bugged him
when he found out that here was
something I wanted to talk about
and I couldn't approach him. That really bothered him.

I: Because he saw himself as different
than you saw him? He saw himself
as approachable and open?

J: Yeah, and he wanted to be, he wanted
to be the person that you could always talk to. He said that he doesn't
think that us talking about this is going to do him any good. He says
that it's not going to help him at all
but he wants to do this for me, to try
and help me. I don't really agree
with that. I think that it's going to
help him too, but he doesn't see it
that way right now.

I: It may take him a while to see the benefits for himself, but you think it will
help both of you to talk openly
about your brother's death?

J: Yeah. He's just a person that is real set
in his ways. You know, the kind that
just keeps everything in; they deal
with everything themselves. And
that's the way I was brought up. But
then I came to a point where I
couldn't deal with this by myself.

I: You got to the point of wanting to talk
about your brother's death with your
parents?

for talking about the death.

Parents' perceptions of their
level of openness may vary
from their children's perceptions; self-awareness is important for adults who want to
help grieving children.

Optimally supporting children
in their grief is a shared journey between adults and children where each share and
grow.

Shows a level of strength.

J: Right. The family doesn't really have many communication problems. I mean, we're all very close, but it's just this topic that's difficult to talk about. My dad would tell me how they as parents didn't know what to do, and he regrets it now. He can remember times where my mother would be upstairs crying and my dad would be down watching us, and then she would come down and he'd go up and cry. Now looking back he can see that they were never there for my sister and me. And me and my sister have taken it really differently it seems.

I: In what ways is it different? How has it been for your sister?

J: Julia is 3 years older than I am. She was in the middle between Mark and me. She sees everything really different. I don't have any memories of my brother alive because I was only 5 or 6 years old when he died. My father thinks I should remember. He says he thinks I have the memories but it's just that they're all blocked up. That might be true, because he said that after Mark died I was really quiet and withdrawn for a long time. My sister remembers a lot, but her memories are different from the way my parents remember things. She remembers that she was the one that always got blamed for things. Mark and I were always together; my parents have said that Mark and I were really close. Julia was the troublemaker, and she got punished all the time.

I: And this is what Julia remembers? Always being the one in trouble?

J: Yes, and that she and Mark weren't so close. It really bugged me when I found out that Mark and I had been

Even families that are expressive and open about many issues often have difficulty talking about death.

Parents are often overcome with their own grief and surviving children can feel neglected. Parents may feel that it would be detrimental to cry in front of their children.

so close. That's probably something that I would rather not have known because that just makes me feel really bad. Just knowing that we were really, really close when we were young, and that he was such an important part of my life and I have no memories of it at all. That's probably the thing that's hardest for me now.

Closeness between siblings often means that the surviving sibling will have difficulty adapting to the loss.

I: What about photographs of the two of you when you were little? When you see them, does it help you remember Mark?

J: My grandmother has pictures in Arizona. I haven't seen them yet. We barely have any around the house. We have a few other things that he had, some trophies and poems that he wrote but I haven't seen any pictures of him. My grandmother is the person in the family that kept all the family albums. Everybody sends her pictures, so she's got the family archives. I can recall a few pictures of all three of us; maybe it was Halloween and we were all dressed up. But I can't remember any pictures of just Mark and me. We don't know for sure if there are pictures. My mother and father say that maybe there are pictures around and we can get them if that will help me remember something or help me deal with it.

Photographs often serve as a vehicle for family members to remember and talk about the deceased child. It seems unusual that they don't have photos, when they were so proud of him, but some families take few photos, sometimes for financial reasons, for example.

I: You would like to find those pictures, if there are any?

J: I would. I am still hoping we will find some.

I: You will find out from your grandmother?

J: Yes, I have written her a letter.

It might help the entire family to look at these together—doing so might serve as a vehicle for open communication about events in the family.

I: How about you and Julia? Have the two of you talked about Mark and what his death was like for each of you?

J: Julia is a lot like my father. They both have the problem where they can't be open about this unless they've been drinking a little.

I: That loosens them up a little?

J: Right, and I think that's kind of distorted. I've talked to my sister only a few times, and its because it seems like she resents Mark so much. She sees how Mark was. Mark was a perfect child, and Julia thought she was always judged against Mark. Mark was always a straight A student, and he was sociable. He was real popular with everybody, and everybody liked him. Julia always felt that my parents judged her against that. Then I came along, and I was good in school too. Julia felt like she was stuck in the middle. She feels that she can't be good enough, that she can't match up to Mark. She can only remember me and Mark being together all the time and being the best of friends and she was left out. She has a resentment to Mark.

Being compared unfavorably to the child who died contributes to surviving siblings feeling as if "I am not enough."

I: That she still carries with her?

J: Right. My father told me that Julia told him that maybe it would have been better if *she* had died. My dad said that was completely crushing to hear. I think that's sort of the resentment she has for Mark.

Siblings who feel as if they are "not enough" may wish they were the ones who should have died—a terrible, lonely feeling.

I: That sounds like a heavy load to carry.

J: Yeah.

I: Is this something you have ever felt?

J: No, but I think I've never felt judged for what Mark has done. I've never had that feeling, and I think that's because I've always been a good student and all. Though I wasn't very sociable, and a lot of that is because of the way I reacted with Mark's death.

I: How's that related to Mark's death?

J: Well, I had friends through grade school, and then I got to junior high. That's when I started to be interested in my brother's death and I started to read books on death and dying.

I: There probably weren't many other kids who were interested in the same thing.

J: Right. I never felt ashamed to go into class, having a book on death and reading it before class. In junior high especially is the time where kids see you're reading a book on death, and they have their preconceived ideas about how weird that is. I've never considered myself a sick-minded person, but if you're like that in junior high, people get these preconceived ideas and then whatever you do you're not going to break them. And they don't give you the chance to break them. So, I never had close people through school. I always had people that I could talk to about everyday stuff. I played basketball in school and I had friends there, but there was never anybody that I felt I could call up on the weekend and say why don't we all go to the movie or why don't we do something. If something wasn't going on, I was just kind of in my house.

> Bereaved siblings, particularly adolescents, often feel different from their peers as a result of their experience with a loved one's death.

> Feeling of being alone, isolated. A referral to a bereavement group could have been helpful, but no such groups existed in Jan's rural hometown.

I: So you spent a lot of time by yourself?

J: Yeah. I just felt different than the other kids somehow, and I think it was because I was always thinking about Mark. Later on, I felt more comfortable with people I didn't go to school with. I got a job at 16, and I used to love to go to work because nobody knew who I was. They didn't know about Mark and about what I was interested in. That's where I met my friend. She was start-

> Having one understanding person with whom to talk openly often facilitates the grief process.

ing to work there too, and she was the first person that I felt I could open to and talk to. She was the first person I talked to about Mark. It seemed easy to talk to her. I don't know what it was; I never really cared why.

I: The chemistry between some people that enables you to talk.

J: So, yeah it was, I could talk to her. I explained a lot of things to her, and I just felt real comfortable.

I: Was this the friend that helped you get to the cemetery?

J: Yeah. That's something that I had wanted to do. Growing up for 6 years and not knowing anything. It was 6 years that I was thinking about my brother's death and thinking of all these questions that I could never find an answer for. I'm sure I thought about it as a young child too, but I don't remember those years. I couldn't go to the cemetery because I didn't have my driver's license. I didn't get my driver's license until late. I knew the cemetery, but I didn't know where in the cemetery because I had never been there. Finally I got my driver's license and that was around the time when I was talking to her. I felt I could go out and do something on my own. That was two summers ago. That's when I went and saw the grave, so it was something that I had wanted to do but I never felt I could until then.

Six years seems like a long time to be harboring questions while feeling unable to ask them. Some siblings never get to the point of asking questions.

Jan showed such persistence and determination!

I: And what was it like for you when you went to Mark's grave?

J: It was good. I wished I could have gone a long time ago.

Visiting the actual gravesite often facilitates the grief process.

I: You said that you remembered seeing your brother in his coffin. So, that means you were at his funeral even though you didn't go to the cemetery?

J: Yes, my parents told me that they decided it would be important for me to go to the laying out, and I went to that, but I didn't go to the funeral or the cemetery. I went back to my grandmother's place, and I can't remember any of that but this is what they told me. They said that nobody else in the family wanted me and my sister to be there. They thought that was a wrong thing; they felt pretty strongly that we should not be there. It was an open casket and my father didn't want an open casket, but my mother's grandmother insisted on it and my father today holds a really strong resentment for that. He said that he could never forgive something like that, but myself I, I think I'm kind of glad that it was an open casket because that allowed me to see my brother.

Children usually prefer to be included in funeral events, and resent being excluded.

Perceptions of other adults can influence parents' decision about allowing children to attend the funeral.

Family members may differ in their perceptions of events.

I: And you wouldn't have otherwise.

J: Right, and that's, that is the only, the only image that I have of him. I've seen school pictures of him, but this is the only one that I have that's my very own memory.

Seeing the child's body can provide concrete images that are helpful in creating special memories for siblings.

I: And that's a special memory that you have.

J: Yeah.

I: When does this memory become most clear? How often do you think of this memory?

J: All the time. Well, maybe not that memory exactly, but I think about Mark all the time.

I: Like when?

J: Well, I consider myself a pretty high risk taker. I'm not sure that I associ-

Bereaved siblings often consider themselves risk takers as

ate it with my brother's death. I think it's a combination of other deaths. I've had two of my grandfathers die since my brother died. And I had a friend that died. It almost seems like death just became a regular thing for me in my life. I became a risk taker because it's just something that you're used to—you're going to die. My brother died when he was so young; I guess when you're going to die that it's just when you're supposed to die. There's a sense of almost why hold myself back because if my time is up anyway. . . . Being around death so much, I think it kind of casts away the strong fear of death. I don't feel that I fear death as much as a lot of other people. Like I said, I was suicidal before and I think also that that's one of the reasons why I'm like I am. I think once you reach the point where you're ready to commit suicide, if you come back, you're never going to think the same.

a result of their experience with death and their resultant philosophy of life.

May be perceived as a fatalistic view; also may be a realization that death is inevitable.

This is serious; must be explored. Important to explore any mention of suicide to see if it is a current possibility.

I: What was that like for you?

J: Being almost ready to commit suicide? It was horrible. I can remember in seventh grade, I had a paper route and I can remember the day that I was walking around and I was thinking that I'm not even sure I believe in God. And just from learning from the church that if you don't believe in God, you're going to go to hell, you're going to be a devil worshipper. And I kept thinking if that's what I am, was it even worth going on? I can remember throwing papers and thinking this conversation to myself and having this battle inside my mind as whether I should kill myself or not. Every single day that went on, it was the same thing. There was

Struggling to understand death and one's reactions can be overwhelming for young people and very lonely.

How hard and sad for this young girl! If only she'd had someone to confide in—a counselor or teacher at school, for example.

not a day that went by that I didn't think of killing myself.

I: That must have been very scary. And lonely too.

> Trying to be supportive.

J: Yeah, it was awful.

I: Did you go as far as thinking how you would do it?

J: Oh, yeah. I had it all worked out. I thought of all kinds of different ways, but then you got to the point where it was like you were either going to do it or you're not going to do it. And, as I see it, one thing stopped me from killing myself and it was my mother. I couldn't put her through the death of another child. I knew the way it affected her before, and I saw that when I was growing up, and there was no way that I would want to do that to my mother again.

> Important to uncover what prevented her acting on the impulse/wish.

I: So it was a desire to protect your mother from going through the grief of losing another child that kept you from killing yourself?

> Acknowledge her empathy/ compassion for her mother.

J: Yeah, that was it.

I: Do you still have thoughts of suicide?

J: No. I don't think I have the fear of death that most people have. But I don't sit here and say if I die tomorrow that's just fine and dandy. I don't say I don't care if I die tomorrow. I don't want to die now; there's a lot of things I want to do, but its the thing that if I do die, I'm not going to die regretting things I've done. Even without the religion base, I'm not worried about what is going to happen after I die. Mark has done it, and he'll be there, wherever. I think a lot of people are so afraid of death that's why they don't talk about it. People just don't know how to respond, and I think it's because

> Experiencing the death of a brother or sister impacts upon siblings' attitudes toward death. Many seem to develop a "comfort with" or "acceptance of" death as part of life. The thoughts of suicide are part of her past struggle. Now, it's a good sign that she is planning for her future.

they're uncomfortable and because
it's frightening.

I: So you are more comfortable with death
than young people who haven't had
the experience you have had?

J: Yeah, for sure. When people say how
many brothers or sisters do you have,
what I say depends on how I'm feeling that day. I'll say, I have one of
each, but my brother died. That's
kind of like a conversation stopper
right there, and that kind of puts up
a big buffer zone because they don't
know what to say. Or, they ask,
"What has affected you most in life?"
I end up saying that my brother died.
It's like a big stopper.

> The startled reactions of oth-
> ers to honesty about death are
> ongoing.

I: So the answer to that question—"What
has affected you most in life?"—it
would be your brother's death?

J: Yeah, yeah, for sure. Like I said earlier,
it's guided the way I think. It's
guided my interest in philosophy;
it's provided a reason why I can't be
involved in a Christian religion. It's
not an everyday thing, but I'm always thinking about it. Certain
things will bring it right out; it's always like right on the base.

> The impact of a sibling's
> death can be profound and all
> encompassing.

I: Like an integral part of who you are.

J: It has the most profound effect. Like
the biggest effect would be my idea
that whatever happens is going to
happen. That makes me deal with
things in a different way than other
people do. If something doesn't happen the way I want it to, well, that's
fine and I just move on. I don't have
emotional highs and lows.

> A child's death can strongly
> impact on siblings' general
> outlook on life.

I: You are pretty steady in the way you
deal with life's challenges?

J: Yeah. Steady even keel. As far as
friends or boyfriends and stuff, there
aren't real happy times or real low

> She has developed an accep-
> tance of what she cannot
> change.

times. I take things as they come along. That sometimes affects my relationships with other people because they don't understand that. I want to talk about things that matter. I want to deal with things when they happen.

I: Not waiting until years later?

J: Yeah, exactly. My dad didn't deal with things in his life when they happened. Like my brother's death. I want to really do it. I feel I can talk to him about my brother now. I want to fix what went wrong for me, and I am doing that.

> Opportunity for sharing and talking about sibling's grief can occur many years after the death.

I: It sounds as if you feel you are making changes in how you relate to your dad and in the things you talk about with him.

J: Yeah, and it's good. My dad is quite insightful. He gave me those couple of pages to read, and there was a side of my dad that I never saw before. I never knew what was going on with him. The way he wrote and the way he talked, he was like a big time writer. I told him that this was better than any of these books that I'd read. I got to see a side of my father that I never knew existed. All because he was so closed. So, if you can tell other parents about what happened to me and my dad, maybe it will help other kids. The most important thing is to talk to kids, tell them what's happening—at the time and later too, all the time. Don't try to hide them from death and from all the emotions. Because if you keep things in the closet when kids are little, you just have to clean it out later and by then there's an awful lot of junk stored in that closet.

> Parents do their best to support their grieving children, but they are influenced by their own grief and their own life histories and past experience with grief.

> This is exciting—the fact that she and her father are developing a new relationship.

> The best advice often comes from the bereaved sibling. To assist siblings in optimal ways, include them, offer explanations, and reassure them at the time of the death and thereafter.

> She wants to share what she learned for the benefit of others—such altruism is a frequent motivation for talking about one's own experience with a sibling death.

CONCLUSION

Jan's story very clearly highlights the long-term experience of many bereaved siblings. At the time of Mark's death and afterward, there was little discussion in the Thomas family about what had happened. In families when a child's death is not discussed openly, the surviving children are often left with unanswered questions about what happened, and oftentimes about their role in and responsibility for what happened. In Jan's case, she did not seem to feel responsible in any way for her brother's death, but she did not have a clear understanding of the illness that caused his death. Because Mark's name was seldom mentioned, Jan was left with the impression that he "should" not be talked about. Moreover, Jan felt that to raise the subject carried the potential of upsetting her mother or making her father angry. In such families, children tend to keep their thoughts and feelings to themselves, and are thereby deprived of the information and comfort that parents might be able to offer. But the parents too are distressed, and often, out of their perceived need to protect their surviving children from additional distress, they try to hide their own sadness—as Mr. and Mrs. Thomas did when they took turns going upstairs to cry away from the children. When families can openly talk about what happened and about their reactions to events, then children learn that sadness is a normal and natural response and that there is comfort in sharing the sadness.

Jan's story and that of her sister, Julia, exemplify how the quality of the relationship between siblings affects the bereavement experience of the surviving child. Jan had a close relationship with Mark (though she didn't remember it as such until she was told so by her sister and parents). Earlier work has shown that closeness between siblings, as rated by the parents, impacts upon the grief experience of siblings. Even though Jan and Mark were neither close in age nor of the same gender, they shared a special bond that was obvious to their parents and to Julia. At the same time as Jan felt even more compelled to learn about her brother's death because they had been so close, she also felt comforted by this knowledge and by her recollections of him. Julia, on the other hand, had felt "left out" of the special relationship Mark and Jan had shared. It seemed there had been times that Julia had resented her two siblings. Moreover, Mark was a good student, an accomplished athlete, and popular, and Julia felt inadequate by comparison. Her sense of inadequacy persisted after his death to the point of her stating that she wished that *she* had been the one to die. Her father was very dismayed over this comment, but the lack of open communication and reassurance to Julia that she herself was special in her parents' eyes more than likely contributed to her feelings of "I am not enough."

In my interviews with other siblings who have experienced the death of a brother or sister in their childhood, I learned that some of them continued throughout many years of their lives with their questions unanswered. Then, by attending a lecture or presentation on sibling bereavement or reflecting on their inner lives with a counselor for some seemingly unrelated reason, they would realize the impact of their sibling's death. As they continued to explore their experience of sibling bereavement, they would often gain additional insights about their own behavior, such as having suicidal thoughts (as Jan had). Jan demonstrated an inner urge to explore and find out more on her own. She showed remarkable persistence and determination, knowing at some level that finding out the answers to her questions was important for her. As a result, she experienced greater peace of mind, as many bereaved siblings do when they have the opportunity to examine their earlier experiences.

My interview with Jan was for research purposes. However, as a clinician who has worked with and talked to many bereaved siblings, I have learned that such interviews also serve therapeutic purposes. At the conclusion of each research interview, after the tape has been turned off, I ask about the experience of participating in the study. Frequently, people indicate that this is the first time they have ever told their story; such was the case with Jan, though she had written about various aspects of her experience in the Death and Dying class. More often than not, individuals say that they enjoyed the opportunity to just "tell their story" and to have someone "interested in what I have to say." Through the telling of their story, they often gain new insights and perspectives. With Jan, she referred back to her concluding comment about keeping things in the closet when kids are little and having to clean it out later, but by then there's a lot of junk stored in that closet. Jan felt that the interview had been another step in "cleaning out the closet." And, as is the motivation for many siblings to participate in a research project of this type, Jan hoped that sharing her experience would somehow benefit other children so they would have "less junk stored in the closet."

DISCUSSION QUESTIONS

1. Discuss some of the typical reactions of a 5-year old to death. How do Jan's memories of her brother's death resemble or differ from these?

2. Since different family members often have very different responses and feelings about the death of a child or sibling, what type of counseling is appropriate? Discuss the pros and cons of family/individual and group counseling with regard to Jan's family.

3. How would you assess Jan's capacity for dealing with future losses? Do you consider her to be "at risk," and why or why not?

4. How could Jan's experience be used to provide guidance to parents about how to support their well children when another child is seriously ill?— About how to support their bereaved children following the ill child's death?

5. What approach might be appropriate in helping Julia, Jan's older sister, in dealing with her experience of sibling bereavement?

REFERENCES

Balk, D. (1983a). Effects of sibling death on teenagers. *Journal of School Health,* 53(1), 14–18.

Balk, D. (1983b). Adolescents' grief reactions and self-concept perceptions following sibling death: A study of 33 teenagers. *Journal of Youth and Adolescence* 12, 137–161.

Balk, D. (1996). Attachment and the nations of bereaved college students: A longitudinal study. In D. Klass & P. Silverman (Eds.), *Continuing bonds: New understandings of grief* (pp. 311–328). Washington, DC: Taylor & Francis.

Ball, J. (1976/1977). Widow's grief: The impact of age and mode of death. *Omega: Journal of Death and Dying,* 7, 307–333.

Binger, C. M. (1973). Childhood leukemia: Emotional impact on siblings. In J. E. Anthony & C. Koupernick (Eds.), *The child and his family: The impact of disease and death* (pp. 195–209). New York: Wiley.

Binger, C. M., Ablin, A., Feuerstein, R., Kushner, J., Zoger, S., & Mikkelsen, C. (1969). Childhood leukemia: Emotional impact on patient and family. *New England Journal of Medicine, 2804,* 414–418.

Blinder, B. J. (1972). Sibling death in childhood. *Child Psychiatry and Human Development, 2,* 1969–1975.

Brent, D. A, Perper, J. A., Moritz G., Liotos, L., Schweers, J., Roth, C., Balach, L., & Allman, C. (1993). Psychiatric impact of the loss of an adolescent sibling to suicide. *Journal of Affective Disorders, 28,* 249–256.

Brett, K., & Davies, B. (1988). What does it mean?: Sibling and parental appraisals of childhood leukemia. *Cancer Nursing, 11*(6), 329–338.

Cain, A., Fast, I., & Erickson, M. (1964). Children's disturbed reactions to the death of a sibling. *American Journal of Orthopsychiatry, 34,* 741–745.

Carey, R. G. (1977). The widowed: A year later. *Journal of Counseling Psychology,* 24, 125–131.

Cobb, B. (1956). Psychological impact of long-term illness and death of a child in the family circle. *Journal of Pediatrics, 49,* 746–751.

Davies, B. (1988a). Shared life space and sibling bereavement responses. *Cancer Nursing,* 11, 339–347.

Davies, B. (1988b). The family environment in bereaved families and its relationship to surviving sibling behavior. *Children's Health Care, 17,* 22–31.

Davies, B. (1995). Sibling bereavement research: State of the art. In I. Corless, B. Germino, & M. Pittman (Eds.), *A challenge for living: Death, dying and bereavement* (Vol. 2, pp. 173–202). Boston: Jones & Bartlett.

Davies, B. (1999). *Shadows in the sun: The experiences of sibling bereavement in childhood*. Philadelphia: Brunner/Mazel.

Davies, E. (1983). *Behavioral response of children to the death of a sibling*. Unpublished doctoral dissertation, University of Washington, Seattle.

Doka, K. (Ed.) (1989). *Disenfranchised grief: Recognizing hidden sorrow*. New York: Free Press.

Fulton, R., & Fulton, J. (1971). A psychosocial aspect of terminal care: Anticipatory grief. *Omega: Journal of Death and Dying, 2*, 91–100.

Futterman, F. H., & Hoffman, I. (1973). Crisis and adaptation in the families of fatally ill children. In E. F. Anthony & C. Koupernick (Eds.), *The child and his family: The impact of disease and death* (Vol. 2, pp. 121–138). New York: Wiley.

Gibbons, M. B. (1992). A child dies, a child survives: The impact of sibling loss. *Journal of Pediatric Health Care, 6*, 65–72.

Hilgard, J. R. (1969). Depressive and psychotic states as anniversaries to sibling death in childhood. *International Psychiatry Clinics, 6*, 197–207.

Hogan, N. S. (1988). Understanding sibling bereavement. *The Forum, 12*, 4–5.

Hogan, N. S., & DeSantis, L. (1992). Things that help and hinder adolescent sibling bereavement, *Western Journal of Nursing Research, 16*, 132–153.

Hogan, N. S., & DeSantis, L. (1996). Adolescent sibling bereavement: Toward a new theory. In C. Corr (Ed.), *Handbook of adolescent death and bereavement* (pp. 173–195). New York: Springer.

Kaplan, C. P., & Joslin, H. (1993). Accidental sibling death: Case of Peter, age 6. In N. B. Webb (Ed.), *Helping bereaved children: A handbook for practitioners* (pp. 118–136). New York: Guilford Press.

Krell, R., & Rabkin, L. (1979). The effects of sibling death on the surviving child: A family perspective. *Family Process 18*, 471–477.

Lauer, M. E., Mulhern, R. K., Bohne, J. B., & Camitta, B. M. (1985). Children's perceptions of their sibling's death at home or in hospital: The precursors of differential adjustment. *Cancer Nursing, 8*, 21–27.

Martinson, I., Davies, B., & McClowry, S. (1987). The long-term effects of sibling death on self-concept. *Journal of Pediatric Nursing, 2*, 227–235.

McClowry, S., Davies, B., May, K., Kulenkamp, E., & Martinson, I. (1987). The empty space phenomenon: The process of grief in the bereaved family. *Death Studies, 11*, 361–374.

McCown, D. (1984). Funeral atendance, cremation and young siblings. *Death Education, 8*, 349–363.

Mufson, T. (1985). Issues surrounding sibling death during adolescence. *Child and Adolescent Social Work Journal, 2*, 204–218.

Nixon, J., & Pearn, J. (1977). Emotional sequelae of parents and siblings following the drowning or near-drowning of a child. *Australian and New Zealand Journal of Psychiatry, 11*, 265–268.

Parkes, C. M. (1975). Determinants of outcome following bereavement. *Omega, 6*, 303–323.

Pollock, G. (1962). Childhood parent and sibling loss in adult patients. *Archives of General Psychiatry, 7*, 295–305.

Pollock, G. (1978). On siblings, childhood sibling loss and creativity. *Annual of Psychoanalysis, 6*, 443–481.

Rosenblatt, B. (1969). A young boy's reaction to the death of his sister. *Journal of the American Academy of Child Psychiatry, 8*, 321–335.

Rosenzweig, S. (1943). Sibling death as a psychological experience with reference to schizophrenia. *Psychoanalytic Review, 30*, 177–186.

Stehbens, J. A., & Lascari, A. D. (1974). Psychological follow-up of families with childhood leukemia. *Journal of Clinical Psychology, 30*, 394–397.

Stephenson, J. (1986). Grief of Siblings. In T. A. Rando (Ed.), *Parental loss of a child* (pp. 321–338). Champaign, IL: Research Press.

Tooley, K. (1973). The choice of a surviving sibling as "scapegoat" in some cases of maternal bereavement: A case report. *Journal of Child Psychology and Psychiatry, 16*, 331–339.

Vachon, M. (1976). Stress reactions to bereavement. *Essence, 1*, 23.

Webb, N. B. (1993). Assessment of the bereaved child. In N. B. Webb (Ed.), *Helping bereaved children: A handbook for practitioners* (pp. 19–42). New York: Guilford Press.

6

❦

Suicide in the Family

SANDRA L. ELDER
DON KNOWLES

Suicide is a tragedy. By its very nature, a suicidal death may raise strong feelings in survivors, such as extreme guilt and self-blame, stigmatization, and feelings of rejection by the deceased (Silverman, Range, & Overholser, 1994/1995). Reactions vary depending on the age of the child or adolescent, the relationship to the deceased, circumstances prior to the suicide event, and the time since the death. The number of children and adolescents experiencing a family member's suicide is difficult to determine in part because of underreporting. In the United States, an estimated 30,000 suicides occur each year, yielding an estimated 180,000 survivors (McIntosh, 1996). In Canada, the suicide rate was 21.5 per 100,000 for males and 5.4 for females in 1995 (Harrington, 1998). Among children 5–14 years of age, the number of suicides was 229 for the period 1993–1997 (Suicide Information and Education Center [SIEC], 2000). S. Goldman and W. R. Beardslee (as cited in SIEC, 2000) estimated that in the United States nearly 1% of school-age children attempted to harm themselves. Typically, suicide rates are highest for ages 30 to 50 years (SIEC, 2000), although the rate for the elderly (Stimming & Stimming, 1999) and adolescents has been high among some populations. Thus, a family suicide involves the death of brothers and sisters, parents, aunts and uncles, cousins, or grandparents.

In this chapter, we review the responses to suicidal death that have been relatively well documented. Our perspective is that, following a suicidal death, the reactions of important adults are extremely important as the child attempts to gain some understanding or meaning about the nature and consequences of the death. We describe the stories of loss of three young people who experienced family suicide in order to present some different meanings attributed to suicidal deaths by different survivors. Finally the role of counseling interventions will be considered.

UNDERSTANDING THE CHILD'S
PERCEPTION OF THE DEATH

The level of cognitive development is a key component of the suicide survivors' ability to conceptualize the meaning of death and to understand why the person took his/her life. Young children's egocentricity and their tendency to think in a cause-and-effect manner may make them believe that something they did or did not do caused the death (Lonetto, 1980). They believe that if they are good the world will be good but if they are bad the world will be bad. So when things go wrong, they may think they are to blame.

If these thoughts and feelings are left unchecked, young children may weave in more information based on their imagination and fantasy in order to complete their story of what happened to their loved one. The fact that young children think in concrete terms and have a difficult time understanding abstraction means that they must rely on their parent, siblings, and other adults to interpret what has happened (Lonetto, 1980). When they are confused and upset, they are more apt to respond to the emotional tone of the person who is conveying the information and to nonverbal information from the person and the situation. As discussed in Chapter 1 (this volume), children tend to mourn in bits and pieces because they have difficulty dealing with the intensity of their grief on a continuing basis.

By the time they have reached the age of 7 or 8, many children have developed the capacity to understand that death is irreversible and that body functions and sensations cease. However, the trauma of a suicide death may make them so unsettled that they may feel responsible, puzzled by the death, anxious about their own bodies, and concerned about what happens after death (Leenars & Wenckstern, 1990).

During preadolescence and early teen years, youngsters begin to think in an abstract manner, more like adults. They are often more capable of managing the emotions of grief than younger children, but their ability is still limited by developmental constraints. The developmental process known as separation–individuation during adolescence involves a shift from a partially dependent to an increasingly autonomous relationship with their parents (Elder, 1993). When a parent dies, important developmental processes may be interrupted. Changes that might normally be expected may be averted, avoided, or may not transpire. Such an arrest of developmental unfolding may put adolescents "on hold" in one phase and thus interfere with the development of skills and energy necessary to meet subsequent phase-appropriate demands (Elder, 1993). Raphael (1983) considers parental death as being "the greatest loss for the adolescent, especially in the earlier years when he or she has not completed the separation process" (p. 145).

After a family suicide, children and adolescents are affected by the reactions of surviving family members, especially in the case of a parental death. They tend to take their cues from these family members. For young children especially, a surviving parent may try to control the amount of information that is transmitted to them. A stable parent or caregiver is able to meet the emotional needs of the child and provide the opportunity to help them release their thoughts and feelings about this kind of loss.

A recent school-based example highlights the importance of considering the child's experiences of a suicidal death and the need to distinguish such reactions from those of the adults around the child. The second author was serving as a consultant for a child assessment project in a kindergarten class in which a 5-year-old's father had recently committed suicide. The teacher asked Knowles, the consultant, to pay particular attention to this boy to assess his well-being. In the initial consultation the teacher reported that the boy seemed withdrawn; the teacher and consultant speculated about the sense of abandonment that he was feeling. Questions arose about the concerns that could lead a father to make a decision to leave a boy to face his absence. Had the family missed signs of the father's being so upset? How could the child tell his friends how his dad had died? Preliminary discussion with the teacher led to agreement that such thoughts and feelings in the boy seemed likely. However, it soon became apparent that most of those reactions belonged to the adults—with little, if any, indication that the child shared these questions. Observation of the child at play and discussion with classmates, together with quiet conversations with the teacher, indicated that he was deeply hurt that his father had died, that he had specific concerns about "looking after Mummy," and that he wished things could be returned to their earlier state.

When a family member takes his/her own life, survivors and those in caretaking roles have reactions that are likely to be considered unique in contrast to reactions to other deaths. Those who work with young children are particularly likely to see the effects of family suicide as "severely traumatic" (Dunne-Maxim, Dunne, & Hauser, 1987) and requiring "urgent interventions" (Hurley, 1991). It is true that many of the reactions to suicide are unique and that child survivors will likely need support (as they do in other forms of death). However, some of the reactions that these children have may be similar to those that other children have as a result of sudden, frightening deaths of family members. McIntosh (1999) commented, "there still seems an attempt or need [in the professional literature] to demonstrate that suicide grief is worse than that of other causes of death. . . . Is it not enough to show that suicide produces a different set of bereavement issues and patterns than for some causes but shares some similarities to others?" (p. 161). His conclusion could serve as a caution against responding to suicidal deaths as if they were *completely* different from other family deaths. Many of the counselor's skills and sensitivities from situations involving other kinds of deaths are applicable in working with suicide survivors.

A key factor to consider when children have experienced a family member's suicide is the mediating role of important adults in the child's life in helping the child find meaning and support. Adults often convey many nonverbal interpretations of the death. Their lack of openness may be confusing to a child because the very nature of suicide is likely to raise many taboos, as well as feelings of guilt and self-blame. Suicidal death, as with other deaths, takes on different meanings as the child develops. For example, concerns may arise about some type of "family destiny" to become depressed and take one's own life. Researchers (Brent, Moritz, Bridge, Perper, & Canobbio, 1996) who looked at the costs of the elevated level of grief that follows a family suicide found a differential effect for children and mothers. Siblings did not show the increased depression or posttraumatic stress as their mothers did. Counseling approaches that consider all family members, rather than only the children, would seem to be warranted. Support for the surviving parent may be a very effective indirect way of providing support to the child. A message that applies throughout this chapter is that it is important to read one's own reactions to the suicide in comparison with those of the young child.

SOME REACTIONS OF CHILDREN TO FAMILY SUICIDE

Family Destiny

A family suicide creates a legacy for the survivor who may, at some point, choose suicide as a means of dealing with personal problems. The concern is based on the perception of similarity between the deceased and other family members, in addition to the belief that physiological and genetic factors such as depression contribute to suicide. This concern may become a constant fear, particularly later in life. One woman found herself doing research into her mother's life after the mother took her own life: "I wanted to know if suicide was hereditary . . . how was I going to avoid going down the same path as my mother?" (Stimming & Stimming, 1999, p. 20). The concern seems to be less prevalent in younger children, but we have heard of children who deliberately threatened to "kill themselves" when things were not going well. While many children make this threat, it carries particular potency in a family that has experienced a suicide. A mother reported that, following her father's suicidal death, "Our youngest son, who is named after his grandfather, said he wanted to change his name because of 'what Grandpa did'" (Stimming & Stimming, 1999, p. 70). Such a comment is an important declaration by a child. What the child had in mind could have been a "family destiny" concern, but it could also have been related to shame, feeling the name would trigger bad memories, or anger toward his namesake. Clearly, more exploration would be warranted.

Similarly, suicidal ideation occurs frequently following a family suicide (Pfeffer, Martius, Mann, & Sunkenberg, 1997)—probably more so than for other types of death. As discussed below, such ideas and fantasies can be frightening to all concerned. Further, they can create concern and awkwardness to the adults around the child. Such awkwardness may lead to an avoidance of the subject; nevertheless, suicidal ideation deserves exploration by the counselor.

One other behavior related to "family destiny" is an increase in self-destructive or risk-taking behavior among some child survivors of family suicide. The behavior seems based, in part, on a feeling of powerlessness from being unable to stop the death and also to the "lesson" that tensions are handled by such an escape. Adult family members must monitor and openly address the topic of risk taking. When this appears to be extreme, professional counseling should be sought.

Stigma/Taboo

Any family death produces feelings of shock and mystery in a young child. Suicide carries a sense of shame possibly because of religious teachings, in addition to the pain in imagining that someone close to us actually planned and completed a suicide. We know about a school district that not only will not allow mention of suicide but also removed the pictures from the yearbook of a young person who committed suicide. This policy seemed based, in part, on the fear that acknowledgment of the nature of the death may be seen as condoning it. Further, there is a concern by those who work with adolescents that "contagion," a series of suicides and attempts by friends of the deceased, might occur. Such concerns are important and real, but silence may increase problems for the survivors.

The silence and distance that result from the taboo and awkwardness surrounding suicide isolate the child. Survivors typically hunger for opportunities to tell the detailed story of the events. In preparing for their recent book, Stimming and Stimming (1999) recruited adult participants to tell their stories of the aftermath of parental suicide, in part to break the isolation felt by many survivors. Even though adults provided the stories many years after the parental death, most participants provided extensive "graphic accounts of how the deceased took his or her own life and the physical devastation caused by the means of death" (p. xxxiii). This situation is an example of what Doka (1989) has called "disenfranchised grief," defined as incurring a "loss that is not or cannot be openly acknowledged or socially supported" (p. 4). Such disenfranchisement typically intensifies feelings of anger, guilt, or powerlessness and, by its very nature, precludes social support.

An important problem and resulting counseling need for child survivors is how to find listeners. One young person reported, retrospectively, "Counselors are cut from the same cloth as the rest of the community. No one wants to hear my witness of suicide in my life" (Stimming & Stimming, 1999, p 39). Other children may wish to communicate their feelings and concerns but do not have the words to do so. Young children, in particular, and those severely traumatized, require counseling approaches that utilize nonverbal expression such as play therapy (e.g., Webb, 1991, 1993a, 1999) or the use of favorite objects or photographs. One 6-year-old, on hearing of his grandfather's death, quietly went to his room and located a wallet that his grandfather had made him. He kept the wallet with him for weeks. In some situations, children keep their story in silence; opportunities for exploration and support are thereby removed. One mother found that she did not have the words to engage her children in discussion of a grandparent's suicide but realized they needed to express their sense of events and their concerns: "I bought them some paper and crayons for them to draw on. . . . Through their pictures I became aware of their thoughts and feelings" (Stimming & Stimming, 1999, p. 64).

A related issue that comes from the silence associated with the stigma of suicide is the need to "break the silence" when a survivor makes reference to suicidal thoughts or intentions (Goldman, 1996). An important counseling skill is that of "calling" (i.e., confronting) the client to determine what preparations, if any, have been made for the suicide. Practices that inhibit open discussions with survivors are particularly inappropriate in such situations.

Assuming Responsibility

A very frequent response to a suicide is the feeling of unyielding guilt that some action or personal expression of caring might have prevented the death. Many survivors carry vivid memories of incidents where, in retrospect, clues were provided of deep sadness or suicidal intention. Based on their very concrete understanding of their worlds, children may feel guilt in reaction to any kind of family death. One young boy drew the personal conclusion that his noisiness had caused his grandfather's death. When he was asked to explain his reasoning, he explained that he had been warned frequently to be quiet because Grandpa was sick. When Grandpa died, he concluded that he had not been quiet enough. With suicidal deaths, the guilt may be even stronger. His wishes to have grasped the clues, to have behaved in a less troublesome way, and to have shown more patience are typical of suicide survivors. This sense of guilt may be so strong and so scary that survivors are afraid to speak about it.

Responsibility may be assigned by the child to other members of the family in an attempt to understand the suicide. Pressure on siblings by parents becomes transformed into failure to live up to expectations, or into magnification of the "good" sibling compared to the "bad."

We have heard children offer such questions as "If Dad loved me, how could he have done this?" This form of wondering about responsibility for the death would seem to be particularly penetrating to much of the child's life and future relationships. A young adult, in a search for reasons many years after a suicide, concluded that his father did not "love me enough to stay alive for me—lurking deeper, it was actually my fault that he didn't love me" (Stimming & Stimming, 1999, p. 79).

Very different kinds of "responsibility assumption" are the pressures for a child to grow up more quickly, particularly in the case of parental suicide. The surviving parent may need assistance in taking on the family tasks of the deceased or may not be able to afford sufficient supervision of the children. In the case of a deceased sibling, there may be pressures to take on roles and earn accomplishments that the sibling might have done. Such pressures may not be openly felt with clear awareness but underlie feelings that childhood has ended with the suicide.

Family Disruption

The impact and multiple changes following a family suicide provoke strong needs for family support and counseling. In the case of a young child, support to the parents (or to the surviving spouse in the case of parental suicide) is crucial (Heikes, 1997). Parents are likely to be overwhelmed by their own reactions. In fact, children themselves may become aware of these reactions and attempt to protect the parent by "covering up" their questions and fears.

Further, there is a prevailing view (Hurley, 1991; Leenaars & Wenckstern, 1990) that many families in which a suicide occurs show previous disruption and serious problems. For example, there may have been long periods of depression in the family member and frustrating attempts to deal with it. Attachment issues may have been part of this history, particularly forms of insecure attachment. James (1994) described such reactions to parental death, not necessarily just suicide, as hypervigilance from feeling a lack of protection and frightening flashbacks of helplessness. Survivors of suicide loss are often caught in a no-win cycle of events. Their social environment may contribute to their recovery from such a loss. Social supports tend to be associated with a better adjustment to the stress of a sudden and unexpected death (Leenaars & Wenckstern, 1990).

Parents usually must explain the death to children and answer their questions. A mother described the reasons for their grandmother's death as "She was so sad, so sad the pain was unbearable"(Stimming & Stimming, 1999, p. 4). The child then observed that Mummy sometimes gets sad, too, which provoked an awkward but important discussion. A more protective response which typically leads to serious complications (as in the case of David, described below) is to attribute the death (falsely) to some other cause such as sickness or an accident. Such explanations lead to years of cover-up and eventually unintentional disclosure at a time when there may be little support for the child (Webb, 1993b).

Family preoccupation with the suicide may become very extended and fixated. In fact, the event is typically a redefining moment in the family's history. Such prolonged and incomplete mourning is an example of Rando's (1993) "complicated mourning" and is a sign of the need for professional help.

In summary, survivors of family suicide are likely to encounter few opportunities to express either their grief or their questions about the nature of the death. Both children and other members of the family should be offered support, counseling, or therapy. Invitations to such support or therapy need to be skillfully delivered—a combination of compassionate inviting and caring follow-up (Knowles & Reeves, 1993). Practices such as "sending in the grief counselors" in a public way have provoked resistance and contributed to feelings of being strange and unique. Suicidal death requires sensitive exploration of the needs and personal resources of the survivors. The counselor will typically find that everybody does not have the same needs and resources.

When someone close to them commits suicide, children and adolescents are plunged into confusion, emotional upheaval, and pain that affects everyone involved. The intensity of their loss and the complicated path of mourning may leave them with emotional scars that may last a lifetime.

INTERVIEWS WITH SURVIVORS
OF FAMILY SUICIDE

Three survivors of suicide shared their stories of loss with the first author. All of them are males who have experienced the following suicide losses:

• The loss of a mother by suicide when the boy was 7
• The death of a father by suicide when the adolescent was 16
• The death of an older sister by suicide when the adolescent was 15

The adolescents were recruited from a peer support group for bereaved adolescents. This support group was facilitated by the first author and was composed of adolescents between the ages of 13 and 19 years who suffered the significant loss of a relationship. They chose to participate in the 8-week program, and each of them appreciated having the opportunity to share their stories of loss. They gave permission to us to write about their experiences in the hope this might help others understand the impact of this loss on their own lives and that of their family members. The names of all individuals have been changed.

Case of Peter, Age 15 at the Time
of His Sister's Death

Family Information

Mother, age 36, single parent, independent and a very proactive person
Sister, Ellen, age 18 at the time of her death, in her last year of high school, expelled from school prior to graduation; took an overdose of Tylenol and was taken to hospital by ambulance by her maternal grandmother
Peter, age 15, was at his friend's house when his sister was taken to the hospital
Maternal grandmother, age 52, lived on the same street and was caring for the children
Father, age 38, lived in a different city

Presenting Problem

Peter's sister Ellen was taken to the hospital because she took too many Tylenol capsules. Ellen was initially placed in the intensive care unit and then, after 2 days, on the general ward. The doctors told her mother that her prognosis was optimistic. However, she died 4 days after hospitalization. Although the coroner's report stated that the cause of death was a suicide, Peter and his mother have a lot of questions about the cause of Ellen's death. They find it hard to believe that she *intended* to take her life. Peter's mother sought counseling for herself and Peter. However, he did not want to have individual or family counseling, preferring to join a peer support group for grieving teens. When Peter was 13, he moved with his mother and 16-year-old sister. This was difficult for Peter who was shy and often counted on his sister to lead the way in adapting to new places. She was not only his elder sister but also his best friend, whom he relied on to be there for him. Suddenly all that changed for him very quickly and unexpectedly. Everything that he knew was altered by her death; one minute she was there, and the next thing he knew she was gone. His mother worried about how his sister's sudden death was affecting Peter and suggested that he join a peer support group. However, his initial group involvement was not successful. A year later, Peter decided to try another group.

Content of Individual Session

Peter's Comments	Analysis
"I want to talk about my sister. It is weird how it happened. I was at . . . my friend's house when she was taken to the hospital."	Reliving the details of the suicide event; may retell many times in an attempt to accept the reality.
"I waited until the next day to go to see her in the hospital because I did not think that it was serious. I never thought that she might die."	Peter is reliving his misunderstanding of the seriousness of the suicide either through misinterpretation or disbelief.
"When I got to the hospital, she was in the ICU. I didn't know what that meant. My mom told me that she might not make it and to say goodbye to her. I was in shock!"	The abrupt, sudden nature of the suicide removed any real chance for his preparation for her death.
"Sometimes I still can't believe that she is really gone. The other day I saw a girl in a blue dress. My sister had a blue dress, and for a minute I thought it was her."	Remembering things about his sister is triggered by other events in his life that recall those memories. This often causes the individual to think that they are going crazy.
"Now that I am going to graduate from high school, I think about the fact that she never graduated."	Special occasions in his life cause him to think of his sister and perhaps to regrieve this loss.

"She was my friend as well as my sister. I hate how our move to this place affected all of us."	Acknowledging the value of his relationship with his sister; looking for a reason why she killed herself.
"Her death has changed my life a lot."	Am I still a brother? Being an only child and having to make my own choices.
"It makes me angry how some people don't think that we should remember her because she killed herself."	Strong feelings about possible disregard of sister by others.
"I have a friend whose brother died by suicide too. We have something in common, and we understand each other."	How she died is not who she is.
"I want to thank you for giving me the opportunity to share my story."	Telling his story of loss and having someone willing to listen helps the survivor to heal.

Case of Michael, Age 16 at the Time of His Father's Death

Family Information

Mother, age 42, single parent, divorced from Michael's father
Brother, age 18, at the time of his father's death living on his own
Michael, age 16, living with his mother
Father, age 42, shot himself at his house
Grandmother's common-law husband told Michael about his father's death on the phone

Presenting Problem

Michael's father and mother divorced and Michael lived with his mother and had regular visits with his father. His father was having financial problems, had not been feeling well, and had trouble sleeping. There was conflict between his parents and family members prior to his father's death. Michael's father shot himself at his own house.

Michael participated in two peer support groups. He found it very difficult to talk about his thoughts and feelings during the first group. However, in the second group he was able to express some of his thoughts and feelings in the group sessions. It was after his second group that he decided that he wanted to share his story about his father's suicide death.

Michael's Comments	*Analysis*
"My father's sudden and unexpected death by suicide was an eye-opener for me. I felt a lack of stability in my life."	The impact of the death was major, affecting the basis of his life.
"It made me realize that life is short and I need to do what is best for me. Before he died, I didn't care about the choices I made and I didn't respect people. After his death, I put more effort into what I did; I made better choices."	The impact of mortality is seen by Michael as having a positive effect on giving him more direction to his life. Below we see that the transition is not yet complete.
"Some people blamed my mom and my father's common-law wife for his death. It upset me when people blamed my mom for his death. She was accused of hounding my father for money."	The issue of attributing blame raises issues of unfairness.
"The way he died was an embarrassment to me. I had been told that he was not feeling well and that he was having trouble sleeping. The day before he died he tried to give me his leather jacket."	Deeper emotional descriptions here including social reactions and perhaps some guilt about not picking up on the giving away of possessions—a common sign of suicidal intention.
"I try not to think about these things. Sometimes I get angry and get physical when people make comments about how my father died."	The issues have not gone. The perceived judgments of others have become a burden.
"I wanted people to just leave me alone."	The realization that he needed time alone.
"I found that being a part of a peer support group helped me to talk about my thoughts and feelings surrounding my father's death."	Michael recognizes that sharing with others in a supportive climate is an important activity at this time.
"I stopped using drugs to cope with these thoughts and feelings about my father. I decided to make better choices in handling my reactions to my father's death."	We now learn that some changes to improving his life did not come easy; attempts at "numbing" did not work.
"I completed high school and am presently preparing to take further training in golf course management at a community college."	He has moved toward some academic activity and has a plan for moving on with his life and career plans.

Case of David, Age 7 at the Time of His Mother's Death

Family Information

Mother, age 44 years old, separated from her husband, living with her only daughter

Father, age 44 years old, separated from his wife, caring for his two youngest sons

Sister, Laura, age 22, single, living in an apartment with her mother

Brother, John, age 23, married

Brother, Bill, age 5, living with his father and elder brother, David

David, age 7, living with his father and younger brother

Presenting Problem

David, now 40 years old, wrote the following story about his loss:

David's Story (An Autobiographical Account)

"It was in April 1967. I'm uncertain of the exact day. I was 7 years old. I lived with my dad and my younger brother, Bill, age 5, in a large home that was attached to my parents' motel. It was located in a small town. I remember at that time my older brother, John, was married and they had a daughter. My older sister, Laura, was living in a basement suite in an apartment building. My mother lived with Laura. Mom and Dad were always yelling at each other and at us kids. Dad, Bill, and I would travel every weekend to visit Mom and Laura. I still remember my sister's apartment building. It had dull red bricks and a white fence around it. I remember the smell of mildew and of salt in the hallway of the apartment and the smell of eggs and bacon, pancakes, muffins, roses, and the fur of wet dogs. There was pale white paint on all the walls . . . in the halls, the entrance, and in Laura's suite.

"I was woken up from a sound sleep in my warm cozy bed early that morning. I remember my brown digital clock showed in big red numbers that it was 1:33 A.M. Dad asked me if I was awake, and I said sleepily, 'Yes, sort of.' 'Dad has something to tell you,' Dad said quietly. He told me Mom wouldn't be coming home anymore. I remember saying, 'Okay, fine, we can go and see her.' Dad didn't answer me for quite some time. During this time, he developed a tear in his eye and said to me, 'No, we cannot.' I started to get a lump in the base of my throat, tears in the corners of my eyes, and a heaviness in my chest like I was being sat on (this was first time I had experienced this awful feeling). I asked, 'What do you mean? What are you saying?' Dad again tells me that Mom will not be coming home anymore. I asked 'Why? What did I do this time?' 'Nothing,' Dad said. Again there was a long pause. Dad said, 'Mom has passed away. She passed away of lung cancer because of smoking and because her lungs were unable to function properly.' I wasn't able to think what "passed away" meant. I didn't know what Dad was trying to tell me. I told Dad that I didn't understand what he was trying to tell me, and I'm getting scared. He raised his voice at me and yelled, 'She's dead.' I was aware of a feeling of heaviness in my chest; it was growing, it was expanding. God, did it hurt! I have never felt pain like this before. What was happening? It felt like all the wrongs that I had ever done in this world were upon my chest, my body, upon me. I felt that something was out of place. The lump in my throat felt like a softball and as if it was going to explode. I couldn't even swallow. I had a thought. A suspicious knowing that there was something more. Still with a very loud voice Dad tells me to get back into bed. By now I was bawling. I asked Dad for a hug. Dad wouldn't even give a hug. He gave me a quick pat on the back. That upset me even more. He looked and acted as if he was very upset and mad at me. I quickly climbed back into bed so I wouldn't get the belt, and pulled the covers up over my head. I held back my tears the best that I could until Dad left my room, and then I let the pain out and wailed. It seemed like hours had gone by. I didn't know what was going to happen to me in the morning. I was so, so cold, my whole body was shaking from head to toe. I was at a loss. I was not able to think. I was not able to move. I felt I couldn't even breathe. I thought it was now time to be judged and punished for Mom's death. So there I lay, afraid to move. I was so scared and hurt, I was paralyzed. I didn't sleep. I tried, but there was no way I could sleep. I was convinced that I had made Mom smoke more than she should because I was a bad boy. I thought that if I wasn't born at all she would still be here. I was the cause that drove Mom to smoke more. In the past, I had been told many, many times that I was going to put both of them into an early grave, and now I had put Mom there.

"Prior to Mom's death, I was always getting into trouble, so they both told me over and over again. As a boy I was extremely curious and absolutely full of life. I was fascinated with everything and everyone. I wanted to know how things worked and just not from the outside as many people did. I wanted to go inside and see and feel what made things move and tick. I wanted to know how things tasted. I wanted to listen to the noises that things made. I loved the way things smelt. I wanted to be a part of everything. I wanted to be wanted, not thrown to the side or put on the back burner and forgotten. I wanted to belong. I wanted to be loved. And I had driven her to smoke, and now I'd killed her.

"I remember (I can still see myself) lying there after I calmed down a little bit from bawling. I felt the wetness from my tears on my skin through my pajamas. I could taste the salt from my tears that continuously rolled down my cheeks. My pillows, sheets, and blankets were soaked with my tears. My eyes were so swollen I could hardly see. Everything I looked at was blurry. I was unable to focus. When I was able to see again after my tears cleared, the first thing I saw was the huge thick insulated curtains hanging on the far wall at the foot of my bed. I wasn't able to make out any colors, everything else in my room was in shades of blacks and dark grays except the clock radio's red numbers. It now showed 3:45 A.M. The curtains covered the top half of the wall where the huge window was. I was unable to make out what the pattern was. I could see the outlines of the pattern, and I know now that the pattern was of baseball caps and bats; however, that pattern did not then come to mind. I wasn't able to remember. I noticed that there was a weird faintish whitish foggy somewhat of a human shape in the exact middle of the curtains. It looked like it was stuck there, half in, half out, sort of. I wiped my eyes. It was still there. I scrubbed my eyes hard. It was still there. It seemed like it was two people blended together, side by side, maybe one in front of the other and a bit offset. I couldn't tell. Wow! This scared the crap out of me. I whipped the covers up over my head and froze. I held my breath. I waited. Nothing happened. I ever so slowly lowered the covers. It was still there. I looked, I watched it for a while, it felt like hours. It didn't move. It, this image, had some kind of calming effect, it made no sense to me. This thing, what ever it was, somehow was calling me to go to them. Slowly I got off my bed and went over to the curtains. I found myself caressing the curtains. I was pulling the curtains over and around my head; again, I started to bawl again. I embraced the curtains. I clutched on to them with both hands as hard as I could. I found some comfort in having them around me. I could smell Mom on them. I knew she was there, or at least a part of her was. I helped her make those curtains. All of a sudden I felt I was falling—I was indeed falling. I realized that I had put so much energy into clinging on to those curtains that I had pulled them off the wall, the brackets and all. I picked myself up. There was ice on the inside of the glass at the bottom corners of the window and freshly fallen snow that lay over everything outside. It was beautiful. The moon was just starting to break out of the dispersing clouds. Even though I had seen the snow on things before, this time it was different, completely different. I felt it had a purpose. I felt I belonged. I looked outside for a while, crying. I was slowly sinking. My energy was leaving me. I was so tired. I sat down underneath the middle of the window. I thought, oh boy, am I ever in trouble now. I tried not to move, didn't want to make any more noise or draw attention to myself because if Dad finds out, I'm gone for good. I'm really, really frightened. Dad will send me to a correctional institute for sure now. I gathered up all the curtains and placed them around me and over me, all that was showing was from my chin up. From where I was sitting now, I was able to see my room from a completely new viewpoint. Never thought of this aspect before. I had a new perspective of my room. My bedroom was totally immersed with the touch of Mom. Mom painted my room. Mom and Dad had bought me a new bedspread shortly before, and I helped her put it on my bed. Mom made the curtains. There were pictures of Mom, Dad, Laura, John, and Bill in my room. I had toys all over the room because Dad had been gone for the day. I usually kept it clean and tidy so they wouldn't yell at me.

"I fell asleep after some time. I was woken up by Dad's loud voice. Boy, was I startled! It was time to get ready for school. 'School! What! Today!' I tried to say. All that came out of my mouth was some gurgling sounds. 'You have to be kidding!' I thought. I felt like a zombie. I wasn't able to think of what I needed to do to get ready for school. I couldn't even talk, for the lump in my throat was still there. I thought the lump would have been gone by now. I tried to tell Dad that I had had a nightmare and as I started to tell him, only more noise came out. I realized that what had happened last night indeed did take place. I couldn't believe it! I just could not believe it actually happened. I was brought back to reality quickly. 'What the hell happened in here?' Dad yells at me, 'You're grounded!' I thought, 'Well, that's great. This sucks!' 'Get this mess cleaned up now!' Dad yells at me."

Eleven Years Later

David was 18 when he discovered how his mother died. He was talking about his mother's death by lung cancer with his elder sister, Laura, when she told him the truth. She did not realize that David had never been told the truth about their mother's suicide.

Comments

David's story is not finished. He has begun to realize the impact of his mother's death on his life. He is trying to redefine its impact on his own personal development and his relationships with others. Even though none of his immediate family were willing to talk about his mother's death, he continues his search for answers to his questions. Like someone solving a puzzle that has some missing pieces, he is trying to fill his emptiness with information about his mother: "A part of me went with my mother when she died." He has found through his search that his brother's former wife had a very close relationship with his mother. She is willing to talk with him about his mother and to help him learn things about his mother that will help him to heal from this loss. David is beginning to remember things that he thought he had forgotten about his mother. He is amazed to find out that he does have some memories about his childhood. This is both an exciting and painful process for him, yet he is determined to take these steps. He believes that this will not only help him as a person but will also be beneficial to his young daughter. He is stopping the family cycle of silence: "I am different than the rest of my family!" David is actively involved in individual counseling on a biweekly basis. He is trying to understand why he has made some of the choices in his life that pertain to his relationships with others as well as his relationship with himself.

IMPLICATIONS FOR COUNSELING

Our role as effective counselors, caregivers, and caring human beings is to be present, listen, observe, and be willing to companion those who are trying to make sense of the various losses in their lives. We cannot provide the answers to all their questions, but our ability to listen to their stories of loss will help them heal themselves.

According to Goldman (1996), life issues that are not expressed or acknowledged can become locked in "frozen blocks of time" (p. 9). These frozen blocks of time often stop the normal grief and can interfere with the child's ability to grieve. It can feel as if life stops and time stands still. The natural flow of feelings is inhibited. There is no movement forward until the issues are resolved and the feelings are released.

When children become stuck in this frozen block of time, they can become overwhelmed by frozen feelings and the grief process seems to be "on hold" or nonexistent. The child is not in touch with his/her feelings of grief, or those feelings are ambivalent and in conflict with each other. It is as if a wall of ice is between the child and his/her grief. Our job is to help melt that wall.

Five factors contribute to complicated grief reactions in children, following a suicide:

- A sudden or traumatic death
- The social stigma of the death
- Multiple losses
- The relationship to the deceased
- The grief process of the surviving parent and family members

An adult who was 12 years old when her mother died by suicide describes her family as being viewed by others in her community as "the bad family" (Elder, 1995, p. 144). Their grief therefore becomes disenfranchised grief (Doka, 1989).

Often peer support groups can provide support for children and adolescent survivors of a suicide loss. Most survivors of suicidal deaths seem to feel that their experience is different from those with other types of losses, and they often believe that other survivors with similar experiences are more likely to understand their loss. If it is not possible to form support groups that are homogeneous (that is, composed of *all* suicide survivors) the group should have at least two participants with the same kind of loss in order to help survivors feel comfortable, understood, and supported in the group. Children and adolescents do not like to feel different from their peers. If they can meet someone else who has experienced the same kind of loss in their support group, they will not feel so alone and misunderstood. When they receive support and understanding to help them through this traumatic event, they can learn to survive their loss. However, sometimes the reactions of other individuals to suicidal loss interferes with survivors' ability to grieve openly.

The topic of suicide is often approached with great difficulty. Surviving parents, educators, therapists, and other caring adults are unwilling or unable to speak about the issues surrounding suicide. Our difficulty in discussing this topic openly and honestly with the child and adolescent survivors of suicide can create an atmosphere of fear, isolation, and loneliness that significantly adds to the pain of the death of the loved one. Everyone who believes in the emotional well being of our youth must learn to utilize age-appropriate language, teachable moments, and nonjudgmental values in helping to open the discussion. Goldman (2000) states, "What is mentionable is manageable" (p. 6). Breaking the silence that has surrounded the issue paves the way to finding new ways of learning how to cope with this kind of death and to begin the healing process.

When the child survivors are not told the truth about the loss, they will often have to regrieve their loss at a later time in their life and may be unable to move on with their life. An adolescent whose father died by suicide when she was 7 years old was initially told that her father had died in a car accident. She subsequently discovered the truth about his death from a neighbor who thought that she knew what had happened. This adolescent later described the impact of not being told the truth as "having to regrieve her father's death."

Being a survivor of a suicide death creates for any child a loss of his/her assumptive world of safety, protection, and predictability. Children naturally assume their world will be filled with safety, kindness, and meaning as they attempt to answer the universal questions of "Who am I?" and "Why am I here?" Suicide can plunge young survivors into a nightmarish universe of randomness, isolation, and unpredictability, leaving them with a new assumption: "There is no future. There is no safety. There is no connectedness or meaning to my life."

By joining together, caring adults can co-create an assumptive world that restores a child's birthright to presume love, generosity, and value as integral parts of his/her life (Goldman, 1996). Those individuals who provide the necessary support to the child and adolescent survivors of suicide must be aware of the various ways that can be utilized to help them to begin their healing process. These include the following:

- To have a safe place to express their feelings
- To receive help with family problems arising from a suicide
- To help to prevent the development of family secrets
- To be willing to listen to the children and adolescent survivors' stories of loss
- To utilize methods to help the children and adolescent survivors to express their thoughts and feelings through the use of art, role playing, puppets, creating a memory book of the person who died, sand play, and poetry

When children experience a loss, they begin to work on and process well-identified tasks of normal grief: (1) understanding, (2) grieving, (3) commemorating, and (4) going on (Fox, 1988). In complicated grief, however, other emotional issues become imposed like a wall between the children and their grief process, preventing them from being able to go on. The task of caring professionals is to help them melt down their frozen state in order to begin to grieve normally. A safe environment to express thoughts and feelings is essential to their grief process (Goldman, 1996).

DISCUSSION QUESTIONS

1. What kind of approaches would you use to help children/adolescents express their thoughts and feelings about a suicidal death? Consider the relevance of the child's age in the methods you propose.

2. How can a parent support a preschool child who is faced with the suicidal death of the other parent? What can the parent say or do to help the child? How might the parent's response differ for an elementary-school-age child?

3. In your work with children bereaved by suicide, how can you become aware of and deal with the "conspiracy of silence" the child might be facing?

4. Discuss the advantages and disadvantages of support groups for children and adolescents bereaved by suicide. Do you agree that these children may be incorporated into groups with children who have experienced other types of losses? If so, how can the groups leader(s) deal with the possible reactions of other group members about the nature of the suicidal death?

REFERENCES

Brent, D. A., Moritz, G., Bridge, J. Perper, J., & Canobbio, R. (1996). The impact of adolescent suicide on siblings and parents: A longitudinal follow-up. *Suicide and Life Threatening Behavior, 26,* 253–259.

Doka, K. J. (1989). *Disenfranchised grief: Recognizing hidden sorrow.* Toronto: Lexington Books.

Dunne-Maxim, K., Dunne, E. J., & Hauser, M. J. (1987). In E. J. Dunne, J. L. McIntosh & K. Dunne-Maxim (Eds.), *Suicide and its aftermath: Understanding and counseling the survivors* (pp. 234–244). New York: Norton.

Elder, S. L. (1993). *The impact of parental death during adolescence: On the separation–individuation process.* Unpublished doctoral dissertation, University of Victoria, British Columbia, Canada.

Elder, S. L. (1995). Helping bereaved children and adolescents cope with the aftermath of suicide. In D. Adams and E. Deveau (Eds.), *Beyond the innocence of childhood: Helping children and adolescents cope with death and bereavement* (Vol. 3., pp. 137–151). Amityville, NY: Baywood.

Fox, S. (1988). *Good grief: Helping groups of children when a friend dies.* Boston: New England Association for the Education of Young Children.

Goldman, L. (1996). *Breaking the silence: A guide to help children with complicated grief.* Washington, DC: Taylor & Francis.

Goldman, L. (2000, Spring). Suicide: How can we talk to the children? *The Forum, 26*(3), 6–9.

Harrington, G. G. (1998). National strategies for the prevention of suicide. *SIEC Alert, 31,* 1.

Heikes, K. (1997). Parental suicide: A systems perspective. *Bulletin of the Menninger Clinic, 61,* 354–367.

Hurley, D. J. (1991). The crisis of paternal suicide: Case of Cathy, age 4½. In N. B. Webb (Ed.), *Play therapy with children in crisis: A casebook for practitioners* (pp. 237–253). New York: Guilford Press.

James, B. (1994). *Handbook for treatment of attachment-trauma problems in children.* New York: Lexington Books.

Knowles, D. W., & Reeves, N. (1993). *But won't Granny need her socks: Dealing effectively with children's concerns about death and dying.* Dubuque, IA: Kendall/ Hunt.

Leenaars, A., & Wenckstern, S. (1990). Suicide postvention in the school systems. In J. D. Morgan (Ed.), *The dying and the bereaved teenager* (pp. 140–159). Philadelphia: Charles Press.

Lonetto, R. (1980). *Children's conceptions of death*. New York: Springer.

McIntosh, J. L. (1996). Survivors of suicide: A comprehensive bibliography update, 1986–1995, *Omega: Journal of Death and Dying, 33*, 147–175.

McIntosh, J. L. (1999). Research on survivors of suicide. In M. Stimming & M. Stimming (Eds.), *Before their time: Adult children's experiences of parental suicide*. Philadelphia: Temple University Press.

Pfeffer, C. R., Martins, P., Mann, J., & Sunkenberg, M. (1997). Child survivors of suicide: Psychological characteristics. *Journal of the American Academy of Child and Adolescent Psychiatry, 36*, 65–74.

Rando, T. A. (1993). *Treatment of complicated mourning*. Champaign, IL: Research Press.

Raphael, B. (1983). *The anatomy of bereavement*. New York: Basic Books.

Silverman, E., Range, L., & Overholser, J. (1994/1995). Bereavement from suicide as compared to other forms of bereavement. *Omega: Journal of Death and Dying, 30*, 41–51.

Stimming, M., & Stimming, M. (Eds.). (1999). *Before their time: Adult children's experiences of parental suicide*. Philadelphia: Temple University Press.

Suicide Information and Education Center [SIEC]. (2000). Children and suicide. *SIEC Alert, 39*, 1.

Webb, N. B. (Ed.). (1991). *Play therapy with children in crisis: A casebook for practitioners*. New York: Guilford Press.

Webb, N. B. (Ed.). (1993a). *Helping bereaved children: A handbook for practitioners*. New York: Guilford Press.

Webb, N. B. (1993b). Suicidal death of mother: Cases of silence and stigma. In N. B. Webb (Ed.), *Helping bereaved children: A handbook for practitioners* (pp. 137–155). New York: Guilford Press.

Webb, N. B. (Ed.). (1999). *Play therapy with children in crisis* (2nd ed.): *Individual, group, and family treatment*. New York: Guilford Press.

7

Violent Deaths of Both Parents

Case of Marty, Age 2½

TERESA BEVIN

One month after the tragic news hit the papers, Marty was being protected by his grandparents from the fallout of having witnessed his father shoot his mother to death. Police found him covered with blood, cuddled against his mother's body, his arms around her neck, and his cheek pressed against hers. She was still alive, but her heart stopped as soon as they took Marty off her. His father was found in the locked bathroom, shot in the head by his own hand. Two neighbors had seen Marty's father enter the apartment with his key, then they heard three shots, and then another that seemed to come from deeper within the apartment.

Marty's father had a history of abuse as a child, had suffered from depression most of his life, and often talked about suicide. He was frequently absent from the home and spent very little time with his son. During the short periods of time that he spent with Marty, he yelled at him and called him "stupid" for romping or making noises. Marty's mother was an active, hard-working, and intelligent young woman caught in an unhappy marriage to a man who had physically abused her at least twice. She spent all her spare time with her bright and inquisitive 2-year-old son. He was included in most of her socializing, went with her to the grocery store, to the beauty parlor, to church, and sometimes she would even take him to her office, where Marty was spoiled by the staff. Marty's mother was very close to her parents, who were always willing and ready to be involved in the upbringing of their grandson.

BEREAVEMENT IN EARLY CHILDHOOD

Marty's anguish and desolation after these deaths was immediately apparent, but his grandparents thought that because of his young age he would become accustomed to the situation. Eventually, they realized that both Marty and they needed help in coping with the tragic events that had altered their lives so drastically. Through the use of toys, activities, and guided play, Marty slowly began to reaffirm his self-image, leading, it is hoped, to understanding and eventually accepting the finality of his mother's abrupt departure from his world.

The work of several practitioners and researchers provides a framework for understanding this case. Raphael (1983) projects the process of bereavement throughout the entire life span, focusing especially on the bereaved infant and child. Raphael states that a child in the 2- to 5-year-old age range can experience grief similar to that of adults "but others may not perceive his responses as bereavement"; moreover, because others find "his recognition of death and his painful mourning intolerable they may deny him his feelings and their expression" (1983, p. 95).

The work of Malmquist (1986) also bears on this case, particularly as it is centered around the posttraumatic aftermath related to children who witness parental murder. Aside from the obvious trauma connected with the murder of the prime attachment figure, the issue of delayed intervention is mentioned. In Malmquist's investigation of 16 children who had witnessed parental murder, "most of the cases seem to have had a minimal or no psychiatric intervention prior to the raising of legal issues" (1986, p. 321). In Marty's case, the grandparents waited 1 month before seeking help for him.

Krueger (1983) addresses the developmental consequences of loss as they relate to diagnosis and treatment. In reference to pre-Oedipal loss between the ages of 2 and 4, Krueger states that when the child is "unable to register or comprehend the concept of permanent loss," restitutive fantasies are imposed in order to maintain "an idealized image of the parent who is hoped to return" (1983, p. 585).

Terr (1988) discusses how memories of terrifying events during the preschool years may manifest themselves in later years. She observes that studies show that memories of nontraumatic experiences can be later modified, but "studies do not establish what happens to a childhood memory of real trauma" (p. 97). In her study she establishes the differences between behavioral and verbal memory and discusses approximate ages at which a trauma can be recalled verbally. Her findings show that the age of 2½–3 years "appears to be about the time most children will be able to lay down, and later to retrieve, some sort of verbal memory of trauma" (Terr, 1988, p. 97).

CASE OF MARTY, AGE 2½

Family Information

Mother, Galiana Vega, age 25, legal secretary
Father, Martin Vega, age 28, computer specialist
Only child, Martin Vega, Jr. ("Marty"), age 2½
Grandmother, Demetria Gonzaga, age 55, retired teacher
Grandfather, Melchor Gonzaga, age 54, businessman

Religion and Culture

Marty's family is of Spanish origin. His mother's family was originally from Andalusia, and his father's was from Castille. Historically, both families had been actively involved in the Spanish Civil War and were socialist in their ideology. Religion had not played an important part in their lives, except for Galiana, Marty's mother, who had embraced the Catholic church after her marriage, perhaps in search of counsel and solace over her problems with her husband. However, the Spanish Catholic church is rich in tradition, and Marty's grandparents did adhere to this. They observed Catholic holidays and religious customs. This meant that the funeral was Catholic, and a memorial mass was offered 1 week afterward. Normally, children attend these ceremonies, but Marty's grandparents protectively decided to keep him away from it and sent him to spend a week at the beach with family friends.

Presenting Problem

Marty's grandparents were trying to help their grandson with his tragic loss, even as they, themselves, were grief stricken. They distracted him, bought him toys, took him out often, and indulged and pampered him. They had never been involved with any kind of therapy. When they realized that Marty needed more than their love and care, they began to make phone calls in order to find someone who could help them in their first language. Marty's family functioned in Spanish at home, so they had always wanted the child to learn Spanish before English.

By the time Marty came to me, 1 month had passed since the murder of his mother and his father's suicide. Marty had lost weight, appeared lethargic and whiney, and had abandoned his favorite toys. Malmquist noted how common it is that psychological attention is so often late or nonexistent in cases like this, perhaps because of "the need to deny some of the aftereffects of traumatic events" (1986, p. 321). For Marty's grandparents, this negligence is very understandable, since they were identifying with Marty's pain. As Raphael indicated, to avoid painful memories the surviving adults may deny that the child is affected by the loss, and "then he may be left with residual vulnerabilities to separation and loss" (1983, p. 80).

Marty was told that his mother had gone to heaven because God loved her and had called her to his side. Of course, Marty could not conceive of his mother leaving without him. He would call her, look for her all over his grandparents' home, and fantasize that he was talking with her on the phone. He begged his grandfather to take him "home" to the house where he used to live with her. It was difficult for him to fall asleep, and then he would wake up calling her. Tantrums were a daily occurrence, and Marty regressed to baby talk whenever he was frustrated or tired. "It is at this age that the infant is first unconsolable for his 'own and only mother' whom he has lost"; there is no consolation because "no other person can take away the anguish of his screams. . . . He wants simply her" (Raphael, 1983, p. 82). Bluestone notes that "the death of such a loved one leaves the bereft child with a world that may never again be as secure and safe a place as it was before" (1999, p. 225).

Marty became very attached to his grandmother's cat and wanted to sleep with him, perhaps for added security. Once the cat spent the night outside the home and Marty was inconsolable. Krueger warns that the trauma of loss has implications for intrapsychic organization during development, as "the loss frequently provides a sensitizing precursor for any subsequent experience of loss" (1983, p. 582), and this can impact on natural losses that occur in adult life. I was keenly aware of this child's terrible tragedy and his vulnerability as I began my work with him.

First Sessions

The first session was focused on earning Marty's confidence. His grandmother stayed in the room, and Marty seemed comfortable, playing, running around, asking many questions, and behaving like any 2-year-old. His most outstanding quality was that he spoke very clearly and loudly, although not often, giving the appropriate inflection to his questions. He indicated he needed to go to the bathroom at the proper time and gave no signs of disturbance.

For the second session, 6 days later, Marty was alone with me. He cried a little at the beginning, but his attention quickly moved to a clown dressed in bright colors that had not been in the room the previous time. Marty went to it and grabbed it. He played with the clown, moved around the room holding it, and then "walked" it. He later moved from one toy to the next, dragging the clown, then sat on a small chair, sucked his thumb and looked at me, with his arms around the clown. I asked him if he was sleepy, but he did not answer. I moved toward him, patted him on the knee, invited him to play, but he suddenly burst into tears, threw the clown on the floor, and walked toward the door, calling his grandmother.

When the time came for the third session, 1 week later, Marty was throwing a tantrum and had to be carried in by his grandfather. Marty's grandfather told me that every time they drove past a McDonald's restaurant, Marty would scream for them to stop because he had "seen" his mother. She used to take him there once a week for burgers, soda, fries, and to play on the colorful swings. On their way to this particular session, their route took them past a McDonald's. Not only did Marty insist that his mother was outside the restaurant waiting for him, he also said he could see her, and called out to her, punching his grandfather's arm when he wouldn't stop the car.

As stated by Krueger, the lack of cognitive development to comprehend the concept of death as final causes the child to conceptualize the loss as a reversible departure: "It is a common fantasy of the child who loses a parent to expect a return"; this expectancy is first "consciously and later unconsciously experienced" (1983, p. 584). Bowlby (1963) indicates that the typical grief reaction begins with shock, protest, and anger. The individual cannot believe that the person is really dead, and children are likely to remain in denial for a very long period of time.

Once in my office, Marty continued to cry for about 10 minutes. Finally, he noticed a group of toys on a low table and stopped crying. He looked at the toys, then at me, all this while hanging on to his grandfather's shirt. It took a while for him to let go and walk toward the toys. Then Mr. Gonzaga walked out of the room.

Content of Session	Analysis and Feelings
THERAPIST: *(Sits on the floor, close to the toys.)*	Wondering if he will be able to focus. The memory of the "lost" mother is so terribly painful.
MARTY: *(Approaches the table with his hand behind his back. Looks at me.)*	
T: We can play with that. Go ahead.	
M: *(Walks around the table, picking one toy, then another. Sits on a small chair, carefully, checking around for boundaries. Grabs a hammer. Bangs the table. Touches and grabs toys, asking what they are.)* What's this? *(Smiles easily. Moves his chair closer to me, seems to expect directions.)*	
T: *(Moves closer to Marty.)*	

M: *(Gets up, looks for a new toy, wheels a little wooden dog around the room. Stops and looks around.)*

T: There are more toys in that box. *(Points to a large wooden box.)*

M: *(Picks up a set of family figures using both hands, places them on the table. Goes back to the box and picks a toy gun. Presses the trigger several times, pointing in different directions.)*

T: What do you have there?

M: Gun. *(Turns toward me and shoots several times.)* Bam! Bam!   A moment that was expected and feared at the same time.

T: Ouch! *(Takes hands to chest and leans against the wall.)*   I am not sure about what to do here.

M: *(Moves toward me, aims at my head at close range.)* Bam! Bam! *(Frowns, seems to concentrate on what he is doing. He shoots many times.)*   His mother had been shot three times at close range, once in the head and twice in the back.

T: *(Stays still for a few seconds.)*   I doubt whether this is a good idea.

M: *(Moves toward the chair quietly and sits down, placing the toy gun on the table.)*   He seems overwhelmed by the memory of the traumatic event.

T: *(Sits up.)* What happened?

M: *(Shrugs his shoulders.)*

T: *(Walks toward Marty. Sits next to him.)* What happened?

M: *(Sucks his thumb, stares into space. Does not talk again during the session.)*   My heart goes out to him, but I cannot reach him.

Preliminary Assessment and Treatment Plan

Because witnessing the murder of a parent is a rare event, it is very difficult to draw conclusions. The attempt at making any generalization is hindered by the absence of statistical support (Malmquist, 1986). In cases when a child has been the witness of a parent's murder, the differences in circumstances can significantly complicate research efforts. Krueger states that "the loss event is important as well as the loss process: the chain of events preceding, set in motion by, and subsequent to the loss" (1983, p. 583). The perpetrators vary greatly, as they may be known or unknown;

the witnessing may be only auditory or only part of the scene may be witnessed. In some cases, the child may be hurt him/herself. The reaction of the family after the murder is another important variable, both in the way they conduct themselves and the way they handle the child witness, including the period of time that passes before consulting a professional.

In Marty's case, not only did he see his mother die violently, but his own father committed the murder. Despite the father figure's "distance" from Marty and his mother, a young child focuses a great deal of attention on the male identification model. In addition, this father was dragged from the bathroom, in front of Marty, bloody and limp. Hurley (1991) explored the particular complications in the death of a parent by suicide, in which the grief process is affected by the manner of the loss. The difficulty in treating Marty was compounded by this twist of fate. Another factor in this case is that the grandparents were very close to Marty but their own grief got in the way of the attention they could give him and their ability to perceive or understand his signals. Furthermore, one single shot at a distance can be extremely frightening to anyone, especially a child, and Marty witnessed three shots only a few steps away, saw his mother fall, and then heard another shot. I could not help imagining the fragile psyche of such a young child shattered by the blasts, and I wondered whether Marty's father may have pointed the gun at the child before fleeing to the bathroom and whether Marty witnessed the removal of both bodies. No one will ever be able to gauge the intensity of his fear at that moment.

Marty's sadness, intrusive thoughts, fitful sleep, tantrums, and fear of separation from his grandparents fulfilled the criteria of the *Diagnostic and Statistical Manual of Mental Disorders*, fourth edition, text revision (DSM-IV-TR; American Psychiatric Association, 2000), for posttraumatic stress disorder (PTSD). This case is further complicated by the possible repercussions of the criminal act performed by the father, which Marty attempted to imitate in a session with the toy gun as he tried to communicate what he saw. Though the toy gun was part of my standard play therapy equipment, he chose it among many other toys. He may have found some relief in this replay of the traumatic scene, as stated by Webb: "Through replay of the crisis experience the child transforms the passivity and impotence he or she experienced into activity and power" (1999, p. 33). However, the nature of the criminal act leaves many questions to be resolved as to how such an early memory may manifest itself as the child gets older. Terr found that "repeated and/or variable events (as in child abuse) are less fully remembered than are single episodes of trauma" (1988, p. 97) and that events that are short in duration are recalled more fully than longer events. Consequently, Marty's reenactment of the shooting itself may signal a more vivid memory than the subsequent bloody scenes and may remain imprinted for years to come.

The positive side in the aftermath of these events resided in Marty's grandparents, who were dedicated to him, committed to making him feel secure, loved, and needed. His grandmother often recruited his help in making cookies and always complimented him, saying how grateful she was for his help. His grandfather, in turn, would take Marty with him on his errands, soliciting his cooperation in carrying little bags, holding doors open for him, and also showing a great deal of appreciation for Marty's help. It was obvious to me that Marty might need long-term therapy; my intervention was limited to stabilizing the crisis and referring him to a long-term therapist. It was difficult to find a Spanish-speaking professional, but 2 months from the initial session a suitable referral was located. My focus, then, was to strengthen Marty's self-image, address the finality of his loss, and ultimately, yet very carefully, transfer the case to another therapist who would stay with it for an indefinite period of time. Through play therapy, I was planning to proceed intuitively, because there was very little in the way of research to which I could refer that could help me treat such a young child.

Play Therapy Sessions

The session described below was crucial in Marty's reconciliation with reality. He had been attending weekly sessions for 2 months. Each session was 1 hour in duration. Sometimes one or both of his grandparents would have to be present because he felt insecure and feared he would not see them again if they left the room. The need for their presence, however, diminished with each session.

On this occasion, not only was Marty able to be alone with me without discomfort, but—anticipating his arrival—I seized what I hoped might be a therapeutic opportunity: a dead goldfish. One of my colleagues had a fishbowl with several goldfish in it. One fish had just been found dead, so I asked my colleague to lend me the bowl with the dead fish in it. About 5 minutes into the session, Marty noticed the fishbowl in front of the window. I had placed it on a low table so he could see it up close. I then pretended to be surprised at finding the dead fish.

Content of Session	Analysis and Feelings

THERAPIST: Oh my! This fishy is dead.
(Takes it out of the water and places it on a paper towel next to the bowl where the other fish were alive and well.)
MARTY: *(Looks at the dead fish intently.)*

T: It's dead, see? *(Touches the fish, lifts it, puts it in the palm of her hand.)* Do you want to touch it?

Wondering how he will respond.

M: *(Reaches out, very carefully receives the fish in his hands, stares at it while he strokes it with his index and middle fingers.)*

T: It is dead, Marty, you see? It can't swim anymore, it is like he's asleep, but he can't wake up.

M: *(Keeps stroking the fish.)* No twimmin'.

T: No, no swimming. We have to put him in the earth. We have to bury him. See the others? They are going to be sad because they miss him. He can't swim with them anymore.

M: *(Shifts attention to the live fish while still holding the dead one.)* They sad.

T: Yes, they're very sad because their brother is dead, and now they don't have him anymore. He can't swim, he can't do anything. So we have to bury him. Do you want to help me bury him?

M: *(Nods, with a very serious facial expression, as if in deep thought.)*

T: We are going to need a few things. *(Finds a spoon to use as a shovel, and a tiny box for the fish. Gives the box to Marty.)* That's so you can put him in the box.

Not sure if there is any point in doing this, since the child did not attend the funeral. But his grandparents had tried to explain to him what had happened to his mother's body.

M: *(Puts the fish in the box. Looks up at me for directions.)*

T: Now we can go to the yard to bury him. *(Tries to take Marty by the hand, but he prefers to carry the box with both hands. We go to the yard, to a large planter.)* You see, Marty? This is what happens when somebody is dead. Everybody is very sad, and they have to bury the one who's dead. Do you want to make a hole in the dirt with the spoon?

Hoping at some level that the metaphor will be meaningful to him.

M: *(Nods, gently puts the box on the ground, takes the spoon, and carefully begins to spoon loose dirt out. Makes a huge hole and seems to get lost in the activity.)*

I wonder if he understands the meaning of the procedure.

T: That's very good, you have made a very big hole for the fish. Now you have to put the box in the hole.

M: *(Lowers the box in the hole with care. Once again expects directions from me.)*

T: Now we have to cover the box with dirt.

M: *(With his hands, begins to scoop dirt and put it over the hole.)*

T: *(Helping Marty.)* Now maybe we should find a stone to put here so we know where the fish is.

M: *(Looks around and quickly finds a stone which he puts on top of the small mound.)*

T: Very good. How about a flower?

M: *(Quickly finds a flower and half buries it on the mound.)*

T: Well done, Marty. You know that's what happened with your mommy when she was dead.

M: Shot. Daddy shoot Mommy.

T: Yes, when Daddy shot her, it was like she was asleep and she couldn't wake up. Then Granny and Grampy had to take her and bury her, and they were very sad. It also happened with your daddy.

M: Where's my mommy?

T: You want to know where she is? Where they put her?

Shows no interest in his father.

M: *(Nods.)*

T: We have to ask Granny and Grampy.

Apprehension about the reaction the grandparents may have to this idea.

As I found out later, Marty's grandparents were receptive to the idea. They had not visited their daughter's grave since the burial and thought that such a visit now would be good for all of them. They had started to talk about the funeral and burial in front of Marty, and he had asked many questions about where his mother may be "asleep."

During the following session, Marty seemed cheerful, even when he told me about the visit to his mother's grave:

Content of Session	Analysis and Feelings
MARTY: Mommy has flowers and flowers.	Relieved by his reaction after visiting the grave.
THERAPIST: Did Mommy like flowers?	
M: *(Nods.)* The fishy like flowers.	
T: Do you want to put a new flower for the fishy?	
M: *(Nods.)*	

This did not mean acceptance, but it was a beginning. Marty's grandparents observed that after visiting the grave he seemed less restless and had begun to sleep better. He still looked out the window as if waiting for his mother, and when he heard the turn of the key he would often expect her to open the door. Then he would throw a tantrum out of disappointment.

On a subsequent session, I experimented with some fingerpaints. Marty enjoyed wearing an apron "like Mommy's." He focused on the red fingerpaints, ignoring other colors; he smeared paint on his chest and arms, and remained quietly staring at his arms for a few minutes; he smeared some on a large piece of paper, smelled it, and tasted it. I asked him why he was painting himself red and how he liked the flavor of the paint, but he ignored my questions. His movements were deliberate and slow. After approximately 15 minutes, he insisted on washing himself clean, putting away the paints, and playing with something else. On later sessions, whenever the paints were offered, he rejected them. The red paint seemed to provide Marty with the opportunity to reenact his experience of being covered with his mother's blood.

Mr. and Mrs. Gonzaga continued to visit the grave with Marty and to talk about the incident at home. They reported that Marty would listen without asking questions, as if trying to reach his own conclusions.

The next challenge was termination and transfer. It was time for Marty's new therapist to take over the case. I knew that (fortunately) I had not become a substitute for the lost mother. This was probably due to the nurturing and dedication of his grandmother. However, Marty had felt very comfortable in the last five sessions, had been affectionate toward me, and had obviously given some emotional meaning to the time he spent in session. In order to make the transition as easy as possible, I requested the cooperation of his new therapist.

She attended the last two session with Marty and me to establish a bond. It was explained to Marty that he would be going to her office instead of mine. He was told that I was not going away, that he could visit me from time to time if he asked his grandparents. He did not seem uncomfortable at all and seemed to accept his new therapist quite well.

FOLLOW-UP: MARTY, AGE 10

Marty responded extremely well to his long-term treatment, which was discontinued when he began kindergarten. It is unclear as to whether this was his grandparent's or the therapist's decision, or whether Marty had indicated a desire to stop attending sessions. As explained by his grandmother, school was also instrumental in his recovery. He enjoyed it so much that he often voiced disappointment because he had no school on the weekends. Though he went through a short period of aggressive behavior around the age of 5, his teacher managed to help him through those difficult times by putting him "in charge" of younger classmates, asking him to show them how to use school materials, where the bathroom was, and so on. He was reportedly at his best while helping other children and when given concrete tasks and assignments. His grandmother states that he tells his friends that both his parents are dead and gives no further details. She says that he is "always busy" and involved in many activities, such as Little League and science club; he also takes karate lessons, loves to swim, and is enchanted with the *Harry Potter* books.

When Marty turned 6, he received the visit of his paternal grandmother, who lives in Spain. His paternal grandfather, who had abused his wife and children, died years before the murder–suicide. Marty accepted his paternal grandmother without questions, though he became upset when she cried while holding him during their first meeting. After that, when she came near him he moved away and asked her if she was going to cry. When she indicated that she would not, he was glad to be near her, though he frequently watched for tears. His maternal grandmother indicates that he still becomes very upset when someone he cares about cries in front of him.

By age 8, Marty began to ask questions about his father's childhood and eventually expressed a desire to spend time with his paternal family. His grandparents took him to visit his aunt and uncles in California that summer, and he spent Christmas with them the following year. Since then, he has had regular contact with his father's family and has shown a great deal of attachment toward an uncle who is in his early 20s. He sees him as a role model, and the uncle has responded well, calling him on the phone with regularity and maintaining E-mail correspondence with Marty.

I was subsequently able to see Marty, age 10, and though he apparently did not remember me at all he was polite and friendly toward me. He told me he loves computers and is very good in anything related to science, though he still does not know what he wants to be when he grows up.

CONCLUDING COMMENTS

According to Krueger, "a mourning process is initiated by the perception of loss as well as an acceptance of its permanence and irreversibility. One factor precluding mourning is the maintenance of the fantasy of the retrievability of the loss" (1983, p. 590). After I no longer treated Marty, I often wondered if he had really initiated his mourning process. For children, the mourning process takes years "because children can only tolerate small does of painful feelings" (Bluestone, 1999, p. 228).

In dealing with this case, I often felt I was in the dark because there is a paucity of literature on the subject of the very young child witness to violence. In Marty's case, the violence of the event, the identity of the perpetrator, and the child's age made it impossible to follow any particular guidelines. Marty may need ongoing help as he grows, especially during and after puberty as he understands more deeply how his parents died, as he wonders about the feelings that existed between them, and as he attempts to relate to the opposite sex. At this time there is no evidence that Marty may be at risk of modeling his father's behavior, perhaps because he was too young at the time of the incident to form a lasting picture of his father and his behavior, and because of all the support he has received from his grandparents. Furthermore, he now has a new model in his own young uncle, though they do not live together, not even in the same town. His uncle is providing Marty with a young male confidant and someone he can brag about to his friends, and that seems enough for him at this time. In addition, Marty's grandfather, now in his early 60s, is fit and healthy enough for hiking, fishing, and occasional camping trips, which Marty is reported to love. However, both grandparents may benefit from ongoing assistance to help them convey to Marty that both his parents loved him and that he did not cause, nor could he have prevented, the tragedy that occurred. The outcome for Marty depends strongly on the support of those who love him and their willingness to put time and energy into raising him in a loving home, nourishing him with security, and making him feel important and needed. The added support of his father's family seems to have filled a gap and brought him stability and a sense of belonging.

Many researchers have traditionally believed that trauma behaviors had "no basis in the physiology of the brain" (Doyle & Stoop, 1999, p. 158). Recently, however, an increasing body of research is bearing light on possible neurobiological alterations and their impact on developmental processes in children. Pynoos, Steinberg, Ornitz, and Goengian (1997), propose that the neurobiology of PTSD requires a perspective that goes "beyond the traditional fight/flight paradigm, one that includes the human's capacity for considering protective intervention"; the authors also state that this capacity "should be studied over the course of ontogenesis as it correlates with neurodevelopment" (p. 189). As it relates to Marty's developmental stage at the time of the incident and other factors in his case, these considerations may prove unnecessary. After speaking to his grandmother and seeing him healthy and apparently well adapted, it seems to me that he did arrive at a point of resolution in relation to his loss. But only time will tell just how and to what extent his resilience will hold up in later developmental stages.

DISCUSSION QUESTIONS

1. Discuss the normal grief of a 2½-year-old child related to the death of a parent. What explanations about the death are appropriate in working with a child of this age?

2. If the therapist had not utilized the burial of the dead goldfish as part of her work with this child, what other play therapy materials or experiences might have been introduced?

3. What counseling issues do you consider important in work with the grandparents?

4. At what developmental stages do you consider that Marty might be "at risk" and why? What interventions might serve as a preventive purpose?

5. How would you avoid becoming a substitute for the lost parent while establishing a strong relationship with a pre-school-age child?

REFERENCES

American Psychiatric Association. (2000). *Diagnostic and statistical manual of mental disorders* (4th ed., text rev.). Washington, DC: Author.

Bluestone, J. (1999). School-based peer therapy to facilitate mourning in latency-age children following sudden parental death: Cases of Joan, age 10½, and Roberta age 9½, with follow-up 8 years later. In N. B. Webb (Ed.), *Play therapy with children in crisis* (2nd ed.): *Individual, group, and family treatment* (pp. 225–251). New York: Guilford Press.

Bowlby, J. (1963). Pathological mourning and childhood mourning. *Journal of the American Psychoanalytic Association, 11,* 500–541.

Doyle, J. S. & Stoop, D. (1999). Witness and victim of multiple abuse: Case of Randy, age 10, in a residential treatment center, and follow-up at age 19 in prison. In N. B. Webb (Ed.), *Play therapy with children in crisis* (2nd ed.): *Individual, group, and family treatment* (pp. 131–163). New York: Guilford Press.

Hurley, D. J. (1991). The crisis of paternal suicide. In N. B. Webb (Ed.), *Play therapy with children in crisis: A casebook for practitioners* (pp. 237–253). New York: Guilford Press.

Krueger, D. W. (1983). Childhood parent loss: Developmental impact and adult psychopathology. *American Journal of Psychotherapy, 37*(4), 582–591.

Malmquist, C. P. (1986). Children who witness parental murder: Posttraumatic aspects. *Journal of the American Academy of Child Psychiatry, 25*(3), 320–325.

Pynoos, R. S., Steinberg, A. M., Ornitz, E. M., & Goenjian, A. K. (1997). Issues in the developmental neurobiology of traumatic stress. In R. Yehuda & A. C. McFarlane (Eds.), *Psychobiology of posttraumatic stress disorder. Annals of the New York Academy of Sciences, 821,* 176–193.

Raphael, B. (1983). *The anatomy of bereavement.* New York: Basic Books.

Terr, L. (1988). What happens to early memories of trauma?: A study of twenty children under age five at the time of documented traumatic events. *Journal of the American Academy of Child and Adolescent Psychiatry, 27*(1), 96–104.

Webb, N. B. (1999). Play therapy intervention with children. In N. B. Webb (Ed.), *Play therapy with children in crisis* (2nd ed.): *Individual, group, and family treatment* (pp. 29–46). New York: Guilford Press.

PART III

✍

Death in the School and Community

8

❧

Traumatic Death
of a Friend/Peer

Case of Susan, Age 9

NANCY BOYD WEBB

The death of a friend is a crisis—a danger and an
opportunity—for surviving children. The danger is that the
youngsters will be emotionally overwhelmed by the death. The
opportunity, however, is the possibility of mastering the crisis
and emerging with new emotional strengths. . . . Children who
must deal with the death of a friend are indirect victims, at risk
for emotional and behavioral disturbances both at the time of
the death and in the future.
—Fox (1985, pp. 3–4)

Accidental deaths occur without warning, sometimes striking even a 9-
year-old boy. Many children of this age know about death through their
personal experience of a pet's or a relative's death, and most have witnessed countless television deaths involving cartoon characters and "ce-
lebrities" in news broadcasts. A few 9-year-olds may know a peer who
is terminally ill with cancer or AIDS. For the typical 9-year-old child,
however, death happens to someone who is remote in terms of age,
geography, or state of health. The idea that death could strike a neighborhood friend on a sunny weekday afternoon while being driven to an
after-school activity by his mother is simply beyond belief!

This chapter presents precisely this tragedy: the sudden, accidental, mutilating death of a 9-year-old boy who died instantly when the car, driven by his mother, went off the road into a ditch. The grieving survivors of this terrible accident included not only the dead child's immediate family but also his circle of school, church, and family friends, who were stunned by this sudden, irrevocable loss of a fun-loving fourth-grade student.

What reactions would we consider "normal" for the boy's 9-year-old friend, Susan, who had known him since nursery school and whose mother was an intimate friend of her own mother? Susan did not cry, even at the funeral, nor had she spoken about her dead friend, Carl, since the accident. She refused to enter his house and waited outside in the car while her mother visited Carl's mother. Susan was having nightmares, and her mother was very worried about her because she "was holding all her feelings in." Susan's mother brought her for an evaluation 3 weeks after the accident.

It is sometimes difficult to distinguish between the reactions of "normal" grief and the symptoms of *posttraumatic stress disorder* (PTSD), according to the criteria of DSM-IV-TR (American Psychiatric Association, 2000). The following section discusses the topic of PTSD in children so that the reader can join me in determining whether Susan's response was within the range of "normal" grief or was more aptly diagnosed as PTSD. The case presentation also invites the reader to consider whether or not Susan "needed" therapy and, if so, what kind and for how long. A year after the accident Susan returned for two follow-up play therapy sessions. This permits us to also consider the topic of delayed mourning and its later eruption in anniversary reactions.

POSTTRAUMATIC STRESS DISORDER IN CHILDREN

The diagnosis of PTSD has been used since 1980 to describe a group of reactions that occur following a distressing event outside the range of usual human experience. Table 8.1 outlines the criteria necessary for designating this diagnosis, which "can occur at any age, including during childhood" (American Psychiatric Association, 2000, p. 466). We will examine these criteria with reference to Susan's symptoms at the time of her referral.

A. *Exposure to a traumatic event.* The sudden death of Susan's friend, Carl, whose body was mutilated, certainly meets the criteria. In this particular situation the "mutilation" involved severe damage to the head and involved a rumor that the boy had been decapitated when an object entered the car window. These circumstances

TABLE 8.1. DSM-IV-TR Diagnostic Criteria for Posttraumatic Stress Disorder

A. The person has been exposed to a traumatic event in which both of the following were present:

  (1) The person experienced, witnessed, or was confronted with an event or events that involved actual or threatened death or serious injury, or a threat to the physical integrity of self or others.

  (2) The person's response involved intense fear, helplessness, or horror. **Note:** In children, this may be expressed instead by disorganized or agitated behavior.

B. The traumatic event is persistently reexperienced in one (or more) of the following ways:

  (1) Recurrent and intrusive distressing recollections of the event, including images, thoughts, or perceptions. **Note:** In young children, repetitive play may occur in which themes or aspects of the trauma are expressed.

  (2) Recurrent distressing dreams of the event. **Note:** In children, there may be frightening dreams without recognizable content.

  (3) Acting or feeling as if the traumatic event were recurring (includes a sense of reliving the experience, illusions, hallucinations, and dissociative flashback episodes, including those that occur upon awakening or when intoxicated). **Note:** In young children, trauma-specific reenactment may occur.

  (4) Intense psychological distress at exposure to internal or external cues that symbolize or resemble an aspect of the traumatic event.

  (5) Physiological reactivity on exposure to internal or external cues that symbolize or resemble an aspect of the traumatic event.

C. Persistent avoidance of stimuli associated with the trauma and numbing of general responsiveness (not present before the trauma), as indicated by three (or more) of the following:

  (1) Efforts to avoid thoughts, feelings, or conversations associated with the trauma.

  (2) Efforts to avoid activities, places, or people that arouse recollections of the trauma.

  (3) Inability to recall an important aspect of the trauma.

  (4) Markedly diminished interest or participation in significant activities.

  (5) Feeling of detachment or estrangement from others.

  (6) Restricted range of affect (e.g., unable to have loving feelings).

  (7) Sense of a foreshortened future (e.g., does not expect to have a career, marriage, children, or a normal life span).

D. Persistent symptoms of increased arousal (not present before the trauma), as indicated by two (or more) of the following:

  (1) Difficulty falling or staying asleep.

  (2) Irritability or outbursts of anger.

  (3) Difficulty concentrating.

  (4) Hypervigilance.

  (5) Exaggerated startle response.

E. Duration of the disturbance (symptoms in Criteria B, C, and D) is more than 1 month.

F. The disturbance causes clinically significant distress or impairment in social, occupational, or other important areas of functioning.

Specify if:
  Acute: if duration of symptoms is less than 3 months.
  Chronic: if duration of symptoms is 3 months or more.

Specify if:
  With Delayed Onset: if onset of symptoms is at least 6 months after the stressor.

Note. From American Psychiatric Association (2000, pp. 467–468). Copyright 2000 by the American Psychiatric Association. Reprinted by permission.

were not discussed openly by Susan's family in order to protect their own feelings of horror, as well as those of Carl's family. However, because the rumor about the nature of Carl's injury circulated at school, Susan must have been heard it, and in the absence of open discussion she probably assumed that it was true.

B. *Reexperiencing the traumatic event.* Susan was waking nightly with distressing dreams of being chased by a monster. Although the dreams were not a replication of the accident, they nonetheless caused Susan intense anxiety. She had not had any such dreams prior to the accident, so it appeared probable that they were related to Carl's death.

C. *Avoiding trauma-related stimuli/numbing.* Susan would not enter Carl's house; this appeared to be a way of avoiding memories about him (item 2 in criteria under C, Table 8.1); she was sleeping more than usual (possibly item 1, avoiding thoughts associated with the trauma, or item 5, feelings of detachment from others); she also appears to have restricted affect (item 6), as evidenced in her absence of tears.

D. *Increased arousal.* Susan's mother reported that her daughter was very irritable (item 2 under D, Table 8.1); she also was experiencing some difficulties in concentrating (item 3).

E. *Duration.* The criteria specify that the symptoms must have been evident for at least 1 month. Susan's mother referred her after 3 weeks; however, the symptoms continued for several weeks following the initiation of therapy.

F. *Degree of distress/impairment.* Susan's schoolwork was suffering, and she was exhausted from lack of sleep due to the nightmares.

Preliminary Assessment

There was certainly enough evidence to consider a probable diagnosis of PTSD based on the information reviewed here, which was given by the mother over the telephone. Susan's sessions with me, which will be reported later, confirmed this preliminary impression.

Before proceeding with the case discussion, we will focus briefly on two elements of Susan's symptoms, the nightmares and her isolation of affect, and also on the topic of incomplete mourning and its relationship to anniversary reactions.

Posttraumatic Nightmares

According to Terr (1987), who studied 26 children after their traumatic kidnapping and burial for 29 hours, "children who have been psychologically overwhelmed dream that they themselves die . . . because they no longer believe in their personal invulnerability. They are entirely convinced of their helplessness once they accept the 'fact' during an event that they might die at any moment" (pp. 239–240). Although Susan did not dream of dying, she felt very threatened by being chased by the monster in her nightmares, and that fear awakened her. Perhaps she felt that if Carl could die suddenly, she might be next. Even when a trauma has not been witnessed firsthand it can stimulate nightmares, as happens following frightening television programs and scary movies. It is possible, therefore, that merely hearing about Carl's tragic death proved traumatic to Susan. Terr (1987) states that "horror is contagious. It can be experienced by those who never themselves were directly horrified" (p. 241).

During the latency age of development (elementary school), the bad dreams of the preschool years are usually less frequent and bothersome; Terr comments that "nightmares at this calmer, more organized stage of childhood may . . . often occur at times of severe outside stress" (1987, p. 237). Clearly this seems to be the case with Susan.

Absence of Grief: "Masked" Delayed or Inhibited Grief

Susan's mother was very concerned about her daughter because she was "holding all her feelings in." In Lindemann's classic article about acute grief he refers to the tendency to avoid the sensations of grief "at any cost . . . , and to keep all references to the deceased deliberately from thought" (1944, p. 8). If this is a characteristic of "normal" grief, then Susan's restricted affect should not cause concern. However, in view of the openly expressed grief responses of Susan's family and school community to Carl's death, her lack of reaction seems puzzling. Furthermore, if we interpret the nightmares as the nighttime expression of Susan's repressed daytime anxieties about the death, then these reactions may qualify as evidence of "masked" grief. Worden (1991) defines this term as related to symptoms and behaviors that cause difficulty but which are not recognized by the bereaved individual as related to his/her loss. Susan thus could admit that she was having nightmares, but she could not enter Carl's house, because she would then have to face his grieving mother and other mourners and the reality of his absence. Helene Deutsch suggests that absent grief reactions may occur in individuals whose ego is not sufficiently developed to bear the strain of grief and mourning and who therefore employ self-protective mechanisms to circumvent the process (Worden, 1991). Deutsch's belief is that "every unresolved grief is given expression in one form or another" (1937, quoted in Bowlby, 1963, p. 531). Therefore, it is not really accurate to refer to this type of grief as "absent," since it is present *internally* despite the lack of external signs. Rando (1993) suggests that the terms "delayed" or "inhibited" grief more aptly refer to mourning responses (such as Susan's) that help the mourner avoid the pain of loss.

Anniversary Reactions

When grief is not fully expressed, it may find an outlet in the formation of symptoms such as nightmares, or it may surface at some future time, stimulated by a memory of the loss triggered by a significant date or time of year that stirs up the repressed feelings. The clinical literature views anniversary reactions as manifestations of incomplete mourning (Gabriel, 1992). Susan's inability to deal with her feelings about Carl's death at the time it occurred made her vulnerable to a strong reaction about a year later when her fifth-grade class was reading a story about the tragic death of a young person. This gave her and me another chance to deal with some of her feelings associated with her traumatic loss. Because children's grief is usually sporadic and protracted, this case permits us to appreciate more fully the gradual unfolding of grief, with anniversary reactions "conceptualized as normative and expectable, perhaps, existing on a continuum, unfolding over decades" (Gabriel, 1992, p. 189).

CASE OF SUSAN, AGE 9

Family Information

> Mother, Dina James, age 43, former teacher, currently at home
> Father, Don James, age 43, stockbroker
> Susan James, age 9, fourth grade, active in Girl Scouts
> Becky James, age 7, second grade, described by Mother as "loud and boisterous; takes a lot of my time because she is so 'hyper' "

Maternal and paternal grandparents live on the west coast, as do the mother's and father's siblings. The James family has lived on the east coast for about 12 years. They maintain telephone contact with their western relatives and visit occasionally. Carl's family has been very close to Susan's since prior to her birth, when Dina and Carl's mother taught together in the same school. Susan and Carl were born the same year, and the two young mothers spent many hours together during their children's preschool years. Susan and Carl went to the same nursery school and have been in the same elementary school, although not the same class.

Religious/Cultural Heritage

Susan's family is Protestant and is very active in their church; they attend church weekly, and the girls attend Sunday school. Carl's family attends the same church. All went to Carl's funeral together, where a closed casket, covered with flowers, rested in front of the altar. Because Carl had once expressed negative feelings about cemeteries to his mother, his family selected the option of entombment in a mausoleum for his body, rather than burial in a cemetery.

Background on Referral

The referral came to me, a child and family therapist, through a former social work student who knew Carl's family through the church and who was told by Carl's mother that Susan had become "angry, cranky, and mean."

My usual procedure with a new case is to see the parents alone prior to seeing the child. The purpose is to obtain a detailed history of the problem and to discuss with the parents how to prepare the child for the upcoming evaluation session. In this instance I decided to arrange an appointment for the child with one or both of her parents right away because I viewed this situation as one in which the child was in considerable discomfort, which merited an immediate response in the form of crisis intervention. I therefore spoke with the mother at length on the phone and obtained the information that has already been reviewed. I suggested to Susan's mother that she tell her the day before our scheduled appointment that she had spoken to a doctor who helps children and their families after a death, and that she would be taking Susan to speak with me after school the next day. I advised the mother to not go into great detail about the appointment but to convey through her manner a "matter-of-fact" firmness that the appointment was definite and not optional. In turn, I conveyed to Mrs. James my own conviction that I wanted to see Susan because I knew that it would be helpful for her to speak with someone, although I understood that Susan might find this very difficult initially.

First Session with Child

At the agreed-upon time my buzzer rang and the mother came into the waiting room all flustered, stating that Susan was in the car refusing to come in. My immediate response was to tell the mother that I would go out to the car and speak with her daughter. Without thinking about the 30 degree temperature of February in New York, I left the office without my coat and immediately spotted Susan in the car by the entrance. The motor was still running and Susan was sitting in the backseat. I walked over to the car window, smiled, introduced myself, and invited Susan to come in to the office. She seemed reluctant but nevertheless was aware that I did not have a coat on and that it was very cold. I remember saying to her, "Please come in so we can talk inside; it's freezing out here!" Susan got out of the car and accompanied me into the office while her mother proceeded to park the car. My feeling was, "Well, at least we got to first base. Let's see where things will go from here." Excerpts from the session follow:

Content of Session	*Analysis and Feelings*
THERAPIST: Hi! I'm certainly glad you agreed to come inside. It was *very* chilly out there! I guess you didn't want to come in, but now that you're here we might as well try to get to know each other. *(At this point the mother comes in and I invite her to join us. To Susan)* I know that you've been having a rough time lately. Do you understand why your mom brought you to see me?	This is hard for both of us, but she is probably more scared and uncomfortable than I am. It is *my* job to put *her* fears at rest. Grateful that her mother was able to carry out my instructions and get Susan here. Wondering how Susan will respond.
SUSAN: I'm having bad dreams that wake me up every night. Then in the morning I don't want to get up. I'm tired all the time, even when I go to bed at 8 o'clock.	Sounds like she is worn out!
T: That sounds pretty bad! Can you tell me what the dreams are like?	Stay with *her* concerns.
S: I dream that there is a gorilla in my closet and that he is going to sneak up to my bed and grab me and then take me away and roast me on a barbecue.	
T: That must be pretty scary! Does the dream wake you up?	
S: Yes, and then I run into my mom's bed.	
T: I know that your friend was killed in an accident. You've been through a terrible experience! Can you tell me how you found out about it, and what you were told?	I sense that Susan feels my empathy. She has pretty good eye contact. I am ready to risk asking her directly about the death.
S: Mom and Dad told me. I was home from school with the flu that day.	She does not give any of her reactions. Seems well defended.

T: What a terrible thing to hear! I know
that you and Carl were good friends.

S: I didn't invite him to my birthday
party this year.

Is she denying their friendship or feeling guilty?

MOTHER: Susan had an "all-girls" bowl-
ing party.

T: I know that a lot of 9-year-olds do
that. I'm sure Carl understood.

Wanting to universalize/nor-
malize the situation.

At this point I believed that Susan might be ready to spend some
time alone with me. I invited her mother to wait in the adjourning room
while Susan and I talked alone. I pulled out some drawing paper and
markers, wondering whether Susan would communicate using art.

Content of Session	*Analysis and Feelings*

THERAPIST: Did your mom tell you what
kind of doctor I am?

SUSAN: *(Looking uncertain.)* A therapist?

T: That's right. I'm a therapist. Do you
know what a therapist does?

So far so good. Does she have
any understanding about my
role?

S: *(Shrugs shoulders and looks uncertain.)*

T: I help kids and their parents with their
worries; sometimes we talk and
sometimes we play. I know you have
a lot of worries right now. How
about taking a break from talking for
a while. I usually invite kids to draw
something when they are here. How
about drawing a picture of a person?
*(Susan eagerly selects a piece of paper
and begins drawing a figure of a Girl
Scout; there are a lot of markings
around the figure suggesting rain?/
wind?/turmoil? [Figure 8.1].)* I see
she's a Girl Scout. You draw very
well. Our time is up for today, but
I'd like to see you again and will set
up an appointment with your
mother.

This is obviously a self-
portrait, since Susan is
dressed in her Girl Scout
uniform.

I deliberately do not comment
on the markings since I do not
want to make Susan self-
conscious about her work.

S: Okay. Thank you.

This was a fairly good beginning, considering Susan's reluctance.
Her motivation for accepting help was because of the nightmares, which

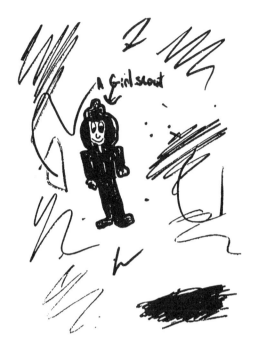

FIGURE 8.1. Susan's drawing of herself as a Girl Scout.

she did not connect to her feelings about Carl's death. Our alliance initially would be around helping her with her discomfort about the dreams.

Sessions 2 and 3

The next two sessions occurred at weekly intervals. Susan reported that she continued to have nightmares. Her description of the dreams varied from saying that they were "scary" to giving fairly good detail. In one dream she was "in a mansion with lots of doors and windows and rooms. I was with my friend, and a monster was chasing us. I was so scared I woke up and ran into my mother's bed." My response was to empathize with her feelings and to suggest to her that "sometimes our daytime worries come back to chase us at night." Susan's usual response to a statement like this was to say that everything was fine and that she wasn't worried about *anything*. In her opinion, her only problem was the nightmares and some headaches she sometimes had in school. My role certainly was not to argue with her but to give her the opportunity to express some of her feelings symbolically in play.

Drawings and Games

In the second session I invited Susan to draw a family. She quickly drew five figures with a pen, then colored their clothes with a green marker and added hats and facial expressions in blue. None of the faces looked happy. In conclusion, Susan drew a circular spiral "whirlwind" around the figures (Figure 8.2). When I asked Susan to tell me about this family she responded breezily, "It's my Girl Scout troop. Can we play a game now?" The game she selected from the wide range of available choices on my game shelf was *Battleship*, a game consisting of two players guessing the location of their opponent's ships and then "bombing" the ships by calling out the precise location; several correct guesses cause the ships to "sink." In my experience, this game is rarely selected by school-age *girls*, and as we played I began to wonder about its significance to Susan. I speculated that possibly the randomness of the "bombs" resembled the unexpected element of Carl's death. My comments to Susan tried to convey this feeling. I made statements such as "Boy, you never can tell when or where a bomb will fall! This is really scary! You never know when your number is going to be picked." Susan's mood during the game was very animated; she seemed to enjoy it greatly and to be totally oblivious to the underlying meaning of the statements I was making.

After completing one game we still had some time remaining in the session, and Susan asked to draw again. She said she would draw a surprise, and indeed it was. She drew a picture of me holding a watering can and watering flowers in a garden. I thanked her for the picture and felt optimistic about our work, despite what I had perceived as

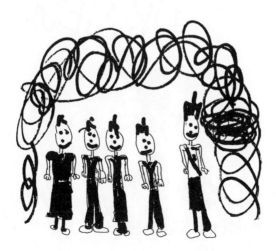

FIGURE 8.2. Susan's drawing of her Girl Scout troop.

unwillingness on Susan's part to talk openly about Carl's death. This was the first picture drawn by Susan in which she used a variety of colors and in which the mood seemed cheerful, including a bright sun shining in the sky (Figure 8.3).

Session 4

Content of Session

Analysis and Feelings

Mother has brought Becky to this session and upon arrival announces that she also has brought some pictures of Carl. I invite Mother and Becky to join me and Susan. Mother spreads out the pictures on the coffee table. Neither Becky nor Susan appears to take any interest.

Mother has told me that she is not concerned about Becky; therefore I do not attribute any special meaning to her presence. I am very interested in seeing how Susan will react to the photos.

THERAPIST: *(To Susan and Becky.)* It must seem strange to look at these pic-

I am watching Susan, but her face does not convey any emotion.

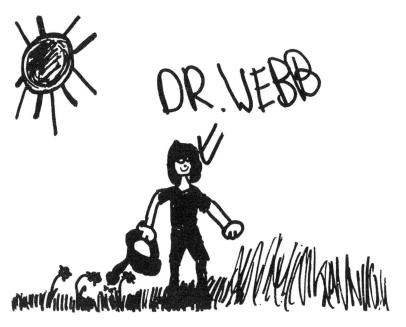

FIGURE 8.3. Susan's drawing of the therapist in a garden.

tures now. I bet it's hard to believe that Carl is dead.

BECKY: He died *instantly* when the car went down the cliff.

Becky can talk about this. It occurs to me that *she* expresses what Susan cannot bear to say.

T: Susan, you're not saying anything. Would you like to speak with me alone? *(Mother and Becky get up to leave without waiting for Susan's response.)*

I want Susan to know that I am there for *her* even though she cannot talk.

SUSAN: *(After the others have gone.)* Can we play *Battleship* again?

She wants to move away from any discussion about Carl.

T: This is your time to use any way you want to. I could see that you didn't want to talk about Carl. It must be *very* difficult for you!

I feel I must at least make some acknowledgment that we are moving away from direct discussion of Carl's death.

As we played the game I was more deliberate in my comments than I had been the week before. The fact that Susan asked for the game again tended to reinforce my hypothesis that it represented to her the random violence of sudden death. I decided to "play this for all it was worth" in the hope that we could talk about Susan's feelings about death in the metaphor of play, since she could not tolerate direct discussion about her traumatic experience.

Content of Session

THERAPIST: *(After Susan has bombed one of my boats.)* What about the people on the ships? What is going to happen to them?

SUSAN: They are swimming. They're going to swim to shore.

T: It's out in the *ocean*. Can they make it to shore?

S: Kennedy swam to an island and then went back to get his buddy. He was very courageous. We had it in school.

T: He was very lucky. What if there had been sharks in the water?

Analysis and Feelings

Deciding to press a bit.

Denial of death is strong.

Am I pushing too hard?

S: He made it to the island okay.

T: Well, I just worry about those people in the boats when they get bombed. I hope someone rescues them.

This denial is very important for Susan. She cannot imagine death, even in fantasy.

As we talked, we continued to play the game and Susan won. She was quite animated. She asked if she could have *two* snacks today because she was "starved." I permitted this, realizing that the game and my comments probably were stirring up anxious feelings. Susan then asked to draw. She drew a picture of her and me playing *Battleship*, with her calling out the winning number and me indicating that she has "hit" one of my ships (Figure 8.4).

Comment on Session

I was struck by Susan's unwillingness to consider the possibility of death, even in a game. Neither she nor Becky wanted to look at the pictures of Carl and to be reminded of his death. I was aware of Susan's anxiety through her almost manic mood; Her eating and her speech seemed more rapid than previously, and she drew and moved from one activity to another with a sense of haste. I believe that she was afraid that if she lingered she might be drawn into a discussion that would overwhelm her. I wondered how long she could keep up this evasiveness.

Session 5

This session occurred 3 weeks after the previous sessions because of a prearranged parent counseling session and a cancellation because Susan had "turned her ankle" and had been advised by her doctor to "stay off her foot."

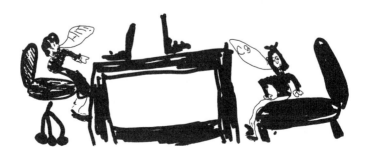

FIGURE 8.4. Susan's drawing after playing *Battleship*.

Content of Session	Analysis and Feelings
THERAPIST: It's been a while since I've seen you. How are you?	Wondering if the break is continuity will result in Susan's "distancing" further from any grief work.
SUSAN: I'm not having any more nightmares or headaches.	How will this affect Susan's motivation to come for therapy??
T: That's great! So your life is sort of getting back to normal, except for your foot.	
S: I'm really mad about my foot, because now I can't do stuff for my Girl Scout camp-out. I'm not supposed to run around.	Could her injury possibly reflect anger turned against herself?
T: How did it happen [that you hurt your foot]?	
S: It just happened. Nothing special. We were doing relay races in gym, and I slipped and twisted my ankle. The doctor X-rayed it, and it's not broken.	Sounds like an accident.
T: Well, I'm sorry you have to go through all of this. As if you didn't have enough to cope with already!	
S: You don't even know the whole story. My guinea pig died, and my friend's father died (conveyed in a very matter-of-fact tone, as if she were reciting events that had little meaning to her).	The reality of death continues. Maybe the cumulative effect will force Susan to talk about her feelings.
T: Tell me about this.	
S: Well, I came home from school and found my guinea pig dead, and we buried it in the backyard. Now I want a bird.	This girl is so literal and cut off from her feelings. I am not sure which death to explore.
T: Were you sad? How did you feel?	
S: It's okay. I'm not going to worry about it.	This is her mantra.

Susan was equally blasé in responding to my expressions of concern about her friend's father's death. When I would reach for a feeling response, Susan would reply with some bit of factual information. She did tell me that Becky had asked, "Why is everyone dying?"—further confirming my hunch that Becky expressed anxieties that Susan felt but could not admit.

Play Therapy Modalities

When I invited Susan to select an activity, she did not ask to play *Battleship* nor did she ask to draw. I suggested that she might be interested in making something out of clay. Her high energy level and sense of tension continued, and I thought that working with clay might relieve some of the tension. Susan made a mushroom out of clay and continued to ask for food during this session. After eating a box of Tic Tacs Susan asked to play the board game *Candyland*, a game usually selected by preschoolers.

Comment on Session

The interruption in treatment had occurred during a number of significant events. Sudden deaths and accidents seemed to recur in this child's life, yet her response remained ostensibly unemotional. She was now "symptom free," which made me wonder, given her great need for denial, how much longer she would be willing to come to therapy. I decided to bring this up with her in the next session, half hoping that she would find some value to continuing therapy. I was pleased that her symptoms had abated and was fascinated by the possibility that the reason for this might have something to do with her participation in play therapy.

Session 6

Susan began this session all smiles. She reported that she had received an A+ on her science test. She also told me about Becky's birthday party the previous weekend and referred to what she wanted to do for *her* next birthday, several months hence. She had had no more trouble with nightmares or headaches. When I asked her about how she felt about coming to see me now, Susan said, "It's okay, but I don't really think I need to come any more." I asked her what she thought the reason for coming had been, and Susan said, "My friend died and my mom thought I was acting different. Now everything is fine; I don't have to run into her bedroom at night any more."

I suggested that we taper off our sessions and plan to have our next session in a month. For the remainder of the session we made squiggle drawings and Susan made up a story about the figures she created. Two of the squiggle drawings and the story follow (see Figures 8.5 and 8.6).

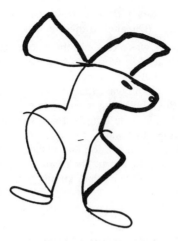

FIGURE 8.5. Squiggle drawing of the rabbit/dog.

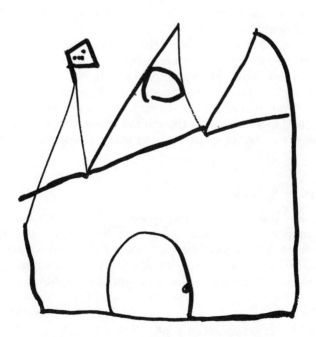

FIGURE 8.6. Squiggle drawing of the castle.

Susan's Story of the Rabbit/Dog and the Castle
(Dictated to the therapist)

Once upon a time there was a castle in the woods. The king was scared of a mean, ugly rabbit/dog who was trying to eat the princess. The princess didn't know that he was trying to get her. The king heard the rabbit/dog talking while he was riding in the forest. The king decided that he had to kill the rabbit/dog in order to save his daughter. When the rabbit/dog is sleeping the king is going to sneak up on him and shoot an arrow through his heart.

The rabbit/dog hears him coming and wakes up and runs away. He will never go near the castle again. The moral of this story: Find a better way to deal with your problems than killing people.

Comment on Session

I was not surprised that Susan wanted to terminate, and in many respects I agreed with her own assessment that her life was more or less back on course. I was somewhat resigned to the fact that Susan could not openly talk about her feelings about Carl's death, and I realized that if I had helped her experience therapy in a positive way she would be more likely to consider it as an option in the future. I reminded myself that children grieve differently than do adults and that for Susan this may be a process that will require many years of "bits of work." I did feel that we had made a good beginning.

With regard to Susan's squiggle story, I noted that the threat of death was an ever-present theme. However, in her story, the princess is protected by her father. Although he contemplates using violence to protect his daughter's life, the threatening creature manages to escape. There is a sense at the end of the story that everyone is safe, although they had been close to danger and even though the rabbit/dog was still at large. I commented that Susan seems to have made a peaceful ending to her story.

Termination Session

The most significant aspect of this session, held 1 month later, was that Susan's mother announced at the beginning that they had all gone to visit the mausoleum that weekend because it was Carl's birthday. Her mother said that she was proud of Susan for agreeing to go, even though she did not want to. My discussions with Susan about this follows:

Content of Session	*Analysis and Feelings*
THERAPIST: I'd like to hear about your visit to the mausoleum.	

SUSAN: It was a big room with names on the walls and something like an altar at the front with flowers.

Susan gives a factual description. Does she realize that bodies are there?

T: Did you see Carl's name?

S: Yes, I put some flowers on a shelf in front of it.

T: What did it *feel* like for you to be there?

Wondering if there is any possibility Susan will describe her feelings.

S: I'll draw a picture of it for you. *(Proceeds to draw, and indicates the place where she put the flowers* [Figure 8.7].)

Susan really "uses" art and games rather than words to communicate.

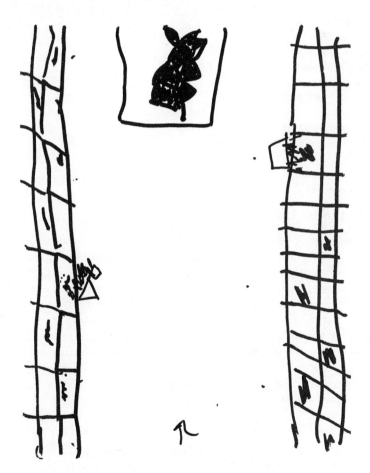

FIGURE 8.7. Susan's drawing of Carl's mausoleum.

T: It must be sad to think that Carl's body is there.

Trying to help her verbalize.

S: *(Brightly, with no hint of sadness.)* Carl's mom told me that his soul is in heaven and that we will all see him again sometime.

T: Still, I'm sure you miss not having him here with you *now*.

S: You can keep the pictures if you like.

She is totally closed off to any feelings of loss or sadness. I am almost concluding that this may be functional for her. She must go on with her life. I am struggling with whether to accept her denial that Carl's death is final and irrevocable. Here it becomes evident to me that the religious view of afterlife may, in fact, discourage open expression of grief.

T: Yes, I'll keep it in your folder with your other drawings. This is the last time we're going to meet for a while, but I'll save your drawings in my file drawer. You might come back again some time in the future if you have worries or just want to talk. If you ever do, ask your mom to call me and I'll always be glad to see you.

Wanting Susan to consider this a real "open door" policy.

S: Okay. Good-bye.

Nine Months Later

Mrs. James telephoned because Susan's teacher had notified her that Susan's school performance had deteriorated seriously in the past 5 weeks. She had evidently stopped doing all of her homework and failed several tests. This was a drastic change for Susan, who typically was a superior, highly motivated student. In discussions with the teacher, Mrs. James learned that the class had read and discussed a very sad story involving the sudden tragic death of a fifth-grader. There had been some references made by one of the students in Susan's class to Carl's death approximately 1 year previously.

I suggested that Mrs. James tell Susan that she was concerned about her and she had called me to make an appointment.

Content of Session

Analysis and Feelings

THERAPIST: *(to Mother and Susan)* Hi! It's been a while. Why don't you both come in together; then I'll spend

Susan smiles at me and seems comfortable.

some time alone with Susan. *(After in office)* It's good to see you. Tell me what brings you here today.

Wanting mother to clarify in Susan's presence the reason for her concerns.

MOTHER: I told Susan I called you because her teacher is worried about her; she failed science, and that's her best subject. The teacher says she had stopped turning in her homework.

Susan watching her mom without expression.

T: *(To Susan)* Don't I recall that science used to be your favorite subject?

Trying to establish some continuity with the past.

SUSAN: Yes. It's already getting better. I'm improving already, since the teacher called.

T: Was something bothering you? Sometimes when we get preoccupied with a worry or concern we neglect our work.

Trying to universalize, to make it easy for Susan to admit worries.

S: I just got so interested in reading I forgot to do my assignments. *(To mother)* You shouldn't let me get so many books from the library, because I just can't stop reading them.

T: Was there any book in particular that grabbed your attention?

S: I just like to read.

M: *(Pulling out book* [Bridge to Terabithia; Paterson, 1987].) Miss Robbins [Susan's teacher] said that this book is about a girl who died in fifth grade in an accident and that it reminded some of the kids about Carl.

I'm glad mom came in since Susan has blocked this out.

I suggested that Susan and I spend some time alone together, and her mother waited in the other room. I commented to Susan that it has been just about a year since Carl's death and that it is *very* common for people to think about someone who died around the same time of the year. In her case, reading that story must really have stirred up some memories.

Susan denied that her lapse in school performance had anything to do with Carl. She kept repeating that her work was already improving and that she would be more careful "not to read too much" in the future. We played the card game *Deck of Feeling*. Not surprisingly, Susan gave rather stereotyped responses. I invited her to draw, and she drew a figure of a Girl Scout with a package of cookies (Figure 8.8). This drawing, in contrast to the first Girl Scout drawing that Susan made in her first session a year ago, had no cloud around the figure and the figure looks happier.

Two Weeks Later

Susan reported that she had made up most of her schoolwork. When I asked her what she thought went wrong, she stated that she "just wanted a vacation from homework."

I told Susan in her mother's presence that I thought it was just too much of a coincidence that she stopped working when she read a sad story about a child dying at the very time of year Carl had died. I said that this might happen to her again sometime and, if it did, she or her mom should react sooner and call me or find someone else to talk with. I clarified my belief that Susan's reaction came from holding her feelings inside and that talking and playing with a therapist really can help.

No further appointment was given, and there was no further contact until 3 years later when I requested and obtained written permission from Susan and her mother to write about her therapy in the first edition of this book.

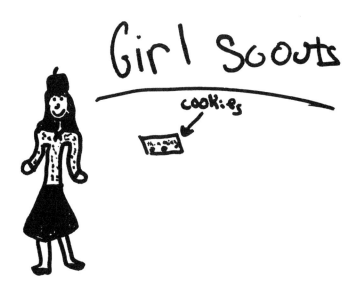

FIGURE 8.8. Susan's drawing of Girl Scout and cookies.

RETROSPECTIVE CRITIQUE AND ANALYSIS

This case is a textbook example of a child who could be classified as a "reluctant griever" (Crenshaw, 1992). This term, coined by Crenshaw to refer to children who have experienced multiple losses and trauma, seemed also applicable to a child like Susan who experienced the sudden traumatic death of her friend and who subsequently seemed totally unable to talk about her loss.

In thinking about my work with Susan in retrospect, I wonder if I might have somehow managed to involve her more in an active grieving process. If I could return again to my early sessions with Susan, I would now invite her to draw a picture of her and Carl doing something together. I would have worked harder to involve Susan in telling me about Carl, what he was like as a person, what they enjoyed doing together, what she liked about him and also what she might not have liked. Since Susan had consistently preferred drawing to talking, she might have been willing to draw some pictures of the two of them together. She also might have responded to a request to draw her view of the scene of Carl's death, as she imagined it to be. Had I followed William Steele's (1998) method of helping a child draw the dead person who died traumatically, Susan might even have been willing to draw a picture of Carl, dead at the scene. The rationale for doing this involves the principle that following traumatic deaths the mourning process becomes derailed because of frightening memories or mental images related to the trauma (Nader, 1997). Nader adds: "Normal grief resolution may be impeded without first attending to the traumatic nature of the death" (1997, p. 17).

As I review my work from a current vantage point, I wonder why I did not engage Susan more in telling or showing me details about her relationship with Carl. Initially, I was careful not to "push" Susan, since she had been so reluctant to come for treatment. In addition to this reality-based caution, I was aware of some personal discomfort based on the circumstances of Carl's death and about the nature of his head injury. This had been described to me in graphic terms by school personnel who felt horrified by the injury. Even in this chapter I have avoided giving details. As I think about this now, it suggests the concept of "vicarious traumatization," a term referring to therapists' reactions to client's traumatic material (McCann & Pearlman, 1990). My *conscious* intent was to proceed at Susan's level of comfort and not to rush her prematurely into painful memories that might drive her away from therapy. However, unconsciously, it is also possible that I was protecting myself from dealing with what I thought would be gruesome details.

In a future situation that generates frightening mental images, I will be more alert to find ways to debrief my own reactions so I will be freer to tune in and explore a child's fears. Although I am not certain that a different approach would have been more successful with Susan, I am certain that an anxious therapist cannot help a child to face something about which she also is fearful. This form of well-meaning and collective collusion avoids confronting the trauma and therefore results in prolonging the inevitable mourning process.

FOLLOW-UP: SUSAN, AGE 20

Seven years after the publication of the first edition of this book I contacted Susan by letter, asking if she would be willing to meet with me one time to discuss her past therapy and to give me permission to include a revision of the chapter about it in a second edition of this book. I included a standard release form in the letter. Within a week I received a telephone response in the affirmative and set an appointment with her. At the prearranged time Susan came with her mother. Susan had recently completed her third year of college and was home, working at a summer job. Previously, she had spent a year abroad, living with a foreign family, learning the language and attending school.

She was an attractive, intelligent young woman who readily volunteered that she had looked up the first edition of this book in the college library and read the chapter about her with great interest. She found only one thing she wished to clarify, and that was my question about whether she and Carl had still been friends at the time she didn't invite him to her birthday party. She said that they were, in fact, good friends, even though they participated in separate activities, like the Boy Scouts and Girl Scouts. She said that they often would sit together and talk at lunch in the school cafeteria.

Currently Susan was dating Carl's best friend, who was a student at a different university in a city close to where Susan had grown up but far from where she is studying. They had been friends for years, and recently their relationship had become deeper. They visited the mausoleum together for the first time at Susan's suggestion 4 years ago. She added that she had gone "many times" with her mother since Carl's death.

Susan's mother clarified the details of how Carl died (and I heard this for the first time during this session). He was sitting in the front passenger seat of the car, and when it went off the road, down an embankment, a roadside barrier came through the front window and into his stomach; Carl bled to death on the spot. Carl's sister, in the backseat, suffered a head injury but recovered. Susan said, "All the rumors at school were that Carl had been decapitated." She stated that she had not asked her mother if this story about Carl's death was true. Susan's mother said that she now regrets not telling her the truth, but she did not do so because she thought it would be too upsetting.

I asked about any ongoing dreams, and Susan said that she used to dream about her mother dying and even herself dying (although she knew even in her dream that she was alive). She says that she used to think about Carl a lot, and now she does less, although she and her boyfriend reminisce about him quite a bit. They wonder what he would be like if he had lived.

Carl's parents had two other children following his death. Susan said that she was able to baby-sit for the younger child, even though it was "weird" to see Carl's sister (who survived the accident) occupying Carl's former room.

I asked if Susan had experienced other deaths in her family or among her friends. Both of her paternal grandparents died several years ago, and she remembers crying a lot at her grandmother's wake, when she would have been 16 years old. This also was about the same time that she began baby-sitting for Carl's younger sister and also the time when she invited her boyfriend to accompany her to the mausoleum. Possibly her grief about her grandmother's death opened the door to help her deal more directly with her grief about Carl.

Susan's mother pointed out that she used to worry that Susan was avoiding forming close friendships after Carl's death, since she always seemed to prefer to be with a group. Susan admitted that she has had more male than female friends over the years, but she believes that this has changed during the past year. She has a close female friend who will be her roommate in the fall when she returns for her senior year in college.

I pointed out that Susan was no longer avoiding her sad memories, and that I thought the fact that she could talk about Carl with her friend and that the two of them could visit the mausoleum indicated that she was able to mourn this tragic loss. I congratulated Susan for her academic success and wished her well.

Susan's ability to express her grief and to talk about Carl and his death can be attributed to a number of factors:

First, the timely play therapy sessions soon after the death helped her to express her feelings in a displaced way and to hear my validation of these feelings through the symbolism of play, even though she could not discuss them directly.

Second, her school, church, and family were open and appropriate in their expressions of grief. The school held a memorial service and dedicated the yearbook to Carl. Susan's mother openly mourned Carl's death and repeatedly invited Susan to accompany her to the mausoleum. The religious beliefs of the family emphasized life after death, thereby giving hope for some future contact with Carl.

Finally Susan's natural resiliency contributed to the positive outcome in this case. She was an intelligent girl, eager to achieve in school, and involved in age-appropriate activities. Her love of reading provided a useful outlet that helped her at times to shut out painful memories.

Susan may, in fact, have been too immature to endure the painful feelings of grief and of trauma at age 9, when Carl died. She may have needed time to absorb the reality of what happened and its meaning to her. Over the years, during visits to the mausoleum, and finally, when she was 16, at her grandmother's wake she gradually began to allow herself to feel the pain of grief.

As therapists we can never be sure how much or how soon to work toward uncovering painful feelings. When dealing with children there are no firm guidelines. Susan has taught me to be patient and to trust the process. A process that began in my office when she was age 9 unfolded gradually until she could permit its full expression when she was 16. I am grateful to her that she wanted to come back and let me know about it. I am optimistic about this young woman's future ability to deal with the stress of losses, despite her vulnerability in this area.

DISCUSSION QUESTIONS

1. Do you concur with the diagnosis of PTSD? If not, how would you assess Susan's presentation of symptoms at the time of referral?

2. Do you believe that Susan's symptoms would have subsided without therapy? Give reasons for your response.

3. How do you feel about the termination in Session 7? Do you think there would have been value to continuing to see Susan? If so, how might this have been structured?

4. What do you predict with regard to Susan's future adjustment? If you anticipate future difficulties, specify at what age and under what circumstances Susan might be especially vulnerable.

5. Do you believe that the therapist avoided Susan's feelings of traumatic grief? Specify where this occurred, and suggest alternative interventions.

REFERENCES

American Psychiatric Association. (2000). *Diagnostic and statistical manual of mental disorders* (4th ed., text rev.). Washington, DC: Author.

Bowlby, J. (1963). Pathological mourning and childhood mourning. *Journal of the American Psychoanalytic Association, 11,* 500–541.

Crenshaw, D. (1992). Reluctant grievers: Children of multiple loss and trauma. *The Forum, 17*(4), 6–7.

Deutsch, H. (1937). Absence of grief. *Psychoanalytic Quarterly, 6*(12), 12–22.

Fox, S. (1985). *Good grief: Helping groups of children when a friend dies.* Boston: New England Association for the Education of Young Children.

Gabriel, M. (1992). Anniversary reactions: Trauma revisited. *Clinical Social Work Journal, 20*(2), 179–192.

Lindemann, E. (1944). Symptomatology and management of acute grief. *American Journal of Psychiatry, 101,* 141–148. [Reprinted in Parad, H. J. (Ed.). (1965). *Crisis intervention: Selected readings* (pp. 7–21). New York: Family Service America.]

McCann, I. L., & Pearlman, L. A. (1990). Vicarious traumatization: A framework for understanding the psychological effects of working with victims. *Journal of Traumatic Stress, 3*(1), 131–149.

Nader, K. O. (1997). Childhood traumatic loss: The interaction of trauma and grief. In C. R. Figley, B. E. Bride, & N. Mazza (Eds.), *Death and trauma: The traumatology of grieving.* Washington, DC: Taylor & Francis.

Paterson, K. (1987). *Bridge to Terabithia.* New York: Harper Trophy.

Rando, T. (1993).*Treatment of complicated mourning.* Champaign, IL: Research Press.

Steele, W. (1998). *Children of trauma: Tools to help the helper* [video]. Grosse Pointe Woods, MI: The Institute for Trauma and Loss in Children.

Terr, L. C. (1987). Nightmares in children. In C. Guilleminault (Ed.), *Sleep and its disorders in children* (pp. 231–242). New York: Raven Press.

Worden, J. W. (1991). *Grief counseling and grief therapy: A handbook for the mental health practitioner* (2nd ed.). New York: Springer.

9

🆂

Sudden Death in Schools

ROBERT G. STEVENSON

A death in a school community causes changes for the members of that community individually and collectively on many levels. In addition to the loss of an individual, other losses impact the school community as a whole. Such losses may include the loss of organization (due to accompanying changes in staff, school schedules, and planned activities), the loss of security (with the realization that we cannot take any day or any life for granted), or the loss of academic and emotional support that may have been provided by the deceased (or by other staff who are now distracted while dealing with their personal feelings of loss).

There is a growing body of professional literature about the impact of a death in the school community (Doster & McElroy, 1993; Elder, 1994; Hickey, 1993; Klicker, 2000; Stevenson & Powers, 1987). One of the points yet to be studied in detail is the different impact based on the role of the deceased in the school. This chapter deals with the sudden death of teachers, counselors, or administrators. The death of a teacher, counselor, or administrator typically causes many upheavals in a school because it constitutes the first in a string of losses with which all members of the school community must find a way to cope. The relationship of the person who died to students and colleagues, the circumstances of the death, and the response of the school community to the death are significant factors in shaping the level of coping in the cases presented in this chapter.

Perceptions of loss differ from person to person, based on an individual's past experience, personal coping style, and relationship to the deceased. Case studies often point to a common pattern of response following a death. Elisabeth Kübler-Ross (1969) developed her model of death and dying based on a pattern of response she and her medical students identified among terminally ill patients. Her model of "denial, anger, bargaining, depression and acceptance" incorporated the earlier work of C. M. Parkes (1959, 1962) and has provided a foundation for numerous procedures and protocols in health care, counseling, and education. Kübler-Ross's model may prove useful in training staff to provide bereavement counseling. It is appropriate to have a staff already trained, since deaths will inevitably occur in every school community.

Sandra S. Fox (1988) of Boston, Massachusetts, developed another grief model that focused specifically on children. Fox defined four basic tasks facing bereaved children. She found that a bereaved child needs to do the following:

1. *Understand*. The child must understand that *death is universal*. All things that live will one day die. It is no one's "fault" that things are this way. This is simply part of life. The child must understand that the deceased person no longer feels anything because a dead body no longer functions as it once did. Finally, the child, apart from the religious beliefs of his/her family, must understand that the physical aspects of death are irreversible: *death is permanent*.
2. *Grieve*. There are many feelings connected with bereavement, especially sadness, anger, and guilt. The child must be able to *both experience and express the feelings that are part of the grief process*.
3. *Commemorate*. The child needs to remember the life of the person who died, both good things and bad, as part of *mourning the real person* who is gone. Where possible, the child should also play some role in helping to decide how the deceased will be remembered.
4. *Move on*. After understanding the loss that has happened and the changes it has caused, grieving the loss, and finding a way to commemorate the life that is now ended and the changes that have occurred, the child needs to move on by *investing emotion in other relationships*. The death or injury to a friend or family member may, at first, present a crisis to a single child. However, when this child returns to interact with teachers and classmates, this crisis extends to other members of the school community. Just as an individual child needs to accomplish these tasks, so too does the school community as a whole.

PROTOCOLS FOR INFORMING STUDENTS ABOUT A DEATH

Procedures published by the National Association of Secondary School Principals for informing students of a death in the school community

(Stevenson & Powers, 1987) employ a protocol that was developed by examining the reactions of students upon learning of the death of a significant individual. These case studies also examined the reactions of administrators, teachers, counselors, and parents to the way in which the information was shared with students.

Informing an Individual Student

The resulting protocol began as a series of questions and suggested responses for educators who must inform a student about a death in their own school. These questions and suggested responses include the following:

Who Should Inform the Student?

Someone who is considered an authority figure should tell the student. An administrator typically assumes this role. Someone who has a close relationship with the student (teacher, nurse, counselor, or fellow student) should be with the student and should be able to remain after the student receives the news.

Where Should the Student Be Told?

The student should be taken to a place where he/she can have *privacy*. The student should be able to sit or to lie down if necessary. The school nurse's office, a counselor's office, or an administrator's office may meet these requirements if that office can be shut off from outside interruptions.

How Should the Student Be Told?

The student should be told what has happened in a quiet, simple, and direct manner. Avoid platitudes or religious symbolism. The child's questions should be answered openly and honestly, but unnecessary details need not be volunteered. Emotions and feelings should not be avoided. Allow the student to begin to sort out confusing feelings and help him/her to see the school in a supportive role. The wishes of the family of the deceased, if they are known, should be respected as much as possible.

How Will a Student React?

After a student has received the news, he/she may have a number of possible reactions. Educators must remember that there is no one "correct" response. Physical contact, such as touching a shoulder or holding a hand, may have a calming effect, but some students are uncomfortable with this. A student may merely wish to sit. This wish should be respected. However, the student should not be left alone. If the student remains silent, inform him/her that it is all right to speak about feelings or to remain silent. The choice is his/hers.

The staff reaction to a student must not appear judgmental. It would be unwise, for example, to minimize any loss, such as the death of a pet. In the overall functioning of the school, the death of a pet may not seem to be a crisis. However, the young person may consider the pet as a lifelong friend who provided companionship and love. A student's particular reaction to *this* news may be difficult to understand until we consider that it does not occur in a vacuum and that other, prior events may contribute to the reaction we now see.

Who Else Should Be Informed?

The family should be aware of what the student was told and the child's teachers, the school nurse, and school counselors should be informed of the situation as soon as possible (Stevenson, 1986).

Informing an Entire School Community

A protocol to address the needs of an individual student is not directly transferable if an entire school community is affected, since the sheer numbers of students make it virtually impossible to cope with the situation on an *individual* basis. Such a crisis requires the cooperation of all school personnel. Coordinating such an effort entails further advance planning. The questions related to how to inform the school community at large are similar to those in the guidelines just presented for work with individual students. However, there are different suggested responses. These responses are related to the complexity of dealing with large numbers of people in a group format. The questions and suggested responses follow:

Where Should the Students Be Told?

It is "efficient" to bring all students together in an auditorium to inform them of a crisis. However, such large group disclosures lack privacy, block the release of emotions, and hinder the identification of students who may need special attention. For these reasons, the larger the size of group presentations, the less beneficial they are for individual students. Whenever possible, students should receive the news of a crisis situation in familiar surroundings with people they know and trust. The classroom offers such a setting.

How Should the Students Be Told?

Preselected trained staff members should be sent to inform all students of the event that has occurred. These people must be chosen and trained in advance, since some educators will not be comfortable in performing such a task. A team of educators, called a "crisis response team" in some districts, should receive training concerning student needs in times of grief and/or stress. The information given to all students should be the same. Information should be given in a calm, direct manner, and the team members should stay to assist the classroom teacher in answering questions and addressing feelings and reactions.

A school nurse is sometimes assigned the role of informing students. However, this removes the nurse from her medical responsibility. Experience has shown that some students experience physical distress and somatic complaints when they become upset following disturbing news. They need the nurse to be available to perform her primary task as a medical professional. Therefore, it is not advisable to assign the nurse a task that would make her unavailable to a large segment of the student body. Designated counselors, social workers, teachers, and/or administrators who can be temporarily freed of other responsibilities should be assigned this responsibility rather than the school nurse.

How Will the Students React?

While it is difficult to predict the reaction of an *individual* student, previous case studies have shown that the reaction of *groups* of students is somewhat predictable. Some students will feel sad or angry and will express these feelings. Other students may feel guilty and seek to withdraw from interaction with peers or teachers. A third group of students may not appear to feel anything at all. Some students in this third group may actually not be affected by the news or feel any personal involvement at that time. However, other students may *appear* uninvolved but are actually seeking to cover up thoughts or feelings with which they are uncomfortable. Still others do not "feel" any reaction and are scared *because* they do not.

It is essential that students be helped to understand that virtually all of these reactions are "normal" because there is no *one* response that is appropriate for everybody. What may cause concerns in the student him/herself and among staff who are unfamiliar with the broad range of grief responses is the intensity of individual reactions. A school protocol must provide for those students who need individual assistance. Again, there are people already in the schools who have been trained to perform this task. These are the school counselors and social workers. However, some school counselors are forced to be so involved with college counseling and mandated testing programs that their skills as counselors may not have kept pace with current practice. To maintain and enhance staff skills in this area, training and workshops should be provided for counselors, social workers, school nurses, and interested teachers on a regular basis.

Who Else Should Be Informed?

All staff members must be kept informed of the details of important related events. Parents must be kept informed of the actions taken in school and of actions that affect their children. Other community leaders (religious leaders, health professionals, uniformed services, and political leaders) should also be part of the information network. All communication must be two-way. School officials and teachers must solicit and be responsive to input from parents and the community as a whole. In times of crisis, no section of the community should be denied a chance to assist affected young people.

What Issues Can Complicate Student Reaction and/or School Response?

Certain events have been found to produce complicated student reactions to loss. For example, suicide can produce a grief reaction that is different from that which follows a death caused by an illness or an accident. Those who are alive after someone whom they loved, knew, or identified with has died as the result of a completed suicide are called *survivors of suicide*. The grief of these survivors is different for one or more of the following reasons (Doka, 1989; Stevenson, 1990):

- The death is sudden and seldom anticipated.
- It is often violent.
- It takes place in the presence of other stresses.
- It accentuates feelings of "regret" and/or "guilt."
- It may cause survivors to experience a feeling of loss of control over the events in their lives.
- It may evoke a reaction from society that is often negative or judgmental.
- It may cause survivors to feel they are being "avoided" by others.

Counselors should be prepared to reach out to classmates and friends to offer special counseling following a suicide (Webb, 1986).

A death from AIDS can also complicate the grief reaction and create a situation in which young people may have special needs. AIDS-related grief can produce the following complications:

- *Isolation.* Friends or family members of the deceased may be avoided through fear or misunderstanding,
- *Lack of social support.* Memorials or other rituals that typically follow a death are not always available after an AIDS related death (Doka, 1989).
- *Feelings of guilt.* Social sanctions may cause special feelings of guilt for friends of the deceased or for those who believe the deceased may have engaged in "high-risk" behavior.
- *Anger/violence.* Strong emotions may be released within the school community and, if no outlet is provided, these feelings may produce incidents of violence (Stevenson, 1991).

DIFFERENT RESPONSES
TO SUDDEN DEATHS

There is an extensive literature available to assist educators to help grieving students (Adams & Deveau, 1995; Fassler, 1978; Fox, 1988; Grollman, 1995; Klicker, 2000; Matsakis, 1998; Mills, Reisler, Robinson, & Vermilye, 1976; Ross, 1986; Schafer & Lyons, 1976; Stevenson & Stevenson, 1996; Webb, 1993; Wolfelt, 1990). Some offer specific curricula, such as Deats and Lenker (1989), who developed a curriculum for addressing youth suicide through literature. There are also sources that address responses to the death of a teacher (Doster & McElroy, 1993) and the death of a counselor (Hickey, 1993).

However, the reactions of schools to the death of a teacher or administrator vary widely. For example, administrators in two upper-middle-class suburbs in New York State each directed their school to react in a very different fashion when a staff member died. In one district, staff members were ordered not to speak of the death and no memorial of any type was allowed. In the other, the death was addressed in classroom meetings with students. The flag was lowered to half-staff for 1 week. There was also an in-school memorial service planned by staff and students together that everyone in the school community had the opportunity to attend.

Each principal believed that he was acting in the best interests of all members of his school community. Each has said that if the same situation were to occur again, there is little he would do differently. Both men recognized that the sudden death of a teacher would have an immediate impact on students and staff. Both wished to prevent further pain and disruption in the school community. However, their decisions as to what actions were appropriate are so different and so apparently contradictory that to be understood they need to be examined in detail. To do this we must understand the demographics of each school community and answer several questions:

- How has this school community responded to past deaths, losses, and the grief that followed for its members?
- What were the circumstances and cause of *this* death?
- What did the administrator in charge hope to achieve and to avoid by making the decisions he did?
- Were there "parallel losses" that may have had an impact on these decisions?

This information can help the reader evaluate each case and decide what responses would be most appropriate when a teacher dies.

Case 1: The Brookside School

The Brookside School is a suburban high school district of approximately 6,500 students from upper-middle-class/upper-class families of two adjacent towns in New York State. The predominantly Caucasian student population has significant numbers of Asian American and African American students. Four of every five students attend college immediately after graduation, and more than half of the remaining students pursue some form of continuing education or career training. Ms. Barry was a 52-year-old Caucasian female who had taught English for 30 years and had been in that district for over 20 years. She was known throughout the community and was considered to be a skilled and caring professional. Her attendance record was excellent and the 200+ sick days she had accumulated gave evidence of the fact that she almost never missed a day of school. One October, she was forced to miss some time for medical tests. She did not discuss the nature of the tests or the results with anyone at the school.

When she began to take several sick days a month, her department chairman and principal became concerned. Her chairman scheduled an appointment with her and asked if there was anything that he or the administration could do to assist her. Would she want some extended time off? She explained that she had developed a "condition" with some medical "complications." She continued to explain that her medication sometimes caused a reaction and that was the reason for her absences. She thanked him for his concern but stated that no time off would be needed. The absences continued and by March Ms. Barry's absence had become a problem for both the students and the administration.

On the Sunday morning of spring break, the school's principal, Mr. Pomeroy, received a phone call telling him that Ms. Barry had been killed in a one-car traffic accident. The school had a protocol in place for dealing with the death of a student, but in this case none of the outlined steps was implemented. There was no phone chain activated to inform the staff of the death of their colleague. There was no faculty meeting before the start of school on Monday. The only official acknowledgment of the loss was a memo placed in every teacher's mailbox informing them of the death and stating that they were not to discuss the death of Ms. Barry with the students. There was no memorial service, no lowering of the flag, nor any official notice taken of the change that had just occurred in this school community. The immediate school response was brief and detached, with no place permitted for student or staff emotion. A permanent substitute teacher was in the classroom by Tuesday, and from that point on it was to be "business as usual." In April, the principal refused to allow any dedication or memorial to Ms. Barry in the school yearbook. The staff wished to donate some books to the school library in memory of their colleague, but the principal vetoed this also. The staff donation went instead to the local library in the town where Ms. Barry lived. The principal told Ms. Barry's students who wished to do something to mark their teacher's passing that it "was not necessary."

It was clear that the principal was the key individual in directing and controlling the school community's response (or lack of response) to the death of Ms. Barry. The principal was asked about his apparent lack of compassion for the losses experienced by the students and staff. He justified his decision by saying that he was aware of the emotional distress in the school community. However, the circumstances of the death made it seem that Ms. Barry may have committed suicide. He said that he wished to avoid glorifying this death to avoid the possibility of other suicide attempts by a distressed staff member or an impressionable student. Past events showed that Principal Pomeroy also had a history of avoidance in dealing with death-related issues in school. He had been an administrative assistant when there were four separate student suicides in neighboring districts in the space of 4 months. Nothing was done in his district to assist students or staff who were troubled by these events. The following year, tutors, other staff members, and friends were visiting two of his students who were battling life-threatening illness at home. Mr. Pomeroy asked several staff members to tell each of the students that he would stop by. However, he was unable to keep his word. After several months, both students died without having been visited by Mr. Pomeroy.

The principal had always considered himself a student advocate.

Students knew that he would even go so far as to believe them before asking a teacher if there was another side to the student's story. Rather than make him popular with students, this apparent lack of objectivity caused students and teachers alike to see him as lacking in leadership qualities. In this situation, Mr. Pomeroy used a coping style that is common among administrators who do not exhibit strong leadership. It is characterized by denial and avoidance. Its logic runs something like this: "If my students have problems that affect their educational performance, I must try to help them. I am not sure what the 'right thing' is to do. Therefore, I will do nothing to avoid doing the 'wrong thing.'" This style is acceptable only if there is no problem to be addressed. In this situation, Mr. Pomeroy directed his energy and resources to attempting to show that (1) there was no problem with which students needed assistance and (2) inaction was a safer response than action that might be harmful. The Board of Education supported Mr. Pomeroy's decision.

A result of this inaction was a sharp split between Mr. Pomeroy and the majority of his staff. The staff felt that a teacher could be present one day, be gone the next day, and no notice would be taken of the absence. The change would not be acknowledged. The implications of this reasoning were serious. If an individual's absence did not deserve recognition, then his/her presence also had little meaning or value. Teacher absences began to increase, and many of the faculty members were reluctant to take on the additional responsibility of clubs, sports, or after-school activities.

The mood of the students became sad and apathetic. The Brookside guidance department has graduating seniors fill out a questionnaire and sends a similar questionnaire to its alumni, 5 years after their graduation. They are asked about a number of items that may have had an impact on their years at Brookside. In this questionnaire, the majority of seniors (52%) stated, "No one here cares about me." In the alumni questionnaire, the staff had received high marks from the students for their caring approach that seemed to make every student matter. Only 11% of the alumni had checked the statement "No one here cares about me," and 73% had checked the statement "In this school every person matters."[1] The change in student attitude was also marked by an increase in violent incidents, both student–student and student–teacher. The number of students transferring to private and parochial schools doubled the previous average in each of the following 2 years. In past years the average number of transfers had been 12 per year. In the 2 years after Ms. Barry's death there were 25 and 27 transfers to local private/parochial schools. These numbers would appear to indicate a negative attitude among many of the school's students. This negativity does not appear to have spread

---

[1]The guidance department at each school supplied all statistics.

outside of the school community, since the number of students transferring into the school from all other schools remained constant. There were 14 transfers per year in the year of Ms. Barry's death and in each of the subsequent 3 years.[2]

The administration did not believe that there were any grief-related issues that needed to be addressed, but the staff disagreed. The teachers' union brought an outside consultant to the school for an in-service training day. It was suggested that the existing protocol for informing students of the death of a fellow student be expanded to include other deaths such as those of a teacher or administrator. A second recommendation acknowledged the difficulty that some individuals have when forced to cope with death-related situations. To avoid the complications caused when the primary decision maker is the one so affected, it was suggested that a "crisis committee" be established to implement and evaluate the recommended protocols. Despite a positive reaction from the teachers and from several parent representatives who attended the in-service day, none of the recommendations were implemented until 3 years after Ms. Barry's death. In the summer of that year, Mr. Pomeroy announced that he was retiring to take a college instructor's position in a neighboring state. His successor, from outside the district, implemented all recommendations as soon as he assumed the principal's job.

Discussion

This case illustrates the impact that one death and one administrator's response to it can have on an entire school community. The unanswered questions regarding the circumstances of Ms. Barry's illness and death complicated the situation by increasing the principal's anxiety. The inability of the chief decision maker, in this case the principal, Mr. Pomeroy, to effectively deal with grief-related issues further complicated the situation. Finally, teachers and students were concerned that if such a situation arose again, it would be handled in a similar manner. Improved communication was fostered among all groups within the school community (administrators, teachers, students, and parents). This dialogue led to the implementation of new expanded protocols and the creation of a "crisis response committee" with specific responsibilities, a clear chain of command, and the authority to modify the response as needed in an individual case.

Research on the impact of grief on the educational performance and behavior of students identifies the following factors:

---

[2]No statistics were available showing whether transfers into the school were from local private/parochial schools or other public schools.

- Increased feelings of anxiety and stress
- Impaired memory and/or ability to concentrate
- Expressions of fear of the future and the possibility of other losses (Stevenson, 1994)
- Physical and emotional fatigue
- Increased visits to the school nurse with somatic complaints (which may be psychosomatic in origin)
- Poor academic performance
- Acting-out or punishment-seeking behavior prompted by feelings of anger or guilt related to the deceased
- Increased absenteeism
- Emotional numbing

A response that is seen as uncaring or ineffective, as in this case, may cause long-term negative consequences within the school community. This has even caused some students and teachers to have such a negative reaction that they chose to leave the school by transferring to other schools in the area. A response that is judged to be "caring," even if it may not be the "best" response possible or meet some external standard of the "ideal" response, can have a positive effect throughout the school community.

One factor in creating such a response is the comfort level of the staff in discussing topics related to loss and grief. In-service training can be provided for all staff members and representatives of the local parent organization to familiarize the participants with the grief process. These programs identify possible behaviors and help participants to differentiate between what responses are "normal" and what responses may indicate a pattern of complicated or destructive grief. Children do not experience grief in the same way as do adults. Professionals need to know how children experience grief and what reactions this may cause for the child and the school community (Webb, 1993; see also Chapter 2 in this volume).

The death of a family member may have a great impact on an individual or a class but at the same time may have a lesser impact or no effect on other members of the school community. In contrast, the impact of the death of a student creates a situation of "community grief" in which the entire school community can be affected.

Case 2: Jefferson High School

Jefferson High School is a suburban high school in a community that is in some ways similar to the Brookside School. This district also serves two towns. The 1,100 students were predominantly Caucasian, with a few African American students (less than 15) and Asian American students (about 36). There were also students who were recent immigrants from eastern Europe (11) and from East Asia (61). The Asian students represented a subgroup within the student body who often kept to themselves. An ESL (English as a second language) teacher encouraged this separation. This instructor promoted activities that kept the Asian students within their own group during the school day and at an after-school club. She did little to encourage them to take a greater part in the variety of activities offered to all students.

However, one teacher reached out to these students. Mr. Connor, an Irish American in his mid-40s, taught English classes to special students, including Asian ESL students. He always was willing to go the extra step (or two, or three) in helping the Asian students improve their language skills. He realized that some of the students had a much better grasp of English than they were willing to admit. This had allowed them to take less challenging classes and to get good grades with little effort. They indirectly used the ESL teacher, the head of guidance, and a sympathetic administrator to exert "pressure" on any teacher who tried to hold these students accountable with a "real" grade. Mr. Connor insisted that these students show a serious effort in developing their English language skills. He refused to give "charity" grades. He also learned key words and phrases in Korean, Japanese, and Chinese so that he could better instruct these students. All of Mr. Connor's students thought he was one of those special teachers they would remember, both for what he did for them and for what he taught them to do for themselves. The Asian students had a special bond with him that was different from any of their relationships with the other teachers. For 3 years, Mr. Connor worked with the Asian students and his work was beginning to pay real dividends. Not only were these students moving ahead rapidly with the mastery of the English language, but they were beginning to take a more active role in other areas of school life.

When Mr. Connor did not show up on the first day of the new school year, a few people were concerned. However, this was a day for staff only and the students would not be there until the next day. Perhaps, it was thought, something had developed that required his attention. The principal left a phone message on Mr. Connor's answering machine asking that he call as soon as he returned home. Everyone expected that he would be present the following day. When he did not show up that day, Mr. Connor's sister went to his apartment. There was no answer to her knocking. When she used her key to enter, she found Mr. Connor dead on the living room floor. Scattered around him on the floor were papers that he had prepared for the start of class. It was later determined that he had died of a massive coronary and that he had been dead for approximately 72 hours.

The administration, upon learning of the death, immediately notified all staff members, who then notified the students in their individual classes. The school protocol for notifying students of a death had been in place for several years and was now implemented. A teacher was dispatched to the Connor family home to express everyone's concern and support. He also offered to serve as an intermediary for the family, screened phone calls, and informed the school of the family's wishes regarding a possible memorial service. The school's flag was immediately lowered, and students and staff remembered their teacher and friend. Two teachers were so overcome with emotion that they could not remain in class. Coverage was provided for the classes by other teachers and by administrators with planning or lunch periods. When the family requested that the funeral be kept small, for immediate family and friends, plans began for a memorial service at the school. The service took place 3 days later, on the day after Mr. Connor's funeral. The service was held during the last period of the day, and attendance was optional. Students, teachers, and community members filled the auditorium.

The Asian students who had grown so fond of Mr. Connor showed up for the service as a group and were welcomed by their classmates and teachers. One of them delivered a very moving tribute to their beloved teacher. A gift of suitably inscribed books was made to the school library and to each of the town libraries. The books were all hardcover, since Mr. Connor saw books as valuable tools and a treasure to be shared with others. He had never been comfortable with the temporary nature of paperbacks. After a week, the flag was again at the top of the flagpole and the school moved on. Later that year, there was a special page about Mr. Connor in the school yearbook that brought both tears and smiles from those who paused again to remember him. The entire school community was sad, but there was no apathy or anger. Students spoke of a new "closeness" with their classmates. Observers believed it was brought about by Mr. Connor's example. There was no increase in disruptive behavior and no transfers to other local schools. Feelings had been openly acknowledged and validated. Mr. Connor's students missed their teacher. The new instructor was one who had been a substitute in the district and was already known by the students. She continued to speak of their former teacher, and the highest praise she would offer after some special achievement was that "Mr. Connor would be very proud of you."

Discussion

Why was Case 2 so very different from Case 1? There are several factors. As in the first case, there had been previous deaths in this school community.

Several years earlier, a long-time coach had died of a heart attack while teaching class. Another popular teacher was killed in a freak hunting accident. In both cases the school responded with openness and support for all students and staff members. The Federal Emergency Management Agency (FEMA) has developed a crisis response model utilizing four phases: preparation, response, recovery, and mitigation.[3] Mitigation involves studying a crisis and the actions taken during and after the crisis to evaluate effectiveness for the purpose of improving responses in the future. It is never possible to prevent all possible losses, but it may be possible to lessen, to mitigate, the negative impact of those losses. Administration and guidance personnel practiced "mitigation" at Jefferson High School long before it became an integral part of the FEMA crisis response model. At Jefferson, effective leadership was shown by the school principal, but he did not have to carry the weight of decision making alone. The members of the crisis response team, consisting of administrators, guidance counselors, the school nurse, and several volunteer teachers, made several key decisions. They had previous experience working together. Information was shared with all staff as it was available and, when appropriate, with students and their families. As in Case 1, the Jefferson High School Board of Education supported the decisions made by the school administration. This time, however, there was input from the entire school community and it was within the framework of a protocol previously reviewed and adopted by the Board. This principal's goal was the well-being of the members of the school community. His actions, and those of the crisis response committee, acknowledged and validated the grief of many of the students and staff caused by this loss.

Clearly, the personality and actions of the principal are key elements in understanding the reaction of the members of the school community to a teacher's death. What then might occur when it is the principal who dies?

Case 3: The Death of a Principal, Mr. Vitale

The community was in the suburbs of a major east coast city. The town's population was predominantly blue-collar, Italian American, and Roman Catholic. The principal of the local public elementary school was Mr. Vitale. He was well liked and admired by staff members and the community at large. His young students loved him. He was the type of man

---

[3]FEMA's Emergency Management Institute has published a series of independent study courses that outline the latest information on emergency response. Two titles that give special attention to the cycle of crisis response and "mitigation" in particular are *Emergency Preparedness USA* (IS-2, 1998) and *Mitigation for Homeowners* (IS-394, 2000).

who seemed to have answers for any problem that might arise, and he always found time for the problems of individuals. He knew every one of his hundreds of students by name. One evening he and his wife knelt for their evening prayer. As he started to rise, he suddenly fell to the ground and died of a major heart attack. There had been no warning, no period of illness or weakness. He was just gone. Many researchers believe the grief following a sudden death can be more difficult for survivors of the loss than a death that follows some time after the onset of illness or injury caused by an accident (Rando, 1984; Worden, 1991; Webb, 1999). Everyone knew that this would be a difficult time for the entire community. Virtually every student in town remembered having had Mr. Vitale as a principal. They and their families were deeply saddened by this death.

The key people in decision making were the district superintendent, who stepped into the role that normally would have been filled by the principal, and the head of guidance, who acted as his chief adviser. As had been done at Jefferson High School, there was notification of students on their entry into school. Early in the morning, parent phone chains reached as many families as possible. Many of the students learned of the death of Mr. Vitale from their parents. When the students arrived at school, they were told about what had happened by their classroom teachers. For some this was a reinforcement of the reality of the loss. For some students it was the first time they had heard of it. Since the emergency phone chain had not reached every family and some parents were in shock, not all parents had been able to tell their children of Mr. Vitale's death. It then became the responsibility of the school to handle this task. Counselors were available throughout the school building to meet with students. Substitute teachers were available to cover classes if needed. However, no teacher requested to be relieved. The school flag was lowered. The funeral home where the wake took place was filled to overflowing for 2 days. On the day of the funeral, students were excused from school to attend. Once again the crowd filled the church and spilled out onto the street.

Following the funeral a committee was formed to decide on a suitable memorial to this man who had done so much for this community. After much discussion and many suggestions, the decision was one upon which all could agree. Work was begun, and 6 weeks later there was a ceremony that again saw almost the entire town in attendance. The elementary school where Mr. Vitale had worked for so many years was renamed in his honor, and his name will remain over the main entrance of the school so that everyone can see, and many can remember, all that he did.

This may not sound like a controversial step, but it could have been. In a regional high school district adjacent to this one, the Board of Education refused to consider renaming an athletic field after a former school official. The Board actually passed a regulation that prohibited naming any building, room, or field after any current or former staff members. One Board member said they were concerned that this would start a practice that might not be in the school's best interests. The controversy split the members of that community, and it was several years before the decision was overturned.

This case shows that an effective leader and a clear chain of command are necessary when a death affects a school community. The school principal often provides that leadership. However, another district administrator can step in and assume the leadership role if the principal is unable to do so.

Comments

A teacher's death has an outcome that differs from the death of a family member or someone outside of the immediate school community. A teacher's death prevents students from using the school as a safe haven. After the death of a family member, some students use the time in school as a chance to see that some parts of life have not changed. School time can give grieving students a break from the rituals of grief. However, when a person from *the school* dies, no such opportunity exists. In this situation, the "break" comes when students are away from the school. Thus some students may absent themselves more to avoid having to deal with the feelings produced by reminders in school.

Teachers need guidance in determining what to do with a deceased child's empty desk and the child's books or personal space (such as a locker). Some schools have found counselor-led support groups to be most helpful. Sandra L. Elder (1994) has led school-based support groups for more than 20 years. In her experience she has found that school-based support groups can do the following:

- Demonstrate to young people that they need not be alone or feel that they are "outcasts"
- Provide information about and frameworks for making sense of death-related events and the experience of grief
- Help students to identify, validate, and "normalize" strong feelings and other experiences associated with loss and grief
- Provide a safe place and permission to confront and express feelings
- Emphasize the positive legacy that can evolve from a lost relationship with a loved one

- Suggest constructive ways in which to remember or memorialize the life that has now ended
- Demonstrate in nonjudgmental ways that life and living do go on

Similarly, administrators may need to make decisions about the desk, bulletin boards, and classroom decorations left after a teacher's death. They must be willing to draw upon community resources and, if arranged by mutual consent, to utilize the staff made available by partner schools. They must also be willing to support any new person brought in to take over the responsibilities of the deceased teacher.

CONCLUSION

It is important to remember that each of the three cases cited involved a *sudden* death. An anticipated death, following an illness or accident, provides the "luxury" of time to plan a coordinated response that will be available to all concerned parties—staff, students, and parents. From the cases cited, it seems clear that effective administrative leadership can ease the emotional toll that a death will take on the school community. This leadership would include shared decision making in deciding on appropriate response(s), a clear chain of command, and open communication among all concerned parties. Those responsible for sharing information with students should consider their ages, levels of emotional maturity, and the circumstances of the death. Available resources from the community and from other schools should be located and the appropriate contact people identified. Schools that agree to share staff during and immediately after a crisis, including a death, are referred to as "partner schools" (Stevenson, 2002). Finally, protocols to guide the school's response should be in place, with Board of Education approval, before a death occurs. If there is to be a dialogue or disagreement about appropriate action, this can take place when such guidelines are adopted. Having an approved protocol in place can assist all parties in providing quick and effective support to the entire school community.

This chapter has presented examples of some people who made poor choices and some who made good choices following deaths. There are no villains; however, unfortunate results sometimes come from actions taken with the best of intentions. That is one of the chief reasons for advance planning and discussion of proposed procedures following any death in the school community, including that of a teacher, counselor, or administrator. It is essential for all schools and for all educators to be prepared.

DISCUSSION QUESTIONS

1. If you were a school counselor, how would you respond if rumors began to circulate that Ms. Barry had committed suicide. What considerations should guide you in dealing with students who are concerned about her death and want to talk about it, despite the principal's decision to downplay her death?

2. Ideally, what do you believe *should* be done with the empty desk, locker, and books of a teacher who dies?

3. What provisions can be made to assist a substitute teacher who must take over a class and find a way to work with the students after their teacher has died?

4. When a teacher has died, if staff members from another school are made available to assist during a period of recovery, how might they be used most effectively?

5. What memorials, if any, do you believe are most appropriate in a school when a teacher dies? Who should be the one(s) to decide on such details?

REFERENCES

Adams, D. W., & Deveau, E. J. (1995). *Beyond the innocence of childhood.* Amityville, NY: Baywood.

Deats, S. M., & Lenker, L. T. (Eds.). (1989). *Youth suicide prevention: Lessons from literature.* New York: Insight Books.

Doka, K. (Ed.). (1989). *Disenfranchised grief: Recognizing hidden sorrow.* Lexington, MA: Lexington Books.

Doster, G., & McElroy, C. Q. (1993). Sudden death of a teacher: Multilevel intervention in an elementary school. In N. B. Webb (Ed.), *Helping bereaved children: A handbook for practitioners* (pp. 212–238). New York: Guilford Press.

Elder, S. L. (1994). Support groups in the schools. In R. G. Stevenson (Ed.), *What will we do?: Preparing a school community to cope with crises* (pp. 147–168). Amityville, NY: Baywood.

Emergency Management Institute. (1998). *Emergency preparedness USA.* Jessup, MD: FEMA Publications.

Emergency Management Institute. (2000). *Mitigation for homeowners.* Jessup, MD: FEMA Publications.

Fassler, J. (1978). *Helping children cope: Mastering stress through books and stories.* New York: Free Press.

Fox, S. S. (1988). *Good grief: Helping groups of children when a friend dies.* Boston: New England Association for the Education of Young Children.

Grollman, E. A. (Ed.). (1995). *Bereaved children and teens: A support guide for parents and professionals.* Boston: Beacon Press.

Hickey, L. O. (1993). Death of a counselor: A bereavement group for junior high school students. In N. B. Webb (Ed.), *Helping bereaved children: A handbook for practitioners* (pp. 239–266). New York: Guilford Press.

Klicker, R. L. (2000). *A student dies, a school mourns: Dealing with death and loss in the school community*. Philadelphia: Accelerated Development.

Kübler-Ross, E. (1969). *On death and dying*. New York: Macmillan.

Matsakis, A. (1998). *Trust after trauma*. Oakland, CA: New Harbinger.

Mills, G. C., Reisler, R., Robinson, A. E., & Vermilye, G. (1976). *Discussing death: A guide to death education*. Palm Springs, CA: ETC Publications.

Parkes, C. M. (1959). *Morbid grief reactions*. London: University of London Press.

Parkes, C. M. (1962). *Reactions to bereavement*. London: University of London Press.

Rando, T. A. (1984). *Grief, dying and death: Clinical interventions for caregivers*. Champaign, IL: Research Press.

Ross, E. B. (1986). *After suicide: A ray of hope*. Iowa City, IA: Lynn.

Schaefer, D., & Lyons, C. (1986). *How do we tell the children?* New York: Newmarket Press.

Stevenson, R. G. (1986). The Shuttle tragedy: "Community grief" and the schools. *Death Studies, 10*(6), 507–518.

Stevenson, R. G. (1990). Teen suicide: Sources, signals and prevention. In J. M. Morgan (Ed.), *The dying and bereaved teenager* (pp. 135–139). Philadelphia: Charles Press.

Stevenson, R. G. (1991). AIDS related grief: Helping young people to understand the impact of societal values on the grief process. *Illness, Crises and Loss, 1*(2), 56–59.

Stevenson, R. G. (1994). Dragons as amulets, dragons as talismans, dragons as counselors. *Death Studies, 18*(3), 219–228.

Stevenson, R. G. (Ed.). (2002). *What will we do?: Preparing a school community to cope with crises* (2nd ed.). Amityville, NY: Baywood.

Stevenson, R. G., & Powers, H. (1987). How to handle death in the school: Ways to help grieving students, *Education Digest, 7*(9), 42–43.

Stevenson, R. G., & Stevenson, E. (1996). *Death education in schools: A comprehensive resource for educators and parents*. Philadelphia: Charles Press.

Webb, N. B. (1986). Before and after suicide: A preventive outreach program for colleges. *Suicide and Life-Threatening Behavior, 16*(4), 469–480.

Webb, N. B. (Ed.). (1993). *Helping bereaved children: A handbook for practitioners*. New York: Guilford Press.

Webb, N. B. (Ed.). (1999). *Play therapy with children in crises* (2nd ed.): *Individual, group, and family treatment*. New York: Guilford Press.

Wolfelt, A. (1990). *Helping children cope with grief*. Muncie, IN: Accelerated Development.

Worden, J. W. (1991). *Grief counseling and grief therapy: A handbook for the mental health practitioner* (2nd ed.). New York: Springer.

10

❧

Treating Children after Violence in Schools and Communities

KATHLEEN NADER

The witnessing of violent death can have powerful and diverse effects on a child. Issues of human accountability, trust, and betrayal may complicate the child's course of response and recovery, and the witnessing of violence may intensify or add to the trauma's challenge to the child's moral development and sense of ongoing safety (Garbarino, 1999; Garbarino, Kostelny, & Dubrow, 1991; Nader, 2001; Nader & Mello, 2000; Parson, 1997; Terr, 1991). After repeated traumas, prolonged captivity, or when there are multiple bloody deaths, symptoms may become more pronounced or altered (Herman, 1992; James, 1994; Nader, 1997; Nader & Mello, in press; Ochberg & Soskis, 1982; Terr, 1991). For example, trauma victims may become attached to those with whom they have endured the experience (Nader, 1997; Nader & Pynoos, 1993). After prolonged captivity or siege, traumatized children may develop a mixed attachment or a complex hatred toward the perpetrator or others. Even a few minutes can be a very long time under siege when there are bloody injuries and intense fears. Grief resolution, rage, and other intense traumatic impressions sometimes must be addressed more than once, and even after some progress has been made in treatment (Frederick, 1985; Nader, 1994, 1997; Nader & Mello, 2000). The therapist must attend to the child's conflicting feelings, attachments, hatreds, and other issues of traumatic experience and response. This chapter emphasizes the importance of processing aspects of trauma in order to free the child to grieve. It demonstrates movement of a child's focus from the traumatic experience to the overlapping issues and, finally, to grief.

THE INTERACTION OF TRAUMA AND GRIEF

After a traumatic death, the child must contend with the symptoms of trauma, of grief, and of the interaction between the two (Eth & Pynoos, 1985; Nader, 1996). Traumatic grief often differs from normal bereavement in the intensity of symptoms, the nature of remembering and reexperiencing, and the complex aspects of recovery and the child's ongoing development (Nader, 1996). Preoccupations with aspects of a traumatic event may prevent or delay grieving.

Children may be so overwhelmed by the intensity of their grief and trauma that they cannot speak or show emotion. For example, when a sniper started shooting children on a playground, Sarah, 8 years old, saw friends fall bleeding, ran in terror to save her own life, and left friends behind to die. When she later was referred for therapy in a school-based intervention program, she did not speak. (See below. The following case reconstructions are based on therapist notes and audiotapes. Certain details have been changed to protect confidentiality, but the dynamics/emotional responses are presented as recorded.)

Content of Session

THERAPIST: *(Sarah has finished drawing.)* Now, can you tell me the story that goes with your picture?

SARAH: *(Silently staring at picture.)*

T: Can you tell me about your picture?

S: *(Silent, long pause; a few times she sighed as if beginning to speak, but remained silent.)*

T: *(After a long pause, pointing to the child in her picture.)* Who's this?

S: *(Sigh and gulp; silence.)*

T: *(After waiting, pointing to item.)* Can you tell me what this is?

S: *(Sigh; gulp; silence.)*

Therapist's Rationale

The child was asked to draw a picture and tell a story about it as per the method described in Nader (1993). Drawing paper, colored pencils and markers were provided. This is my first session with her as training consultant. She remained silent in earlier sessions with her therapist. Child is very constricted and may need assistance getting started.

T: Sarah, would you like to sit on my lap while you tell me about your picture?

Not a common occurrence in this treatment; an intuitive action.

S: *(Nods affirmatively, vigorously; gets right up and climbs on therapist's lap facing the table and the drawing.)*

The child is unable to speak and may need the physical support and comfort of the therapist.

T: Can you tell me about your picture?

S: *(Looks at picture, sighs as if to speak and is silent.)*

T: Are you crying?

S: *(Nods affirmatively, vigorously.)*

Sarah's body is moving as though she is sobbing quietly. Her affect remains flat and there are no tears or sounds, but her body is crying.

The therapist put her arms all the way around Sarah and allowed her to sob silently for the next 15 minutes until Sarah sighed and her body stopped crying. At the end, the therapist talked about how sad and horrible Sarah's experience had been and told her she may need to cry like this again before she could speak about what had happened. The therapist verbalized how tiring it was to cry that hard and told Sarah she could rest or play for the rest of the session. Sarah went to rest in the nurse's office.

Traumatic reexperiencing may interfere with the processes of grieving in a number of ways. Dreams may recall fear or horror instead of assisting grief resolution (Nader, 1996). Normally cherished symbols or reminders of the deceased may become reminders of horror. Spontaneous play may be unrewarding, dangerous, or distressing or provide only temporary relief (Terr, 1979; Nader & Pynoos, 1991). In normal bereavement, remembering the deceased is a part of the course of adaptation, reorganization, and recovery. It may engender pleasurable as well as sad thoughts and generate play that assists the child in accepting, working through, and redefining the relationship with the deceased (Raphael, 1983; Webb, 1993, 1999). In contrast, following *traumatic* death, attempts at remembering the deceased may lead to traumatic recollections such as thoughts of disfigurement or the manner in which the death occurred. Specific individual traumatic impressions may require resolution before additional resolution or grieving can occur. For example, Charlene was 14 years old when she and her family were held hostage in a bank robbery. To encourage and maintain the loyalty of some of the hostages, each hostage was taken into a backroom for conversation or to be shot. Hostages remained otherwise bound and lying behind desks or counters so that they could not see one another. They were told that the other hostages had been released, although they actually had been shot. In therapy several weeks after her initial trauma work, Charlene began some grief work. Later, she began to have dreams in which she bid farewell to her deceased father and brother; she did not dream of her mother. On one visit to "the room," she had seen her mother's bloody scarf on the floor. This part of her experience had to be resolved before she could grieve her mother's death.

Injured children may need some physical recovery and time to process aspects of their response related to their injuries, issues of safety, feeling damaged, and specific rage before grieving is possible. For example, Edgar, a 10-year-old, was badly injured in a shooting at his school. He was not able to return to school or enter treatment until months after the shootings. Even after his physician approved his return to school and entry into therapy, he remained anxiously attached to his mother and refused to go to school or treatment sessions. He engaged in screaming fits with his mother, insisting that he wanted to stay home. In therapy session, he clung to his mother's arm and screamed at her to take him home (and occasionally that he hated her). Edgar did not respond to any question or comment from the therapist until the therapist began to calmly engage him regarding his anger:

Content of Session	*Therapist's Rationale*
THERAPIST: You must be so angry!	Just stating the emotion out loud at this point. Not expecting him to discuss it. He is overwhelmed by his rage, fear, and sense of damage.
EDGAR: *(turns head to therapist and screams)* No! *(turns back to tugging and screaming at his mother).*	
T: You must be so angry to have this horrible injury.	
E: *(screaming at therapist)* No! *(back to scream and tug).*	
T: You must be so so angry that no one protected you.	
E: *(screams at therapist)* Shut up! *(screams and tugs at Mom).*	Definitely hit a nerve here, but he is not ready to process something this loaded.
T: You must be so, so hurt and angry.	
E: *(screams at therapist)* Shut up! *(back to tug and scream at Mom).*	
T: *(lightly wads up a clean Kleenex and tosses it at Edgar).*	Giving him a way to harmlessly express his rage, to focus his rage off of his mother, and permitting him to disconnect a bit at a time from his
E: *(kicks Kleenex back at therapist and continues screaming and tugging at Mom).*	

T: *(throws lightly wadded Kleenex back at Edgar).*   mother who is also anxiously attached to him.

E: *(lets go long enough to throw it back at the therapist, then returns to screaming at Mom).*

This process continued until the child spent 10 minutes focusing equal time between the therapist and his mother, and then a few minutes focusing more time interacting with the therapist. A new Kleenex was needed twice. Lightly wadded, it had little power when thrown and could not hurt anyone (a nerf ball might have worked as well). The child was congratulated on a good session expressing his anger well without hurting anyone and was allowed to go home early. Subsequent sessions included more of the same until his mother, at the therapist's suggestion, was gradually moved outside of the therapy room. A system of reentry into the classroom included having his mother at a desk at his side and then gradually move to the back of the room, then to an adjacent room, followed by the school office, and then home. His classmates were assisted to deal with Edgar's changed behaviors and enlisted to help, rather than hinder his recovery. Other than brief mention of two dead friends, grief work did not begin until a few months later.

DIRECTIVE PLAY THERAPY

Directive play therapy facilitates the abreactive reprocessing of the traumatic impressions and emotions. Terr (2001) suggests that, except when the stress can be worked out in a child's mind from play unmodified by words, the therapist must begin to enter into the child's play in order to help the child to reinterpret and modify it. Using directive methods while recognizing the child's own rhythms, timing, needs, strengths, and weaknesses, the clinician can expedite the child's resolution of difficult aspects of traumatic response and experience. This process often results, in a single session, in the release of emotions and the reduction of specific related symptoms. Deeper levels or variations of traumatic emotions (e.g., of attachment, rage, or fear) may require additional directive attention in later sessions or as they unfold with life experience.

Successful directive treatment requires knowledge, training, practice, and skill in order to avoid worsening symptoms and more dangerous outcomes (e.g., psychosis, suicide) (Nader, in press). The clinician must develop the ability to anticipate the child's needs, strengths, stamina, and timing. Confidence, good concentration, and high levels of energy are important assets to this form of treatment. When skillfully accomplished, directive or facilitative play therapy can be of great assistance to the traumatized youth.

In nondirective play therapy, the clinician may enter the child's play at the child's request. For example, the child, as director, may assign the therapist the role of victim, perpetrator, rescuer, witness, or another character. Directive play therapy may also permit the child to direct the action or assign characters. The direction given by the clinician may be as simple as a request to focus more intensely and/or in more detail on one scene or to tell or retell a specific episode (or all) of the traumatic experience using replicas to demonstrate. Facilitation may also be more complex. For example, the therapist may establish a rhythm with the child in which he/she (recognizing clues from the child's symbolic drawings or actions) follows in the direction the child is moving and then adds, magnifies, assists, or even carefully pushes the child through processing a set of memories and emotions.

As is true for nondirective play therapy, during directive play therapy with traumatized youths the treatment room is equipped with a variety of toys. Toy replicas of all aspects of the event (e.g., toy people, buildings or blocks, tables, weapons) enable the youth to play or demonstrate scenes from his/her traumatic experience. If appropriate toys are not available, we usually build them or provide materials for the child to quickly construct them (e.g., wax paper or plastic to use for glass). An additional variety of toys permits the child to deviate from focusing exclusively on traumatic scenes when life issues become intertwined with traumatic issues.

Age and Developmental Issues

Treatment of childhood traumatic stress must consider the affect of age on traumatic experience and response as well as the effect of trauma on the child's continuing development (Nader, 2001). Developmental issues influence children's experience, symptomatic presentation, behavior in treatment, and course of recovery (Pynoos & Nader, 1993). Moreover, competence achieved in one phase affects each subsequent phase (Combrinck-Graham, 1991). Because of trauma-induced regressions, post-trauma precocious development and the interaction of age and other factors (e.g., culture, child traits, previous experience, aspects of the trauma), the effects of age on traumatic experience and response (and vice versa) are complex (Nader, 2001).

Age may affect the perception and meaning attributed to aspects of the traumatic experience and affect the aspects of the event that take initial prominence. For example, the importance of a parent to the child's survival may influence the initial focus of a young child's experience.

Issues such as adult competence and the child's ability to intervene may become a part of elementary-school-age children's responses. For adolescents, dependence versus independence and invulnerability versus vulnerability may be among the issues that take prominence (Nader, 2001).

During treatment sessions, traumatized individuals may engage in play at older ages or may relapse into more juvenile play than would normally be expected. Nevertheless, adaptations are often made for age groups in play therapy. In general, these adjustments may include, for example, the following: (1) for preschoolers, increased focus on play with a clinician verbalizing reactions and sequences for the child; (2) for younger school-age children, more use of play and drawing combined with cognitive review and discussion; and (3) for adolescents, greater emphasis on discussion, perhaps with role play or demonstration. For older youths and adults, demonstration of scenes from the event may exhibit the qualities of traumatic play or play therapy. Although directive play therapy may assist the treatment process for school-age youths, providing appropriate toys is indicated for preschool children and is usually sufficient to instigate specific traumatic play.

Length of Treatment

Moderately to severely traumatized children have benefited from 2–16 sessions of trauma/grief-focused therapy (Goenjian et al., 1997; Nader, 2001). In addition to the symptoms of posttraumatic stress disorder (PTSD), intense traumatic impressions may affect the youth's quality of life and may result in undesired patterns of thought and behavior. Moderately to very severely traumatized children, especially those exposed to life threat and multiple bloody deaths or injuries, often require 1–2½ years of treatment to fully resolve their traumatic reactions. Specific characteristics of the youth or aspects of the trauma may increase or decrease the length of treatment regardless of exposures. Additional sessions may be required over time as a result of developmental factors, the interaction of trauma factors and life events, or as traumatic impressions take on new meaning for the youth/adult (Nader, 2001).

TRAUMA/GRIEF-FOCUSED THERAPY

Trauma/grief-focused therapy (Nader, 1994, 1997, 2001, in press; Nader & Mello, 2000; Nader & Pynoos, 1991; Pynoos, 1993; Pynoos & Eth, 1986; Pynoos & Nader, 1993) combines play with other methods (e.g., abreactive, cognitive-behavioral, or group therapy). Within a framework of play therapy, this method includes the following:

- The review and re-review of aspects of the experience
- Directed and spontaneous reenactments of traumatic episodes
- Bringing subconscious traumatic impressions to clear consciousness and permitting the assignment of new meaning
- Emphasis of intense traumatic moments prior to redefinition

Treatment addresses the child's personal symbolism and personal experience of the trauma. The clinician responds to the changing ambience created by the emotional tone of the traumatic segment and the child's demeanor, affect, body language, and personal needs. Closure is achieved at the end of each session. When possible, school, family, and group work provide important adjunctive treatments (Nader & Mello, 2000). This treatment method has effectively reduced symptoms of PTSD and prevented the escalation of depression (Goenjian et al., 1997; Nader, 2001). Sessions vary in the amount of spontaneous play and of direction given by the therapist. The following examples primarily include more directive sessions.

The initial session (Pynoos & Eth, 1985) examines the child's experience and worst moment. The focus of this and subsequent sessions are tailored to the child's readiness and needs. Drawings, verbalizations, behaviors, assessment measures, and the reports of adults and friends provide clues about areas of importance (Nader, 2001, in press; Nader & Mello, 2000). For example, when a sniper opened fire on a school playground, Angie, an 8-year-old girl, ran for safety while her sister tried to hide under an outdoor lunch table. The sister was shot in the face and killed. Angie, who was now receiving the focus and attention her naughtier sister had previously received, spent periods enjoying the attention, and then periods acting naughty. Her mother thought she was trying to replace the sister. There were no apparent signs of grief. Angie talked about her late sister as though talking about the weather. In sessions with another therapist, she had maintained this tone throughout. At the beginning of the session, Angie was asked to draw a picture of her choosing. Gentle probing helped to elicit the meaning of her drawing:

Content of Session	*Therapist's Rationale*
ANGIE: Done!	
THERAPIST: All done?	
A: Uh huh.	
T: Now tell me the story that goes with this picture.	
A: I was at my grandfather's house . . . hold and *(mumble)* one here and one here.	

T: You were at your grandfather's house?

A: Yeah, and I'm holding two ropes.

T: And what are you going to do with those ropes?

A: I'm trying to make it into a jump rope.

T: You are trying to make them into a jump rope?

A: *(Nods.)*

T: But right now they are not—kinda not anything, huh?

A: Uh huh.

T: And they need to be tied into one so they can be something?

A: *(firmly)* Uh huh.

T: Um hum. So this is you?

A: Um hum. *(Silence).*

T: And you have blond hair and blue eyes and you're smiling, and you have hands full of love, look at that. *(Angie is nodding and saying uh huh throughout and laughs after the therapist said her hands are full of love.)*

T: These hands are full of love, aren't they.

A: Uh huh.

T: Why are those hands full of love?

A: Because I'm happy.

T: What are you going to do with all that love?

A: I'm going to give my mom *(softly)* hugs and kisses.

T: Your mom?

A: Uh huh.

T: And who else gets some of that love?

A: My grandpa and my daddy.

T: Your grandpa and your daddy.

A: Uh huh.

T: Anyone else?

I repeat the child's statement to confirm that I heard it correctly, and to encourage her to continue.

I anticipate that she is representing her divided self/emotions, her lack of integration of aspects of trauma/grief. It also could represent her now "broken family."

Child has made a pink roundish area over her heart and (it looks like) in one hand cupped under her heart.

Seems shy about this. May feel guilty that she now receives the love and attention her sister received.

A: Probably, I guess I give some to my grandmother too.

T: *(Softly)* Your grandma too.

A: Uh huh.

Note the absence of her sister on this list even though she has reluctantly included Grandma.

T: *(pointing to picture)* You know what? It looks like you're about to fall off this thing.

A: Ha! *(smiling and rocking a bit but silent).*

T: Is *this* the bottom of the hill *(pointing)*, or is *this* the bottom of the hill?

A: This is the bottom of the hill *(a long drop down).*

T: So you're on the top of the hill. And you're kind of leaning over.

A: Uh huh.

T: And are those ropes keeping you from falling?

A: Mmmmmm.

T: No?

A: *(mumble)* It's like I slide over the mountain and hold on there.

T: So if you let go of the ropes you are going to fall?

A: Uh huh.

T: Oh, you'd better hold on to those ropes, huh.

A: *(Laughs.)*

She's drawn herself beginning to fall off solid ground—a risk she would have to take in order to reintegrate her divided self and mixed feelings. The attempt would put her in emotional peril—holding on by two large threads.

T: How are you going to get them tied together if you're holding on that tight?

A: Use rocks on each end.

She is resourceful; knows how to protect herself.

T: You use rocks on each end of the ropes, and they are holding you up on the mountain so you don't fall— because you're leaning, you're almost about to fall, huh?

A: *(Nods.)*

T: What is this purple thing here?

Again verbalizing her readiness to take this leap and her fear of its danger.

A: That's the, uh, the other part of my dress.

T: It's your dress? And underneath there? What is that?   Her body shows through.

A: That's part of my body.

T: Okay. So, this is a little girl who has on a covering, but I get to see through it, right.   Defining transparency to mean that I get to see inside her.

A: *(Nods.)*

T: I get to look inside, don't I?

A: Uh huh.

T: I bet there's lots of stuff inside there, isn't there.

A: Uh huh.

T: And I bet some of that stuff inside is as beautiful as this love in your hand, huh?   Giving her one option to claim or disclaim as the two parts.

A: In my heart.

T: In your heart *(with tone and nodding to show understanding)*.

A: Uh huh.

T: And I bet some of it doesn't feel so good?   I give her the chance to admit some negative feelings.

A: Uh huh.

T: What part of it doesn't feel so good.

A: *(as though she can hardly breathe)* Ah 'o know.   Saying, "I don't know."

T: You don't know?

A: *(letting out her held breath)* nn nn.   Trying to stay general with options and also trying to elicit her definition of what the picture is showing. With this confirmation, I move to "sad" from "not happy."

T: And this little girl is part happy and part not happy, isn't she?

A: *(firmly and nodding affirmatively)* Um hum.

T: She has kinda sad eyes, doesn't she?

A: Um hum.

T: 'Cause she's got something real sad in her heart?

A: *(barely eking it out)* Um hum.

T: What is that?

A: My sister.

T: Tell me about your sister.

A: Sha ... ta ... *(mumbling)* killed my sister.

T: Who did?

A: A shooter came and killed her, she *(silent)*. . . . It's not her fault, because, I don't know why. She was doing, she wasn't doing wrong things. She was like only *one* thing was her fault, she went under the table.

T: The part that was her fault was she went under the table?

A: Uh huh.

Although this is difficult for her, I know that our therapeutic relationship has steadily increased. I have faith that this relationship and my attunement to her rhythm and needs will see her through. Add to list of mixed feelings: anger at sister for not protecting herself. This later becomes a main focus.

Review of Traumatic Episodes

In trauma/grief-focused therapy, the youth may review, on multiple occasions, the traumatic experience or its episodes. This is accompanied by recognizing, verbalizing and underscoring the child's traumatic impressions (e.g., episodic or sensory impressions), emotions, desires for action (or inaction) (i.e., to intervene, flee, rescue or be rescued, prevent harm, self-protect, ward off, calm, etc.), and his/her successful actions (and inactions). The abreactive processing of experiences generally leads to a sense of relief, animation, increased expression, and resolution of related symptoms. Play and drawings are used, with discussion and role play or demonstration for older children and adolescents. Miniature replicas of the trauma site are provided so that youths can re-create and demonstrate the experience. This treatment method honors the intensity of traumatic impressions, identifications, emotions, and fantasies and facilitates their resolution (Bevin, 1999; Nader, 1997, 2001; Nader & Mello, 2000; Pynoos & Eth, 1985, 1986; Pynoos & Nader, 1993; Webb, 1999). Symptoms may temporarily increase as numbing and avoidance are reduced.

Review and re-review of aspects of the event may include a slow-motion retelling of segments of the experience, backing up and moving forward to recapture lost details and/or to facilitate the reintegration of memory and emotion toward release. In essence, a magnifying glass is placed on each memory segment. Angie, who depicted her conflicting emotions, was asked to describe the shooting. The following description includes the reviewed and re-reviewed segments about her escape; segments removed from the session are indicated by brackets (e.g., [snip]). This review process freed her to express a fuller range of attitudes and emotions, and to more fully grieve:

Content of Session	Therapist's Rationale
THERAPIST: I know you told people before what happened that day. But, I'd like you to tell me. Would you mind telling me?	She has talked to other therapists before. I want to remove resistance to telling her story again.
ANGIE: nn nn. We were eating lunch, right?	
T: Um hum.	
A: And, and then the glasses start opening and I got scared. I went underneath. I started to go underneath the table; no, I couldn't get under the table so I try to stay underneath one of the tables, but no, I was just on the side on 'em. Then she said "Run!," and I stand off the table, off the table onto the floor, off the table and into the kitchen.	Her description reflects her experience. She is speaking urgently and rapidly, and is correcting herself as she goes. The experience was one of urgent, rapid, trial and error escape.
T: Who said, "Run!"?	
A: Uh, one of the teachers. Run to the kitchen, and she got cut on her foot.	*(Asterisks under "Therapist's Rationale" denote when I, the therapist, made a mental note that this part of her experience would need review in the future.)
T: She did? [SNIP]	
T: (Pointing to toys.) Can you set up the playground for me?	
A: Uh huh. (Places replicas of cafeteria tables, benches, children, basketball court, and other things on the playground.)	
T: Okay, now where's the school building in all of this?	It is important to slow her down and examine the details of her experience as she remembers them.
A: (Points at where the building is.)	
T: Right here?	
A: (Nods.)	
T: And where's your table?	
A: (Points to her table.)	
T: Right here?	

A: *(Nods affirmative.)*

T: *(Moves table.)* And weren't the tables like this against the wall?

> Based on faulty assumption from knowledge of the event.

A: No, this way *(as she turns them back the other way).*

T: And where's the cafeteria, right here?

A: Right here.

T: Uh huh.

A: *[Describes the layout of playground and cafeteria.]*

> Getting details of the scene as the child remembers them.

T: And where were you sitting?

A: Right in here *(points to a table perpendicular to the building).*

T: And where was your sister?

A: *(Up to now she has been speaking firmly and loudly about her experience. Now she speaks very softly.)* Right in here. She was sitting right there *(a different but nearby table).*

T: By the little fence?

A: Uh huh. . . . *(pause)* Yeah, I was close to her.

T: Do you and your sister usually sit together?

A: Yeah.

T: How come you didn't sit next to her that day?

A: 'Cause she had friends she had to do, and she didn't feel like sitting by me, but she said someday; I'll sit by you next week.

T: So she had other friends she wanted to talk to.

A: Uh huh.

T: How did you feel about her not wanting to sit next to you that day?

> Reaching for what probably are very mixed feelings.
> Aware that she is reluctant to express negative feelings.

A: Sad.

T: You felt sad?

A: Uh huh.

T: Were you mad at her?

A: nn nn.

T: Not mad but hurt?

A: Uh huh.

*(As explained above). Note another set of hurts from her sister.

T: Um hum. So, who was sitting all along here?

A: [Describes the line up of friends sitting on either side of her and her relationship to them. She was eating an egg salad sandwich.]

T: And what were you doing before the shooting started?

A: Talking. [Describes details of their talking about wanting to be nurses and of the shooting starting.]

T: Were you scared?

A: No! Not 'til the glass fell. I thought it was firecrackers.

T: Tell me about when the glass fell.

A: The popping was happening, and then the glass flew. What?! And I got so scared. So I go underneath the table, then (demonstrates with the toys what's happening with the glass and demonstrates what she's saying as she says it). Then I did other things.

As is common, the child gives few details. The sniper shot at the children sitting at lunch. The bullets went through the tables. One bullet hit and shattered a window. The child has moved the piece of glass directly toward herself.

T: Show me how the glass went.

A: Little pieces came, big pieces came. (Demonstrates using torn waxed paper.)

T: Show me the first piece of glass you saw.

A: It was this one (medium piece). It was, like, flying.

T: Flying at you?
[A long segment here: Angie describes and demonstrates the glass flying at her.]

*

T: On the bench right next to you?

Important to get as many details as possible.

A: *(Uses herself-doll to demonstrate all of this.)* Yeah. And I was sitting on half of it, and I moved and I saw more glasses was coming down, then I ducked my head a little bit, and then I tried to get under the table—half under here and coming up a little bit when I couldn't get under. Then I stayed here, and the teacher yelled, "Run, run for the kitchen." Then we all ran, and then I stepped on here and here and here and on the tables. Then I got half to the kitchen table, then I was standing and Joey kept going and peeking out there. He could have got hurt. And that's all, and we all standing there and I was crying *(inhale)*, and that's all.

She speaks rapidly.

Individual segments here and in brackets will need a future session even though described in some level of detail here.

[*Long segment: child describes glass flying at her, being unable to scream, trying to hide, escaping, her friend putting his head out, and her mother hearing about her sister being badly injured.*]

T: So when you were right here, you were mostly worried about yourself because *(emphasizing)* you could get hit with a piece of glass?

Starting to define her choice to run/focus as the necessity it was.

A: Uh huh.

T: And you tried to hide from it and then you tried to run, and you did run.

A: Mmm huh.

[*Another segment includes the child talking about the bloody image she had in her mind when her mother told her about her sister.*]

*Will need a future session.

T: Let's put you right back in this cafeteria and right at this table, and here is this glass coming at you. And [Sister], where is she?

Introducing her sister into the process.

A: *(Gets a doll to represent her sister, and moves it up and down along the bench.)*

T: Okay, you're not sure exactly where she is, but it is somewhere on this table?

A: *(Nods.)* Yes *(mumbles something).*

T: If you could do anything at all, what would you do right now?

A: Get [Sister] out of this seat and she'd run into the kitchen.

T: How would you do that? Show me how you'd do that.

A: *(Laughs a little and rummages through dolls.)* Can't find one. *(Rummages through until she finds the right two dolls that she wants to be her and her sister).*

Choosing new dolls seems to mark a transition in her play and thinking.

T: This is you at the farther away table *[from shooting]?*

A: Uh huh. *(Takes a minute to finish setting up so that she has the piece of glass and the two children in the place she wants them to be.)*

T: Okay, so here comes the piece of glass and what are you doing?

A: I'm trying to get out of the way and then I go like this, and then I can't get under the table. So, I go like this and the glass lands right here and then *(calls out her sister's name).* Do you want me to show you how I'd do it?

T: Uh huh.

A: She's like this. And I come and say, [Sister], get out of the seat. *(Angie is demonstrating as she speaks.)* Now, get up, come on in here. *(She grabs the doll and quickly moves her into the kitchen area.)*

Although engaging in the action more readily, she is still distancing herself, speaking rapidly and acting hurriedly.

T: So where are you?

A: In the kitchen.

T: So you ran to the kitchen? *(Angie nods yes.)* And she's lying down?

A: Uh huh.

T: Is she hurt?

A: No.

T: What about you?

A: I'm a little scratched.

T: You got a little scratch from helping her?

A little badge of courage.

A: Right on my knee.

T: Right on your knee from helping her?

A: Uh huh.

T: So you got a little scratch from helping her and [Sister] is okay. How does it feel to save her life back?

A: Good.

T: Yeah?

A: MM huh.

T: You know what I think? *(pause and wait)*

To punctuate what I will say.

A: nn nn.

T: I think you need to do it over. And this time I think you have to show me how scared you were and how awful noisy it was.

She was still doing it in her essentially emotionless tone and very rapidly.

A: Uh huh. *(Picks up doll.)* Here I am.

T: Here you are.

A: And I go underneath here and I can't get under there and the leaves . . . the leaves . . . and they fall on the table and right there. And I didn't get hurt. Then see another glass. Scared if I see another glass. *(Talks to sister doll)* Are you *(mumbles)* and she goes, "Come!"

T: Who goes "Come!"?

A: One of the teachers in the kitchen. So, I'm standing right here.

T: Uh huh.

A: And [Sister] is shot. [Sister] under here.

T: [Sister] is all shot under here? *(Angie nods)*, and how do you know that?

A: Because I *(pause)* . . . window *(mumbles)* and I thought I saw it. And this is like this *(still moving things around)*.

T: But you couldn't really see [Sister] if she was under there, right?

A: Yes, only I *(pause)*.

T: But you are trying to see her?

A: Yeah.

T: So this is what it looked like, and you know what I want you to do this time. I want you to show me how very scared you were and how you would rescue [Sister]. Can you do that?

A: MM huh. And I was scared about [Sister]. *(Starts the demonstration over again.)*

T: Now what's happening inside of you?

A: My heart's beating really fast.

T: Your heart's beating very fast.

A: My skin's frightened.

T: And how does frightened skin feel?

A: Kinda itchy. And my eyes are trying to close.

T: How come?

A: 'Cause I don't want to see.

T: So your heart's beating very fast, and your eyes want to close 'cause they don't want to see . . . *(brief pause)*, and your skin is feeling very scared.

A: And itchy. *(Therapist nods. Angie continues to demonstrate.)*

T: Mm hm. And here comes the glass. And you see [Sister] over here. Now, what are you going to do?

A: *(Hesitates and does not move her doll toward her sister.)* I move my feet over here.

T: You're having trouble moving yourself over there, aren't you?

*Will need future clarification. Have already decided to focus on issue of Sister not saving herself, and Angie not saving Sister. It will be important later to explore the mixed desire to see and to avoid seeing what happened to Sister. She trusts me and I trust myself to see her through repeating this with more emotion now. Making it through this will energize her.

Indeed!

I know how frightening this experience was for her, but I also know how much better she will feel when she is moved carefully through it while reexperiencing the emotions.

A: *(laughs a little)* Uh huh.

T: How come?

A: 'Cause I don't want to get hurt.

T: 'Cause you don't want to get hurt, right. Well, you know what you and I really know?

A: What?

T: That you really couldn't go over there, could you? 'Cause you would have gotten shot.

A: *(Sighing with relief and showing some delight.)* Uh huh.

T: You did the right thing, you ran to the kitchen. Did you know that?

A: Uh huh.

T: That's how you saved your life.

A: *(Smiling and sighing as though relieved.)*

T: Now this time when you do it, it'll be just pretend, and so let's do it the way you really want to do it. Do exactly what you want to do.

A: *(in a whisper)* Get up, get up, get up, get up . . . *(she is saying "get up" repeatedly, softly).* See here. *(Takes both herself and sister dolls and runs them into the kitchen.)*

T: I think you need to say it *more forcefully* to her than that.

A: [Sister] get off, the bullets are going to hit you. Get off that seat *(again says it softly).*

T: Oh, and you said it so softly and sweetly, like you're not even scared or mean it. I thought you were scared!

A: *(Whispers)* I am.

T: Well, now, say it like your scared and like you really mean it.

A: *(Softly)* I can't say it like that. *(Again, softly)* [Sister], you'll get shot.

I have a very good sense of what she can do.

Note how seriously she is taking the play.
Continuing to reinforce her wise choice.

Gradually freeing her to fully express and feel what she really wished she could do, including her anger at her sister for not protecting herself.

Trying to faciliate a full reenactment.

T: Can you yell at her?

A: Yeah. "You'll get shot!" *(she yells it).*

T: Tell her what you want her to do.

A: *(Again, softly)* get off the chair.

T: *(Forcefully)* Now tell her what you want her to do.

> My tone is both modeling and permission.

A: Get off the chair and go to the kitchen, *now (forcefully). (Grabs herself doll and Sister doll by the arm and jerks Sister across the table and into the kitchen).*

A: *(Drops sister when she gets there.)* She fell.

T: She fell. Is she all right?

A: *(sigh of relief)* Yeah.

> She may be expressing some of her anger here, but it is not time to confront that issue directly.

T: That was hard making her do all of that, wasn't it?

A: Mm huh *(nodding, smiling, and sighing).*

T: It was. You look like you're a little relieved 'cause you finally got her to listen to you.

A: Uh huh. *(Big grin. Looks pleased and relieved.)*

T: Uh huh. Why don't you come around here and see how she's doing in the cafeteria. I wonder if you could say anything you wanted to to your sister, what would you say?

> Permitting resolution of unfinished business.

A: *(Forcefully)* [Sister] you should have run. Because if you had of run you could have saved yourself. . . . *(Pause)* Lucky I told you to run.
[Session continues below.]

Conflicting Emotions and Attitudes

During a traumatic experience, things may happen that cause mixed feelings toward one of the participants in the event (e.g., the perpetrator, a family member, a friend)—especially if he/she has died or been injured.

After a woman who had been wronged (and was trying to make it public) held them hostage, children felt sorry for the woman and were also angry for being terrified and witnessing her bloody suicide. The boy whose father brutalized him, his mother, and his siblings was somewhat sad but more relieved at his father's death. For these youths, it may be necessary to remove any hindrance to the separate and full expression of each emotion. This can be done, for example, by placing the person at a more comfortable emotional distance during role play, by allowing the child to divide her/himself into separate parts—each to express one of the separate emotions—or by facilitating the full expression of the appropriate emotion in the reenacted episode. For example, Carl, an 11-year-old boy whose father shot someone in front of him was sad for losing his father to incarceration and horrified at his father's behavior. Toward the end of his first session the therapist asked him what he thought should happen to his father for what he had done. Until then he was unable to grieve the loss of his father from his life or address the trauma.

Content of Session	Therapist's Rationale
CARL: *(sadly and shruggingly)* He should go to jail.	
THERAPIST: Can you draw me a picture of what you think should happen to him?	The child's response was not expressed with any conviction. Processing needs assistance.
C: *(Draws picture of father in jail, but the bars are wide enough apart for him to slip out.)*	
T: Look how far apart those bars are! I bet you wish your father didn't have to be in jail. That he could just walk right out and come home.	Sometimes assisting this recognition provides relief and frees the child to pursue related issues.
C: *(Bowing his head toward his chest)* He killed someone. He *has* to go to jail.	
T: Let's pretend for a minute that the person you saw shoot the man was not your father. Show me what you would want to do to him for what he had done and for making you watch.	It is clear that the child will not be able to fully grieve the loss of his father from his life until he has seen him properly punished.
C: *(Sits up straight; eyes brighten; draws picture of father at court, himself as judge with a gavel in his hand; he takes pretend gavel—toy hammer—hits it on the table.)* It is *wrong* to kill people. You	

have to go to jail for the rest of your life. . . . *(brief pause)* You shouldn't let children see you kill people 'cause it is makes 'em scared and gives 'em nightmares *(brief pause)* and bad thoughts. Now! Go to jail! And don't come out! *(Picks up picture of father in jail and starts adding bars; makes them very close. Then sighs deeply and relaxes.)*

Youths may also become angry at a friend or acquaintance, for example, who prevented their running to safety, caused their injury or aggravated the assailant. Sandy, a high school student, was really angry with—but also sorry for—a classmate, Bobby, who kept trying to come into the room while another student held her class hostage. The hostage taker became agitated, pulled the boy into the room and shot him, killing him.

Content of Session	Therapist's Rationale
SANDY: *(Is holding a doll by the legs, representing Bobby, the classmate, after demonstrating how he kept tugging at the door while the shooter held it closed. She talked about how angry she was at him.)*	
THERAPIST: Pretending that Bobby was sitting here in front of you in the form of that doll, tell him how you feel about what he did.	
S: *(Looks at Bobby doll.)* You shouldn't have done that. *(Looks up at therapist as though hoping to get away with that.)*	Her heart was not in it.
T: *(rolling eyes)* Wow, you really told him.	I said it unemotionally and rolling my eyes to let her know that she had not gotten away with it.
S: But he got shot. I can't get mad at him.	
T: Let's separate the part of you that is angry with him from the part of you that is sorry for his death. Here, is another Bobby *(taking another doll that looked the same)*. Put one in each hand. First tell this Bobby how angry you are with him. You can talk to the one you are sad about in a minute.	Began with anger; in this case it seemed likely that sorrow would not be fully expressed if stated first.

S: *(to Bobby doll)* You stupid dufus. You
   could have gotten us all killed. *(Slaps
   the Bobby doll. Starts banging his head
   on the table). (Giggles. Smiles. Sighs.)*

T: *(Nods. Waits in case there is more.)* Is   I didn't feel she was finished.
   that all?

S: *(Thinks. Bangs him on the table again.)*   The process should permit full
   You pig!! How do you think I felt   expression.
   watching you bleed all over the
   floor! *(Begins to sob.)*

Creating the proper emotional distance and the expression of each set of
emotions could have been accomplished in a few different ways depending on the needs of the youth in treatment. Sandy could have been asked
to use two dolls that represented the two different parts of herself, could
have used one doll for herself and one or two for Bobby, or (as above)
talked directly to the dolls representing Bobby. The last of these approaches allowed Sandy to hold onto the Bobby she was concerned for
while still keeping that emotion away from her angry feelings.

Mixed attitudes may result from preexisting complicated relationships prior to the event as well as actions during the event. The following
is a continuation of Angie's session:

Content of Session   *Therapist's Rationale*

ANGIE: *(Starts to set up a funeral and she
   lines up a bunch of people. She names
   off a bunch of people.)*

THERAPIST: Are these all your sister's
   friends?

S: These are *my* friends.

T: All your friends came too.   Feeling very compassionate to-

A: Yeah, all these people. They probably   ward her. Waiting to see if
   miss her. *(Pause.)*   she will get to her personal
                                                 feelings.
T: You think these people all miss her?

A: *(Nods. Continues to create a funeral setting.)* Here's Mother. *(Continues to set
   up.)* There's everyone.

T: Here's everyone, and here's your sister. Now what?

A: Some people walk up and just sit
   right here.

T: And they look?

A: Uh huh.

T: Do you want to do that?

A: Yeah. So here's the first one, my mamma. Mumble, mumble, mumble, mumble (*as though the doll was talking*).
(*Makes two lines of people and moves them up, one from each line at a time, to the front, to mumble something toward the dead sister.*)

A: I can hear what Jonathan is saying.

T: What's he saying?

A: "You big fat Mamma."   Said huffily, with disdain.

T: He says, "You big fat Mamma"? And why did he say that?

A: I don't know (*laughing*). Because (*mumbles something like because his mamma made him go*) so he said "big fat Mamma."
(*Continues to move one from each line forward at a time, making a few remarks*).

T: You know what I think? I think it's   The child has not moved her
hard for you to say good-bye to your   self doll forward in all of this.
sister.

A: (*Laughs a little*) Uh huh.

T: But it's your turn, isn't it?

A: Yeah. (*Laughs but does not move self doll forward*).

T: It's really hard, isn't it?

A: Uh huh. . . . (*pause*) I'll use my mom.

T: That's a good idea.

A: (*Mumbles good-bye's and moves one row of the dolls up one at a time but not her self doll*) Nya nya nya nya (*makes noises like they are talking without saying anything clearly*). Good-bye, [Sister].

T: Well, let's just assume that all those   I decide to shift the focus trying
other people have had a chance to   to get her to express her own
go up. What happens to her body?   grief and good-bye. She had
                                            more trauma work to do first.

A: *(Places her sister under a barricade, not unlike the table, except using solid blocks instead of the thin table replicas, and she barricades her sister into it.) (Softly)* "shut up" *(back to normal tone)* He's saying "shut up" because he is saying bad things.

May also be talking to the therapist.

T: He's saying bad things about her? *(Angie nods.)* Is that because there are good and bad things about her, or because he is just like that?

Child is now expressing both sets of emotions.

A: He's just like that. *(Continues to move children from one of the lines up, to the place where she placed her sister, to say something).* "Shut up." That's because they're all saying bad things about her. How ugly she was.

She is still checking it with "Shut up."

The first line of people were saying pleasant good-bye's. Now, they are saying "bad things."

T: How ugly she was.

A: *(Moves the next child up)* "'cause she's fat." They're all calling her fat, big Mamma. *(Continues to move that row of people up.)* These guys don't care about her. *(Therapist nods.)* *(Angie moves the next child up.)* I don't like [Sister], she's big, she's fat, she's ugly. *(Looks at therapist.)* That's it, that's all the people. *(Places Sister doll under.)*

She is checking to see my reaction.

T: Okay. Now is she being buried?

A: Me and Mamma are gonna go bury her.

T: You're going to bury her body?

A: Yes.

Angie is a Protestant Christian and believes the soul goes to heaven.

T: And where is [Sister] that's inside the body?

A: Right under here *(points under the barricade that she built for Sister doll).*

She is setting it up so that Sister is fully present.

T: Sorta' like being under the table?

A: Yeah, like the, being under the table. *(Continues to move things around and fortifies the casket table.)* Okay, right in there.

*May need to process the segment under the table in a later session.

T: You know what? Look how you built this table. You made it so big and thick that no bullet could go through it, huh?

A: Uh huh.

T: It just can't even be shot through. I bet you wish that table that she was under had been so sturdy that no bullet could have gone through it?

Underscoring the desire indicated in the play.

A: Uh huh *(delightedly)*.

T: Look how much you wished that! You built her a table that nothing could go through.

A: *(Big smile)* Mm huh. *(Child is still smiling, sitting straighter, chest swelled)* and now if you want to see her, you just go here and open this like this.

A fantasied desire to be able to be with her at any time desired.

T: And she's under a table where nothing can ever hurt her. Isn't that nice?

A: Uh huh *(smiling really big and with a totally different demeanor than in the beginning of the session)*.

T: Oh, yes. And *you* built it.

A: Yes. Me and my mamma. *(Child is really beaming and does some proud-of-herself kind of movements and laughing.)*

T: And that made you happy, didn't it? Building her a table that nothing could go through to hurt her.

A: Yeah, and now we go wheeeee, and me and Mommy go inside the table and go wheeeee, and then we have to get out and so we get out and close the door. *(Child seems joyous at this point.)*

Showing some sense of completion. More permission to enjoy it.

T: And that was really fun, building that table.

A: And we did it in only one day. *(Brings herself back to the table-coffin and brings her mother back to the table, and goes wheeee each time. She takes one friend at a time to see the thing that she*

built and goes wheee.) And now me
and Mommy are going to see it.
Wheeee. We built the thing.

T: And it's important that people see this
table that can't fall down.

A: There go *(mumbles)*. And nobody sees
and nobody knows where she's hid-
ing. And Mommy goes, "Where's
[Sister]?" "Does anybody here see
[Sister]? Did anybody here see [Sis-
ter]?" Now she goes under here and
she looks and she says, "[Sister]!"
(The Sister doll then says) "Yes,
Mommy?" *(Mother doll:)* "What are
you doing under there?" *(Sister doll:)*
"Nothing." *(Mother doll:)* "Get out.
Come on out of there." *(She takes the
Sister doll out and slides her over the
top of the indestructible table)*
"Wheee!" *(She takes her self doll and
slides it over the top of the indestructible
table)* "Wheee!" Now let's take another big jump, come on, wheeee!
Come on, Gramps Gramps, Grams,
wheeee!

*[Continues to have her sister and herself slide
and go wheee! Periodically she says
things like "Come on" or "I'm over
here," "It'll be fun," "Don't go so far"
and laughing and giggling.]*

T: Wouldn't it be nice if you could have
had a table like that, that no bullet
could go through. That stopped the
bullets, and you could still have
[Sister].

A: Yep, I'm having fun with her.

Searching is a part of normal
grief. This is one part of the
process permitted by expressing anger and intense desires.

Searching as a part of the
trauma will need future work.

As if she wants to continue to
have fun and change the sadness of death and loss.

Implicitly, she has begun
mourning her loss.

CONCLUSIONS

When a youth is severely traumatized during a violent event, processing
a few or many aspects of the traumatic experience, emotions, and impressions may be necessary before grieving is possible. Issues of betrayal (e.g.,
by a perpetrator or parent perceived as not protecting), personal injury
(i.e., physical or emotional), conflicting attitudes and emotions (e.g., sym-

pathy, love, or dependence vs. anger, fear or hatred), the intensity of emotions and impressions (e.g., of bloody human inflicted deaths, of saving oneself), and continuing issues of self-protection may impede the normal progression of grief. In addition to treatment that includes the clinician's appropriate verbalizations (e.g., interpretations of behavior, emphasis of the child's action and/or emotion), directive play therapy methods can effectively facilitate children's full or partial resolution of their traumatic memories. Play therapy may assist the normal process of grieving in addition to uncovering and assisting the ongoing trauma recovery process.

DISCUSSION QUESTIONS

1. What distinguishes traumatic grief from the normal grief process?
2. How does directive play therapy differ from nondirective play therapy? When and why is it appropriate to use directive play therapy? What background and training would prepare the clinician for this work?
3. When directive methods are used, how can a youth be assisted to deal with conflicting emotions toward someone else who was a part of the traumatic experience?

REFERENCES

Bevin, T. (1999). Multiple traumas of refugees—near drowning and witnessing of maternal rape: Case of Sergio at age 9, and follow-up at age 16. In N. B. Webb (Ed.), *Play therapy with children in crisis* (2nd ed., pp. 164–182). New York: Guilford Press.

Combrinck-Graham, L. (1991). Development of school-age children. In M. Lewis (Ed.), *Child and adolescent psychiatry; A comprehensive textbook* (pp. 157–265). Baltimore: Williams & Wilkins.

Eth, S., & Pynoos, R. (1985). Interaction of trauma and grief in childhood. In S. Eth & R. Pynoos (Eds.), *Post-traumatic stress disorder in children* (pp. 171–186). Washington, DC: American Psychiatric Press.

Frederick, C. J. (1985). Children traumatized by catastrophic situations. In S. Eth & R. S. Pynoos (Eds.), *Post-traumatic stress disorder in children* (pp. 71–99). Washington, DC: American Psychiatric Press.

Friedrich, W. N. (1996). Clinical considerations of empirical treatment studies of abused children. *Child Maltreatment, 1*(4), 343–347.

Garbarino, J. (1999). *Lost boys: Why our sons turn violent and how we can save them* (pp. 120–145). New York: Free Press.

Garbarino, J., Kostelny, K., & Dubrow, N. (1991). What children can tell us about living in danger. *American Psychologist, 46*, 376–383.

Goenjian, A. K., Karayan, I., Pynoos, R. S., Minassian, D., Najarian, L. M., Steinberg, A. M., & Fairbanks, L. A. (1997). Outcome of psychotherapy among early adolescents after trauma. *American Journal of Psychiatry, 154,* 536–542.

Herman, J. L. (1992). Captivity. In J. L. Herman (Ed.), *Trauma and recovery* (pp. 74–95). New York: Basic Books.

James, B. (1994). *Handbook for treatment of attachment-trauma problems in children.* Lexington, MA: Lexington Books.

Nader, K. (1993). *Childhood trauma: A manual and questionnaires.* Unpublished copyrighted material including a manual for use with the Child Post Traumatic Stress Reaction Index (CPTS-RI, © 1992, C. J. Frederick, R. S. Pynoos, & K. Nader) and exposure and coping questionnaires.

Nader, K. (1994). Countertransference in treating trauma and victimization in childhood. In J. P. Wilson & J. Lindy (Eds.), *Countertransference in the treatment of post-traumatic stress disorder* (pp. 179–205). New York: Guilford Press.

Nader, K. (1996). Children's exposure to violence and disaster. In C. A. Corr & D. M. Corr (Eds.), *Handbook of childhood death and bereavement* (pp. 201–222). New York: Springer.

Nader, K. (1997). Treating traumatic grief in systems. In C. R. Figley, B. E. Bride, & N. Mazza (Eds.), *Death and trauma: The traumatology of grieving* (pp. 159–192). London: Taylor & Francis.

Nader, K. (2001). Treatment methods for childhood trauma. In J. P. Wilson, M. J. Friedman, & J. D. Lindy (Eds.), *Treating psychological trauma and PTSD* (pp. 278–334). New York: Guilford Press.

Nader, K. (in press). Innovative treatment methods. In S. Brock & P. Lazarus (Eds.), *Best practices in crisis prevention and intervention in the schools.* Bethesda, MD: National Association of School Psychologists.

Nader, K., & Mello, C. (2000). Interactive trauma/grief focused therapy. In P. Lehmann & N. F. Coady (Eds.), *Theoretical perspectives for direct social work practice: A generalist–eclectic approach* (pp. 382–401). New York: Springer.

Nader, K., & Mello, C. (in press). Shootings and hostage takings. In A. M. LaGreca, W. K. Silverman, E. M. Vernberg, & M. C. Roberts (Eds.), *Helping children cope with disasters: Integrating research and practice.* Washington, DC: American Psychiatric Press.

Nader, K., & Pynoos, R. (1991). Play and drawing as tools for interviewing traumatized children. In C. Schaeffer, K. Gitlan, & A. Sandgrund (Eds.), *Play, diagnosis and assessment* (pp. 375–389). New York: Wiley.

Nader, K., & Pynoos, R. (1993). School disaster: Planning and initial interventions. *Journal of Social Behavior and Personality, 8*(5), 299–320.

Ochberg, F. M., & Soskis, D. A. (1982). Planning for the future: Means and ends. In F. M. Ochberg & D. A. Soskis (Eds.), *Victims of terrorism* (pp. 173–190). Boulder, CO: Westview Press.

Parson, E. R. (1997). Post-traumatic child therapy (P-TCT): Assessment and treatment factors in clinic work with inner-city children exposed to catastrophic community violence. *Journal of Interpersonal Violence, 12,* 172–194.

Pynoos, R. S. (1993). Traumatic stress and developmental psychopathology in children and adolescents. In J. M. Oldham, M. B. Riba, & A. Tasman (Eds.), *American Psychiatric Press Review of Psychiatry, 12,* 205–238.

Pynoos, R. S., & Eth, S. (1985). Children traumatized by witnessing acts of personal violence: Homicide, rape, or suicide behavior. In S. Eth & R. S. Pynoos (Eds.), *Post-traumatic stress disorder in children* (pp. 17–43). Washington, DC: American Psychiatric Press.

Pynoos, R. S., & Eth, S. (1986). Witness to violence: The child interview. *Journal of the American Academy of Child Psychiatry, 25,* 306–319.

Pynoos, R. S., & Nader, K. (1993). Issues in the treatment of post traumatic stress disorder in children and adolescents. In J. P. Wilson & B. Raphael (Eds.), *The international handbook of traumatic stress syndromes* (pp. 535–539). New York: Plenum Press.

Raphael, B. (1983). *The anatomy of bereavement.* New York: Basic Books.

Terr, L. C. (1979). Children of Chowchilla: Study of psychic trauma. *Psychoanalytic Study of the Child, 34,* 547–623.

Terr, L. C. (1991). Childhood traumas: An outline and overview. *American Journal of Psychiatry, 148*(1), 10–20.

Terr, L. C. (2001). Childhood posttraumatic stress disorder. In G. O. Gabbard (Ed.), *Treatment of psychiatric disorders* (3rd ed., Vol. 1, pp. 293–306). Washington, DC: American Psychiatric Press.

Webb, N. B. (Ed.). (1993). *Helping bereaved children: A handbook for practitioners.* New York: Guilford Press.

Webb, N. B. (Ed.). (1999). *Play therapy with children in crisis* (2nd ed.): *Individual, group, and family treatment.* New York: Guilford Press.

PART IV

❧

Interventions with Bereaved Children

11

§

Counseling and Therapy
for the Bereaved Child

NANCY BOYD WEBB

As we have seen in the cases presented in this book, children experience death at home, at school, and in the community at large. Death may occur in their own backyards, in a hospital, on the highway, and in their classrooms. The children may witness death, may hear about it from a relative or school counselor, or may not be told until years later because of the family's sense of shame and inability to discuss the death openly. Sometimes the child may be advised that a death is imminent, so that he/she can say a last "good-bye" to the loved one (see Chapter 3, this volume); some children accompany the family to the funeral and grave-side service. On the other hand, some families give the child no informa-tion at all and may send the child away to avoid his/her knowledge about or involvement with the death (see the example of 6-year-old Christopher Lucas in Webb, 1993).

Obviously, these "death-related factors" and "family factors" will interact with unique "individual factors" and result in different grief responses for each bereaved child. In the "best possible scenario," a boy is informed by his parents that his elderly grandmother is very sick and may not get better, and that it might be a good idea for him to give Grammy a special kiss and tell her that he loves her and will always remember her (Chapter 3 describes a situation like this). Many children in these circumstances feel some anxiety and sadness, and may benefit from brief, supportive counseling from the family's religious leader or funeral director.

By contrast, an example of the "worst possible scenario" might involve the violent deaths of both parents of a preschool child who is too young to comprehend the finality of death and who in all likelihood will require intensive long-term psychotherapy to help him overcome and live with the knowledge that his father shot his mother before killing himself (Chapter 7 describes the initial therapeutic intervention in a traumatic situation like this).

There are countless variations between these two types of death situations: one "timely," anticipated, and of natural causes; and the other, "untimely," sudden, and violent. Because of this wide variability in the circumstances of deaths and in the responses of the child survivors, mental health professionals and community leaders should be prepared to offer a range of counseling and therapy options according to different individual circumstances and needs. These are described in detail later in this chapter. However, before presenting these options I discuss the rationale for professional intervention with bereaved children and the appropriate training for performing this work.

PROFESSIONAL INTERVENTION: RATIONALE AND TRAINING

Is professional assistance necessary and beneficial for all bereaved children? Death is a part of life that every person sooner or later will experience. These characteristics of inevitability and universality could lead to the conclusion that professional help should not be necessary to assist individuals through an essentially normal life passage. Indeed, the support of family, friends, and community does provide sufficient assistance for many bereaved individuals.

However, the situation of the bereaved *child* is different. Many adults feel uncomfortable talking with children about death. Reflecting the attitude implicit in the Wordsworth quotation at the beginning of Chapter 1, these adults prefer that the child remain innocent of knowledge about this terrible fact of life. Many well-meaning adults want to "protect" children from exposure to death, and therefore they refrain from discussing death with children.

Another contributing factor in adult reluctance to talk with children about death can be the mutuality of the loss experience. Frequently, when children are bereaved, the adults in their family also are grieving the same loss. Quite understandably, this means that the adults are less available to comfort the child since they are immersed in their *own* grieving process. Furthermore, the child may not express his/her feelings openly, which may suggest (erroneously) to family members that "the child is doing fine."

With the family members thus not open or available to the bereaved child, who can offer assistance? We know that many bereaved children do not welcome the support of their friends, because being bereaved sets them apart and makes them feel "different." Unlike adults who appreciate and respond positively to condolences from friends, many bereaved children do not like to have their friends speak to them about their loss. Most often, the child's peers are themselves uncomfortable in this situation and do not know what to say. This, then, eliminates another source of potential support for bereaved children. As a result, in many instances the bereaved child has neither family nor friends to console him/her. Even when someone might be available and able to reach out, comforting a bereaved child is not easy because the child is so confused and uncomfortable about his/ her feelings. The bereaved child may be unable to tolerate the pain of talking about the person who died.

All of these reasons argue for the assistance of a trained professional to help bereaved children. However, even an experienced child therapist may find it challenging to attend fully to the bereaved child's varying moods. The therapy must move at the child's pace, using play therapy methods of symbolic communication, in addition to verbal interaction.

Grief Counseling and Grief Therapy

What kind of counseling or therapy is appropriate for bereaved children? Some writers (Worden, 1991) distinguish between grief "counseling" and grief "therapy" based on whether the client's grief is viewed as uncomplicated (i.e., "normal") or pathological (i.e., complicated). Worden specifies the goal of grief *counseling* (for uncomplicated grief) as "helping the survivor complete any unfinished business with the deceased and say a final good-bye" (1991, p. 38); the goal in grief *therapy* (for complicated grief) is "to identify and resolve the conflicts of separation which preclude the completion of mourning tasks in persons whose grief is absent, delayed, excessive, or prolonged" (1991, p. 79).

I think that these tasks do not apply to *children's* bereavement and that we must conceptualize the tasks of children's grief differently because of the child's immature development and ongoing developmental changes. As I discussed in Chapter 1, the child may not understand the finality and irreversibility of death until age 7 or 8, so the goal of saying good-bye may not be realistic until the child is older. Furthermore, when a child has lost a parent, he/she may need and want to retain a relationship with that deceased parent, in fantasy, as a source of comfort and ego integrity. Baker, Sedney, and Gross (1992) state that the "ability to maintain an internal attachment to the lost person may be a sign of healthy recovery, not of pathology" (p. 109). These authors propose that the psychological tasks of bereaved children take a considerable span of time for completion, even in the best circumstances extending for many years following the death. So the notion that delayed or prolonged grief constitutes "pathology" should not be applied to children.

I prefer to use the terms "therapy" and "counseling" according to their more conventional usage: namely, by *therapy* I refer to a process of help conducted by a mental health professional, and by *counseling* I refer to the process of help as provided by religious leaders and educational personnel. The goals and procedures in each method will differ according to the needs of the specific child and according to the training of the helper. There are certainly many similarities in the bereavement work of counselors and therapists. However, the training of therapists in understanding the psychodynamics and psychopathology of human behavior makes them better prepared to help when the bereavement situation is atypical or complicated. In situations of traumatic, violent, or multiple losses, a therapist trained in traumatic bereavement understands and knows about the importance of helping a child deal with traumatic memories before the grief work can proceed (see Eth & Pynoos, 1985, Nader, 1997, and Chapters 7, 8, and 10 in this volume).

Qualifications of Counselors/Therapists

Because of the importance of developmental issues in working with children, the grief counselor/therapist must have a firm grounding in child development. In addition, counselors and therapists who work with children should be trained to use play therapy in order to engage and interact effectively with their child clients. Some verbalization, of course, always occurs depending on the child's age and ability to communicate directly about the painful topic of death. However, therapy or counseling with a child using *only* verbal communication would be foolhardy and probably futile. Therefore, the grief counselor/therapist who intends to work with children must either already possess or arrange to obtain specialized training in child development and play therapy. In addition, bereavement counselors who work with children should have a thorough knowledge of reactions of children in situations of extreme stress, including knowledge about normal regressive as well as dysfunctional reactions.

Training of Grief Counselors/Therapists for Work with Bereaved Children

The task of helping bereaved children is demanding and requires specialized knowledge and experience. Although a scout leader or school nurse may offer supportive help to a grieving child based on his/her intuitive empathy for the child's grief, such a helper might fail to identify the *traumatic* components of a death that indicate the need for a timely referral to a mental health professional.

Ideally, community caregivers such as school, hospital, and recreational personnel should receive in-service training about when to refer to a therapist who specializes in work with bereaved children. The referral must be made, however, in a manner that "normalizes" the need for it. The last thing a traumatically bereaved child (or family) needs is the covert message that there is "something wrong" with him/her! Worden comments that "there is always the risk of making grief seem pathological because of the formal intervention of a mental health worker, but with skilled counseling this need not be the case" (1991, p. 38). "Normalizing" the need for a referral involves making a statement to the child and family that they have suffered a *very* serious loss and that there are people who are specially trained to help in situations like theirs.

A list of training programs in play therapy, in grief counseling, and in trauma counseling appears in the Appendix to this book. The professional associations of each group publish newsletters that list continuing education workshops and training seminars.

COUNSELING/THERAPY OPTIONS

Depending on the age of the bereaved child, the nature of the death, and the availability of different intervention alternatives, the following options may be appropriate for helping a bereaved child:

- Family therapy
- Bereavement groups
- Individual therapy

These different forms of treatment may be available in a variety of settings, such as hospitals, schools, hospice programs, bereavement camp programs, clinics, churches, and through private practitioners. Regardless of the counseling/therapy method and the setting in which it is offered, it is important for the therapist/counselor to respect the unique needs of the child and to be mindful about the child's developmental stage and the timing implications of the child's bereavement process. The following discussion presents the three major forms of professional intervention with bereaved children, giving consideration to the advantages/disadvantages of each approach and to the specific indicators for selecting one approach over another.

Family Counseling/Therapy

As emphasized in Chapter 2, an understanding of the family context is essential to appreciate the unique significance of a particular child's bereavement. A family systems perspective maintains that the response of one family member will reverberate among all family members; in an interlocking system one person's pain becomes everyone's pain. Therefore, to help a bereaved child effectively, the family will need to be involved to some extent. If the death has occurred to a member of the family, *all* will be grieving. In this situation, the therapist/counselor may come to represent the only adult who listens fully to the child's questions and concerns because the other family members are so focused on their own grieving they cannot attend fully to the child.

It is very helpful for the family to attend counseling/therapy together after a death. A family session some 7–14 days after the death allows time for the initial shock to have passed, and yet the family will still be very preoccupied with bereavement issues. The purpose of the family meeting differs, depending on the circumstances of the death and the age of the child(ren). The therapist/counselor working with a bereaved child can utilize the information and observations from the family session to understand the significance of the loss to the family as a whole and observe how they are managing in the face of this experience.

Walsh and McGoldrick identify two family tasks that benefit the immediate and long-term adaptation of both individual family members and the family as a functional unit: (1) shared acknowledgment of the reality of death and shared experience of loss, and (2) reorganization of the family system and reinvestment in other relationships and life pursuits (1991, pp. 8–13). Obviously, the timetable for achievement of these tasks varies greatly, but the above authors believe that if these tasks are not achieved eventually, the family members will be vulnerable to dysfunction. Walsh and McGoldrick's task of acknowledgment and sharing dovetails nicely with that of Baker et al. (1992), whose first-stage task focuses on understanding. The family task of system reorganization, on the other hand, subsumes the child's role into functions of the system as a whole. For example, after a mother's untimely death from cancer, a 9-year-old girl might be expected to fulfill some of the mother's previous caretaking of her 3-year-old brother. In a family session with a counselor/therapist, the father might be helped to realize that this arrangement is not fair or appropriate for the 9-year-old even though the girl had agreed to perform the duties. With the help of the child/family therapist some compromise could be achieved congruent with both the child's and the family's needs. The provision of psychoeducational guidance such as this is an important purpose of a family session following a death. Examples of family interventions with bereaved children following a death can be found in Chapters 3 and 4 of this volume. Table 11.1 summarizes the advantages/disadvantages and special indications for family, group, and individual counseling/therapy options.

Bereavement Groups for Children

Because children dislike being considered "different" from others, bereavement groups should be considered the treatment of choice for the bereaved

TABLE 11.1. Comparison of Counseling/Therapy Options: Webb

	Advantages	Disadvantages	Special indications
Family	Observation of child's role in family	Child's "voice" may not be heard by adults	Early in grief process
	Assessment of "availability" of family members to the child Members share reality of death "Education" of family members re: different pace and form of children's grieving	Family so involved in own grieving, they cannot empathize with child	*Purpose/goals* To establish alliance To assist in engaging child To offer psychoeducational guidance
Group	Relieves isolation of child "Normalizes" death experience Child sees others in later stage of grief who have "survived"	Child may hear "horror" stories from others in group Child may be overwhelmed by intense feelings of other group members Shy child may not participate	Most appropriate for child dealing with tasks of *middle stage* of bereavement
Individual	Child's needs receive one-to-one attention Therapy/counseling can be paced according to the child's individual needs Permits in-depth exploration of idiosyncratic feelings	Sense of stigma/blame for being "singled out" Engagement of the bereaved child is often difficult	For traumatic bereavement For suicide bereavement For complicated bereavement

child. These groups may be school or community-based. They offer the peer support that the bereaved child so greatly craves, since the group helps him/her realize that other children have also lost loved ones to death. Many of the children in Jill Krementz's book (1981/1991), as quoted in Chapter 1, mentioned their fear of being pitied because someone had died in their family.

These sentiments make the rationale for bereavement groups very clear: Everyone in the group has suffered a loss; therefore the group members can offer support to one another, because of their similar experiences.

Short-Term Bereavement Groups

A typical format is a time-limited (8–10 weeks) group that utilizes a planned agenda of drawing, writing, and other group activities and exercises to enable the children to express their feelings about death. Chapters 6 and 12 of this volume each describe the content and process of different bereavement groups. Often these groups are based on the "mutual aid" model of group work (Schwartz & Zalba, 1971). In addition to the peer support that counteracts the bereaved child's sense of isolation, the group is a place where questions can be aired, either verbally or anonymously, through the use of a question box.

Tait and Depta (1993) describe the process of one such eight-session group consisting of 10 children, ages 7–11, each of whom had experienced the death of a parent, stepparent, grandparent, or other family members. There were two co-leaders, which the authors recommend in order to make it possible for one leader to attend to individuals who may become upset during the group sessions while the other leader can continue with the group process. Insofar as bereavement groups may include the recently bereaved with members who are in middle or later stages of bereavement, the groups offer the child a firsthand experience with children who have withstood the pain of bereavement and survived. It also can be very therapeutic for the children who are further along with their own grieving to be able to offer support to more recently bereaved children (Yalom, 1985; Schiffer, 1984). Sometimes, however, a recently bereaved child may feel overwhelmed when exposed to the feelings of others. The therapist needs to be attuned to this possibility and consider delaying entry into the groups for the recently bereaved child. Usually, a group experience is very valuable for either adults or children, but only when the bereaved individual is ready. Sometimes it is helpful to suggest that the person try the group once or twice, rather than automatically rule it out.

In an earlier publication (Webb, 1993) I pointed out that bereavement groups are *not appropriate* for traumatically bereaved children or for children bereaved by suicide. The special needs of these individuals can be more appropriately met initially in one-to-one therapy. Bereavement groups are not usually recommended for the child who is bereaved by a suicide because the child may feel some sense of stigma about the suicidal death. Furthermore, other group members may be unable to feel a sense of connection with the suicide-bereaved child because of the voluntary nature of the death. Like the child who has been exposed to a traumatic death, the child bereaved by a suicidal death needs individual help to deal with the trauma.

School-Based Groups for Children Exposed to Violent Death

Because of the serious increase of violence in our society, children may be exposed to violent deaths on the street corner, on the playground, and even in the school building (see also Chapter 16, this volume, re terrorist attacks). The literature reports research investigations and interventions following a sniper attack on a school playground (Pynoos et al., 1987), the murder of a teacher in her classroom (Danto, 1983), and a massacre of 21 persons in a McDonald's restaurant (Hough et al., 1990). Whether or not the traumatic death occurred on the school premises, the children come together in the school following the occurrences of violent deaths, making this setting the ideal locale for implementing a preventive mental health intervention in a group format.

Pynoos and Nader (1988) describe a clinical intervention protocol that can be implemented in schools for children exposed to violence, trauma, or sudden bereavement. Implicit in this approach is the principle of timely "first aid" intervention because of the possible negative impact of violent crime on children's ego-oriented thought. "After a violent death, especially one witnessed by a school age child, attempts at trauma mastery can complicate the bereavement process and greatly increase the likelihood of pathological grief" (Pynoos & Nader, 1988, pp. 452–543). They view the classroom as an appropriate site for dealing with fears of recurrence of the trauma and for publicly addressing issues related to dying and loss. Terr elaborates further that "teachers can be trained to use art, musical expression, poetry, or storytelling as expressive therapeutic techniques after traumatic events" (1989, p. 6). In the present book, Chapter 9 describes a variety of intervention approaches in schools following students' exposure to death.

In an earlier publication (Webb, 1999b) I described the format of an initial group "debriefing" of children following urban bombings. This ideally includes both verbal and nonverbal approaches such as art and play to help children release the feelings they cannot articulate. Typical debriefing sessions with children in schools begin by asking some leading questions about the crisis event. Children who are able to do so describe the details of their experience and are prompted to emphasize the involvement of all their senses in response to specific questions by the teacher or mental health professional—that is, what did you see, smell, hear, do, feel? (Alameda County Mental Health Services, 1990). When the children have verbally described their recollections, they then are invited to draw what they experienced. Often the graphic memories have a special poignancy and power not evident in the verbal accounts. Group debriefing sessions also aim to put some closure on the traumatic experience by emphasizing the fact of the participants' survival and current safety status. This helps put some distance between the trauma and the present reality.

Individual Therapy/Counseling: Play Therapy

In situations of suicide and traumatic bereavement and in situations of complicated bereavement, the treatment of choice is individual therapy with a therapist who can help the child cope with some of the intrusive memories and fears associated with the trauma. Often this occurs through play therapy, utilizing drawing, doll play, and other methods to help the child express his/her feelings and gain some support. For example, Kaplan and Joslin (1993) illustrate helpful play therapy interventions using clay and a dollhouse with a 7-year-old boy whose sister died after falling into their backyard well.

The rationale on which the practice of play therapy rests is that the child identifies with and projects his/her own conflicts and concerns onto play materials. As Enzer (1988) points out, the play therapy interaction with the therapist encourages the child to experience catharsis, reduction of troublesome affects, redirection of impulses, and a corrective emotional experience.

As I explain in the first edition of *Play Therapy with Children in Crisis,* "in crisis situations, the child has felt helpless and afraid. Through replay of the crisis experience the child transforms the passivity and impotence he or she experienced into activity and power. . . . Just as the mourning adult needs to review over and over the details surrounding the death of a loved one, a traumatized child may repeatedly seek to reconstruct a crisis experience symbolically through play" (Webb, 1991, p. 30). A range of play therapy methods, such as art techniques, doll play, puppet play, storytelling, and board games are all described and illustrated through detailed case examples in the second edition of *Play Therapy with Children in Crisis* (Webb, 1999a). Since death is clearly a crisis, many of these techniques are applicable to work with bereaved children.

Some of the distinct advantages of individual therapy over group or family therapy are that it permits maximum attention to the particular needs of the child, allowing the therapist to move at the child's pace in a careful, in-depth exploration of the child's underlying feelings about the death. As previously indicated, and as demonstrated in various examples in this book, the play therapist uses verbalization judiciously, and only tentatively ventures to make connecting statements between the child's play themes and the child's life experience. This matter of "interpretation" or of "clarification" is one of the trickiest tasks of the play therapist, and one that requires many years of supervised experience to master (Webb, 1989). Terr states that "overinterpretation may be more confusing and wasteful than is play without much direct interpretation. An entire treatment through play may be engineered without stepping far beyond the metaphor of the 'game'" (1989, p. 14).

Combined Approaches: Treatment Planning

Often it is desirable to employ a combination of individual, family, and group therapy/counseling in helping a bereaved child. One approach does not negate the other, and in fact different purposes are served through each modality.

As already mentioned, a family session is often very useful initially, just as it is helpful to see the child individually soon after the death. In the initial stages of work with a bereaved child, the counselor makes an assessment of the nature of the child's bereavement, even as he/she also begins to develop rapport and offer supportive help to the child. Depending on the therapist/counselor's evaluation, the decision may be to recommend a limited number of individual sessions, with a follow-up family session after 6–8 weeks. Referral of the child to a bereavement group might occur following this initial period of individual and family therapy/counseling.

There are no hard and fast rules about treatment planning. If the counselor/therapist found, in the family session, that the family as a unit seemed to be involved in dysfunctional behaviors such as scapegoating, withdrawal, or failing to function adequately to meet their own needs, then the treatment recommendation might more appropriately focus primarily on family therapy; alternatively, individual family members might be referred for individual bereavement counseling. On the other hand, if the family appeared to be functioning adequately despite its bereavement, the treatment plan might be to see the child individually, with parent counseling, or family sessions on an "as needed" basis. Terr states, with reference to working with traumatized children, "Most likely the treatment of childhood trauma will remain a multifaceted one, relying upon *several different approaches used simultaneously or in tandem*" (1989, p. 18; emphasis added). This statement is equally applicable to work with bereaved children.

Community Programs for Children

Because death often occurs in hospital settings, medical personnel have a central role in referring families to community-based programs suitable for their specific needs. For example, the American Cancer Society has a wide range of groups for patients and relatives affected by cancer. Many of these groups are co-led by a social worker and a nurse.

Hospice programs offer other resources. The hospice movement has grown from a single program in the United States in 1973 to more than 2,000 programs at the end of the 20th century (Kastenbaum, 1998). A growing number of services and programs have been developed especially for children and utilize art, storytelling, and play as methods for helping children express their grief. Increased awareness in the professional community about the nature of effective interventions with bereaved children has resulted in varied and age-appropriate services.

Camp programs provide other options for facilitating children's bereavement. Camps for terminally ill and bereaved children and/or family members have flourished throughout the United States for at least 20 years (Maher, 1995). Some of these camps consist of 3-day sleep-away weekend "retreats" for the entire family, whereas others consist of day programs for children over a 1- or 2-week period. All combine recreation with activities specially designed to promote bereavement. Some examples of the latter include a get-acquainted "icebreaker" activity in which children circulate among the group of participants looking for people who meet certain criteria, such as "who has flown in an airplane," "who has been to the cemetery," "who can snow ski," "who experienced a sudden death," and so forth. This activity mixes death-related information about the other campers with more general details about their lives (Hospice Southwest, 2000).

Most of the camp programs feature rituals for saying good-bye (Suarez & McFeaters, 2000), and many times this is in the form of a campfire memorial service that might include lighting candles in the bonfire and giving a brief tribute about the person who died (Moyer, 1988). Clearly these camp programs are very meaningful both for the child and family participants as well as for the professional and volunteer staff.

WHEN NO THERAPY/COUNSELING IS AVAILABLE: HOW DO CHILDREN COPE?

Although awareness is growing about the value and role of bereavement counseling and therapy for children, this need has not yet received sufficient recognition to merit routine attention in the schools. Death is ubiquitous, yet the response to it of most educational institutions occurs on a case-by-case basis. The notion of "psychological immunization" (Kliman, 1968) argues for "small doses" of information about stressful topics such as death for the purpose of preparing children in advance for the certain reality of future exposure. Whereas the *Good Touches/Bad Touches* curriculum (Turkel & Fink, 1986) appropriately informs and guides young children in New York State about the danger of sexual abuse, there is no similar preparation about the far greater certainty that they will encounter death experiences. Children *can* cope without such assistance, but how much better equipped would they be if a standard curriculum in the schools helped prepare them in the elementary grades for the reality that death exists and that it is a topic that can be discussed. There are some excellent children's books that could be used at different grade levels to stimulate such discussion.

Case Example: Amira Thoron—Bereaved, Age 3; "Closure," Age 23

Amira, one of the children portrayed in *How It Feels When a Parent Dies* (Krementz, 1981/1991), was 3 years old when her father died of cancer. Jill Krementz interviewed her when she was 9. Amira holds a picture of her father and reminisces about the few memories of him she can recall. In her account, the 9-year-old acknowledges that she has been fearful about the possibility of both her own and her mother's death. She had nightmares about something happening to her mother, and she would wake up crying because she was so frightened. At that time Amira prayed as her method of consoling herself. She also was beginning to demonstrate some ability to think about her life, apart from death issues. She commented as follows:

> I used to be a real worrywart and worry that I was going to die. But now I realize that the most important thing is to have fun. There are so many things in my life I'd like to do that I just want to try and do them and not worry about dying .... [W]hen somebody dies, it's just like taking away a part of me, but I try to replace them with someone else I know. Now I realize that no one can last forever and I think it's made me a stronger person. (Krementz, 1981/1991, pp. 98–99)

Eleven Years Later

Amira, then a college student, wrote the following letter to Jill Krementz, in which she speaks eloquently of her gratitude for having been asked in the interview about how she felt concerning her father's death:

Jill,

I just wanted to tell you that you were one of the first people to ask me how I *felt* about my father's death. I am so grateful to you and your gentle and caring questions. I really felt you cared.

And it is only now that I am truly grieving and processing my loss [emphasis added]. I want to thank you though, because I do feel *you planted a seed that what I felt and said was worthy of being heard and listened to* [emphasis added].

You gave me the beginning of a gift that I'm really learning and practicing now—that it's only in talking about my thoughts and feelings that I can heal the past and embrace my present with love, energy and courage. Thank you.

I love you.

Amira

This letter is published with the permission of both the writer and the recipient. When I contacted Amira to ask her permission to reproduce it in the first edition of this book, she shared additional information with me relevant to the topic of how children cope with the death of a parent.

Amira asked me to include the fact that she had attended the same boarding school as her father, and she realizes now that she was "looking for him there." She was a high achiever and won several awards at graduation. She recalls feeling very strongly that her father would be present to see her graduate from "his" school, especially since she had done so well.

This realization did not come spontaneously to Amira, but, rather, in the course of a grief-recovery workshop she attended one summer when she was in college. Amira sought out this workshop, traveled some distance to attend it, and credits it with making a tremendous difference in her life. The "step-by-step" program (James & Cherry, 1988/1989) emphasizes moving beyond the memories and pain of bereavement so that the individual can live more fully in his/her present life. Amira believes that since the 3-day workshop she has been more "free" to pursue her *own* interests, rather than following upon the path of her deceased father. Amira movingly described the finale of the workshop during which she was instructed to imagine her father's face as she spoke the following words: "I love you, I miss you, and good-bye."

The Issue of Timing

Impressed as I was with the sincerity and importance of Amira's grief work, I wondered if she might have achieved this state of acceptance about her father's death at a younger age. Those who believe mourning can be complete only after adolescence would see Amira's progression as normative. I asked Amira if she thought that she might have been helped sooner to talk about her father with a school counselor, nurse, clergyman, or teacher. She says now, at age 23, that she thinks she could have been helped sooner. She remembers no one reaching out to ask about her feelings before Jill Krementz interviewed her when she was 9 years old (5 years after her father's death). She is very supportive of my attempt, through this book, to recognize the needs of bereaved children. Amira wrote to me as follows: "I'm so grateful that I can give back some of what was given so freely to me. . . . I am so *relieved* that you, too, believe that children's voices and feelings should be heard. Thank you!"

EFFECTS ON COUNSELORS/THERAPISTS: VICARIOUS TRAUMATIZATION

The rewards of receiving appreciation and thanks from bereaved and traumatized children rarely take the form of warm and spontaneous letters such as those Jill Krementz and I received from Amira Thoron. More often the therapist/counselor is left with varying degrees of uncertainty about whether or not an intervention with a child was useful. Whereas the evaluation of the "success" of psychotherapy is almost always somewhat subjective, in work with the bereaved the therapist/counselor faces an irreconcilable barrier: We can *never* really achieve what the client wants— the return of their deceased loved one. Therefore, the therapist/counselor must have very clear goals about what he/she *can* achieve: not taking away the pain of the loss but, rather, helping the client gradually learn to live despite that loss. We must be able to tolerate tears and pain without becoming engulfed in them, and we must be able to withstand "horror stories" when we know that the child has witnessed traumatic scenes and needs to obtain whatever relief may come with the verbal or pictorial description of that horror.

There has been growing awareness in the field of traumatology about the possible negative side effects of this work. The term "vicarious traumatization" refers to the profound psychological effects that therapists may experience in response to exposure to the graphic and painful material presented by their clients. McCann and Pearlman state that "exposure to the traumatic experiences of the victim may be hazardous to the mental health of people close to the victim, including therapists involved in the victim's healing process" (1990, p. 135). According to these authors, the therapists' reactions may even replicate posttraumatic stress disorder (PTSD), evidenced by intrusive thoughts and painful emotional reactions (p. 144). Chapter 15 in this volume discusses issues and guidelines for therapists working with bereaved children.

When the client is a *child*, the therapist may even be more prone to strong reactions. These can include feelings of protectiveness, sorrow, grief, as well as feelings of "existential insecurity." Dyregrov and Mitchell state that "more than any situation, pediatric trauma and death triggers thoughts about life's meaninglessness and unfairness. . . . Since children are unable to protect themselves, their suffering is seen as unjust and unfair" (1992, p. 11). Dealing with a grieving adult is hard enough; when the bereaved is a young *child*, the therapist may feel a sense of outrage that, if unchecked, can interfere with the therapist's ability to help.

Coping Strategies for the Therapist/Counselor

There are methods that can help the therapist/counselor. Chapter 15 (this volume) discusses this topic in detail. The following suggestions were culled from the literature (McCann & Pearlman, 1990; Dyregrov & Mitchell, 1992; Johnson, 1989; Worden, 1991):

1. Avoid professional isolation through contact with other colleagues who work with victims and/or bereaved. "Debriefing" through talking to others soon after a stressful experience is helpful.

2. Normalize and avoid pathologizing the emotional responses of helpers. McCann and Pearlman (1990) view vicarious traumatization as a normal reaction to the stressful and sometimes traumatizing work with victims. Worden (1991) recommends "active grieving" for the counselor as a way to avoid burnout.

3. Understand your personal limitations and avoid undertaking work that goes beyond your ability to be effective. These limits will differ for different people and may depend on the nature of the bereavement circumstances as well as on the quantity of work focused on bereavement. Johnson states that "too much drain for too long can make any well dry up" (1989, p. 172).

4. Explore your own personal history of losses to identify "any irresolution still present from prior losses" (Worden, 1991). Because of the advisability of counselors to have "worked through" their own grief, someone who has been recently bereaved should not undertake this type of work until some healing and closure has occurred.

5. Recognize the positive consequences that can result from working with traumatized and bereaved children. In addition to identifying the stress of this work, we must admit the satisfactions. It can bring many personal rewards, flowing from the knowledge that we are contributing to a child's ability to proceed appropriately with his/her life.

REFERENCES

Alameda County Mental Health Services (1990). *How to help children after a disaster.* Alameda County, CA: Author.

Baker, J. E., Sedney, M. A., & Gross, E. (1992). Psychological tasks for bereaved children. *American Journal of Orthopsychiatry, 62*(1), 105–116.

Danto, B. I. (1983). A man came and killed our teacher. In J. E. Schowalter, P. R. Patterson, M. Tallmer, A. H. Kutscher, S. V. Gullo, & D. Peretz (Eds.), *The child and death* (pp. 49–74). New York: Columbia University Press.

Dyregrov, A., & Mitchell, J. T. (1992). Work with traumatized children: Psychological effects and coping strategies. *Journal of Traumatic Stress, 5*(1), 5–17.

Enzer, N. B. (1988). *Overview of play therapy.* Paper presented at the annual meeting of the American Academy of Child and Adolescent Psychiatry, Seattle, WA.

Eth, S., & Pynoos, R. S. (Eds.). (1985). *Post-traumatic stress disorder in children.* Washington, DC: American Psychiatric Press.

Hospice Southwest (2000). *Stepping Stones Family Retreat* [Mimeo]. Vancouver, WA: Author.

Hough, R. L., Vega, W., Valle, R., Kolody, B., del Castillo, R. G., & Tarke, H. (1990). Mental health consequences of the San Ysidro McDonald's massacre: A community study. *Journal of Traumatic Stress, 3*(1), 71–102.

James, J. W., & Cherry, F. (1989). *The grief recovery handbook: A step-by-step program for moving beyond loss.* New York: Harper & Row. (Original work published 1988)

Johnson, K. (1989). *Trauma in the lives of children.* Alameda, CA: Hunter House.

Kaplan, C., & Joslin, H. (1993). Accidental sibling death: Case of Peter, age 6. In N. B. Webb (Ed.), *Helping bereaved children: A handbook for practitioners* (pp. 118–136). New York: Guilford Press.

Kastenbaum, R. J. (1998). *Death, society, and human experience* (6th ed.). Boston: Allyn & Bacon.

Kliman, G. (1968). *Psychological emergencies of childhood.* New York: Grune & Stratton.

Krementz, J. (1991). *How it feels when a parent dies.* New York: Knopf. (Original work published 1981)

Maher, J. T. (1995). Camps: A therapeutic adjunct for children with cancer or HIV/AIDS. In D. W. Adams & E. J. Deveau (Eds.), *Beyond the innocence of childhood: Helping children and adolescents cope with life-threatening illness and dying* (Vol. 2, pp. 101–130). Amityville, NY: Baywood.

McCann, I. L., & Pearlman, L. A. (1990). Vicarious traumatization: A framework for understanding the psychological effects of working with victims. *Journal of Traumatic Stress, 3*(1), 131–149.

Moyer, J. A. (1988, March–April). Bannock Bereavement Retreat: A camping experience for surviving children. *American Journal of Hospice Care,* pp. 26–31.

Nader, K. (1997). Childhood traumatic loss: The interaction of trauma and grief. In C. R. Figley, B. E. Bride, & N. Mazza (Eds.), *Death and trauma. The traumatology of grieving* (pp. 17–41). Washington, DC: Taylor & Francis.

Pynoos, R. S., Frederick, C., Nader, K., Arroyo, W., Steinberg, A., Eth, S., Nunez,

F., & Fairbanks, L. (1987). Life threat and posttraumatic stress in school-age children. *Archives of General Psychiatry, 44,* 1057–1063.

Pynoos, R. S., & Nader, K. (1988). Psychological first aid and treatment approach to children exposed to community violence: Research implications. *Journal of Traumatic Stress, 1*(4), 445–472.

Schiffer, M. (1984). *Children's group therapy: Methods and case histories.* New York: Free Press.

Schwartz, W., & Zalba, S. (1971). *The practice of group work.* New York: Columbia University Press.

Suarez, M. M., & McFeaters, S. J. (2000). Culture and class: The different worlds of children and adolescents. In K. Doka (Ed.), *Living with grief: Children, adolescents and loss* (pp. 55–70). Washington, DC: Hospice Foundation of America.

Tait, D. C., & Depta, J. L. (1993). Play therapy group for bereaved children. In N. B. Webb (Ed.), *Helping bereaved children: A handbook for practitioners* (pp. 169–185). New York: Guilford Press.

Terr, L. C. (1989). Treating psychic trauma in children: A preliminary discussion. *Journal of Traumatic Stress, 2*(1), 3–20.

Turkel, D., & Fink, M. (1986). *Good touches/bad touches: A child sexual abuse prevention program.* White Plains, NY: Mental Health Association.

Walsh, F., & McGoldrick, M. (Eds.). (1991). *Living beyond loss: Death in the family.* New York: Norton.

Webb, N. B. (1989). Supervision of child therapy: Analyzing therapeutic impasses and monitoring counter-transference. *The Clinical Supervisor, 7*(4), 61–76.

Webb, N. B. (Ed.). (1991). *Play therapy with children in crisis: A casebook for practitioners.* New York: Guilford Press.

Webb, N. B. (1993). Suicidal death of mother: Cases of silence and stigma. In N. B. Webb (Ed.), *Helping bereaved children: A handbook for practitioners* (pp. 137–155). New York: Guilford Press.

Webb, N. B. (Ed.). (1999a). *Play therapy with children in crisis* (2nd ed.): *Individual, group, and family treatment.* New York: Guilford Press.

Webb, N. B. (Ed.). (1999b). School-based crisis assessment and intervention with children following urban bombings. In N. B. Webb (Ed.), *Play therapy with children in crisis* (2nd ed.): *Individual, group, and family treatment* (pp. 430–447). New York: Guilford Press.

Worden, J. W. (1991). *Grief counseling and grief therapy* (2nd ed.). New York: Springer.

Yalom, I. (1985). *The theory and practice of group psychotherapy.* New York: Basic Books.

12

❧

Bereavement Groups for Children
Families with HIV/AIDS

BARBARA O. DANE

Around the globe, children are direct or indirect casualties of familial illness and death, either as immediate survivors or as witnesses of deaths that involve multiple losses and trauma (Groves, Zuckerman, Marans, & Cohen, 1993). Increasing numbers of American children are members of families in which loved ones have died or are dying of AIDS. Children are very aware of these events, and even when adults try to minimize its importance, the young are sensitive to the experiences of death (Dane & Levine, 1994). Children from families with HIV/AIDS face a particular combination of vulnerabilities that sets them apart and merits special concern. Most young children who are orphaned are not themselves HIV infected but nonetheless are at high risk of economic deprivation, a range of behavioral and developmental problems, as well as the possibility of engaging in high-risk behaviors associated with HIV transmission. When their parents die, these children often need new sources of financial assistance, shelter, food, and medical care, in addition to emotional support and guidance (Dane & Miller, 1992). Children whose families are torn apart by social ills are profoundly affected by the additional crises of parental loss.

This chapter focuses on a bereavement treatment group for latency-age children who are orphans of the HIV/AIDS pandemic. The healing dimension to the experience of being heard and accepted by other grievers is outlined in eight group meetings. Therapists' reflections of planning and co-leading the groups are discussed, as well as stressors the children cope with when a parent dies of AIDS.

The hidden impact of AIDS has had its effects on two groups of children who are uninfected with the virus. The first group is the uninfected children who are siblings of brothers and sisters with AIDS or HIV infection. These may be older siblings, born before their mother contracted HIV, or younger children who escaped maternal–fetal transmission. The second and largest but almost invisible group includes uninfected children whose mother, father, or both parents, another adult relative, or a person unrelated by birth or marriage who has come to be considered a family member either died of AIDS or is living with AIDS or serious HIV disease (Dane, 1996). This latter group of children can rightly be called "orphans."

Children who live in families with HIV/AIDS undergo a particularly wounding experience that encompasses stigma, shame, secrecy, fear of disclosure, multiple loss, and survivor's guilt. When death is accompanied by isolation and followed by instability and insecurity, the bereavement process is more difficult. This is combined with the child's difficulties in understanding the impact of the diagnosis and in coping with the illness and death (Dane & Miller, 1992). Setting the stage for group intervention requires a thoughtful understanding of important issues that children may experience in different ways as family members are affected and die from HIV/AIDS. To understand the barriers to successful mourning and grief with a stigmatized illness, one must assess the family's socioeconomic, cultural heritage, and religious and/or spiritual beliefs. In addition, other factors within the communities in which these children live can help or hinder their attitudes toward pain, illness, and death.

All children orphaned by the HIV/AIDS epidemic share a specific set of concerns related to the death of a parent, but they are by no means a homogeneous group. Because of their vulnerability, children who lose a family member to AIDS face unique issues as they grieve. Often they have experienced the disintegration of their families. They struggle to make sense of a senseless situation and to remain in control, even as they confront circumstances over which they ultimately have no control. In addition to parental loss, many experience multiple deaths of a sibling, aunt, uncle, close relative, friend, or significant other. Many of these orphaned children have little or no safety and predictability in their lives (Dane & Levine, 1994). Parental death occurs within a web of other losses resulting from divorce or separation, mental illness, incarceration, homelessness, or drug addiction within a community plagued by poverty, violence, drugs, and unstable housing. Sometimes mourning the death of a parent is avoided and placed on a "back burner" because of the multiple complicating factors.

Children of HIV/AIDS parents should be considered at developmental risk (Brazdziunas, Roizan, Kohrman, & Smith, 1994) and in need of support services. The chronic illness and death of a parent are uniquely stressful life events (Christ et al., 1994; Rutter, 1987; Saler & Skolnick, 1992). Dohrenwend and Dohrenwend (1981) state that such stressful life events are often associated with increased symptoms of mental health disorder and more multiple negative outcomes. The lives of children whose parents died of AIDS are likely to have been stressful for many years prior to the deaths because adults involved in substance abuse typically lead chaotic lives (Zayas & Romano, 1994). Findings by Christ and colleagues (1993) indicate that the severe stress contributing to increased risk for these children may be even greater before the parent's death than that experienced afterward. Children whose parent died of AIDS often live in secrecy regarding the nature of the parent's illness, thereby increasing their sense of isolation and stigma associated with the illness and death (Doka, 1989). Secrecy and lack of communication also may increase a child's feelings of helplessness, hopelessness, despair, and detachment. Finally, these children often have numerous misconceptions due to their generalized lack of knowledge and insight about the disease, modes of transmission, and course of the illness, which may lead to fantasies about the death. Such children often exhibit symptoms of anxiety and stress (Lewis, 1995).

Although there is no agreement among studies regarding the ages at which children are most at risk of long-term negative consequences from the death of a parent, childhood appears to be a period of special vulnerability. The death of a parent in childhood, whether anticipated or not, may profoundly threaten normal psychological development (Furman, 1974; Siegel, Mesagno, & Christ, 1990). Younger children may also express their wishes, worries, or feelings in ways that may be less familiar than those used by adults—in play, drawings, or by changes in behavior (Furth, 1988; Webb, 1999). These need to be acknowledged and emotional support made available. Preventive intervention programs with children of cancer patients (Siegel et al. 1990) enable them to cope with the stresses of the terminal phase of illness and the acute grief period. Groups for children following a parent's death from AIDS may similarly serve to promote adjustment and support.

RESEARCH ON THERAPEUTIC GROUPS WITH CHILDREN

Group intervention has been effective with a variety of children's concerns: divorce, sexual abuse, bereavement, witness to violence, and academic performance (Masterman & Reams, 1988; Nisivoccia & Lynn 1999; Pelcovitz, 1999; Furman, 1974). It has been suggested that groups are more natural than individual treatment (Davis, 1989; Worden, 1982; Warmbrod, 1986). Beliefs and perceptions of the self are formed from the feedback of significant people in groups: family, friends, and peers. Children function as members of groups in their daily activities—in the family, the classroom, or the peer group. Ormont (1992) emphasized that people are social beings and that their development is influenced significantly by the groups around them. When considering treatment intervention for bereaved children, the support group offers a history of help for children who have suffered loss (Bonkowski, Bequette, & Boomhower, 1984; Epstein & Borduin, 1985).

Johnson and Johnson (1978) reviewed the literature for a definition of a group. They found that various definitions incorporated the following components: "A group may be defined as two or more individuals who (a) interact with each other, (b) are interdependent, (c) define themselves or are defined by others as belonging to the group, (d) share norms concerning matters of common interest and participate in a system of interlocking roles, (e) influence each other, (f) find the group rewarding, and (g) pursue common goals" (p. 7). The authors further state that "any effective group has three core activities: (1) accomplishing its goals, (2) maintaining itself internally, and (3) developing and changing in ways that improve its effectiveness" (p. 8).

A more recent review of the literature, however, reveals a paucity of research on the impact of bereavement support groups for children. The use of support groups with bereaved children is a relatively new phenomenon (Zambelli & DeRosa, 1992). Vastola, Nierenberg, and Graham (1986) describe a group program that they helped develop for bereaved latency-age children at a child guidance center located in an inner city. The authors suggest that a group approach for children who had lost a parent would allow experiences and feelings to be universalized and accepted by others. They further stated that helping to normalize the child's feelings and fantasies concerning the death is a major task. Masterman and Reams (1988) describe models of bereavement support groups for preschool and school-age children who suffered the death of a parent. They report that after their 8-week group treatment, the children in the sample appeared less constricted and angry, and much more able to understand and cope with their emotional reactions to the loss. The parents of these children reported a decrease in problem behaviors at home and school and an increase in communication with their children around bereavement issues that had not been previously discussed. The parents were quite positive about the effects that the group had on their children.

Davis (1989) considers the healing potential of art therapy and group process with grieving children. He discusses how children readily engage in art as a means of expression and how mutual sharing in a group setting provides an opportunity for children to express the emotive content of their trauma. Call (1990) reviews 32 completed school-based support and bereavement groups for children and adolescents that were developed by Cancer Family Care. Group members realized the universality of their experience of feeling their pain and were reassured that they were not crazy. This study underscored that children do not receive adequate support after a family member dies. Participants repeatedly expressed the insensitivity of family and friends and an inability of others to tolerate their need to express their feelings openly and often.

Opie et al. (1992) reports on a pilot exploratory descriptive study that looked at the effect of a bereavement group on the clients' affective and psychosomatic complaints. The study was conducted in two inner-city schools, a junior high school and an elementary school. A significant difference was found between pretest and posttest scores on somatic complaints for the elementary-school-age children only. Tonkins and Lambert's (1996) study of grief group treatment with children represents the first controlled study for the efficacy of such treatment. She found that following a short-term, eight-session grief group treatment, children's grief symptomatology was significantly diminished. Guided by theory, empirical research, and clinical experience, Schilling, Kohn, Abramovitz, and Gilbert (1992) tested a 12-session group intervention for 38 inner-city children who had lost a caregiver. Children rated themselves significantly more depressed at pretest than caregivers did; at posttest this difference diminished. The authors interpreted the reduced gap as indicative of the children's increased ability to express their grief to caregivers—hence, as an indication that intervention was effective. Open communication between parents and children, which permits a sharing of feelings, has been found to facilitate children's ability to mourn (Siegel et al., 1990).

Zambelli and DeRosa (1992) discuss the benefits of bereavement support groups for school-age children after the death of a parent. They believe that these groups may contribute new social meaning to this traumatic event. While statistics report that one out of seven children loses a parent to death before the age of 10, there has been a great reluctance to discuss or identify death and grieving issues in school children. Healy-Romanello (1993) found that grief support groups greatly support the child who has experienced a death in his family. Grieving children often do not have a familial or peer support network. Since other family members are also grieving, the child's family support system may not function as constructively as in the past or it may be nonexistent. Due to the debilitating effect of a death on the entire family, the child may be in need of support from an outside source.

In bereavement support groups children learn to share their feelings, discover that they are not alone, and begin moving through the process of grieving. A time-limited group intervention (Lahnes & Kalter, 1994) was developed for parentally bereaved elementary-school-age children (6- to 12-year-olds), in order to address the difficulties that parentally bereaved children experience both socially and emotionally. New and valuable insights were gleaned from children's thoughts and feelings about parental death and its aftermath. Group participants were described as being remarkably frank and articulate about fears, wishes, and conflicts—a phenomenon that has been usually thought of as beyond their conscious awareness. In addition, children typically talked about having hallucinations of their dead parent. In other contexts this might be considered indicative of serious psychopathology. Themes relating to ongoing fears about safety, stigma, parental dating and remarriage, and the struggle of going on with life reflected the children's psychic pain about their immediate sense of loss, and also clarified their need for help in adjusting to the stresses of having a parent die. Witte and de Ridder (1999) described a group of latency-age children (8–12 years old) affected by HIV disease and provided guidelines for group facilitators that emphasize the importance of the leaders' self-awareness. (See the two chapters on bereavement groups in the first edition of this book [Tait & Depta, 1993; Hickey, 1993].) In summary, bereavement support groups for children can provide a clear sense that others have experienced similar thoughts, emotions, and feelings, which can in turn be a source of support and comfort to them.

PRESCREENING

Many group leaders prefer having a meeting or intake interview with prospective members before forming a group; other group leaders believe that anyone should be eligible to join a group and that the intake interview is unnecessary. An intake interview allows the leader an opportunity to talk privately with prospective members, to learn a little about them and their concerns, and to define some possible goals. The leader also has an opportunity to determine if the child will benefit from a group experience. It also serves as the beginning of a relationship between the leader and the child.

In organizing a group, the leader must consider the appropriateness of each child for the group and assess the family's level of functioning before and since the death. The leader should invite the remaining parent or guardian to participate in the intake assessment process. An intake questionnaire for both parent/guardian and child provides the group leader with valuable information, including the child's attitudes, behaviors, and feelings since the death. Exploration of the child's physical problems, possible changes in eating and sleeping patterns, and school performance gives the group leader a sense of the family's present situation and whether the child is appropriate for group intervention. For some children, individual treatment may be a more appropriate modality, especially if the family has a history of continuous unresolved conflicts or maladaptive coping patterns (Moody & Moody, 1991).

Segal (1984) described children's responses to death as expressions of grief through symbolic communication. He stated that following a death children may respond with denial, assume responsibility for the loss and feel guilty, internalize or act out their anger over the loss, withdraw, repress their feelings, become obsessed with fear about future losses, seek spiritual comfort ("Mom is in heaven"), feel confused about the facts, become dependent, or develop a closer relationship with a friend or sibling to gain emotional support. Segal noted that because these feelings are communicated *nonverbally*, the clinician must become familiar with some primary modes of nonverbal communication in considering whether the child is a candidate for group intervention.

A strength of the intake process is that it allows the family and child to meet the leader(s) and become acquainted with the setting, thereby reducing the child's anxiety in the first session. The child may also benefit from meeting separately with the leader to ask questions about the group and learn about how many members may attend, some of the group activities that may take place, and other issues specific to group affiliation.

GROUP MEMBERSHIP

The number of children in the group depends on their age, maturity, and attention span. Children of 5 and 6 years of age have very short attention spans and are unable to give much attention to others' concerns. Group leaders often limit group size at this age to three or four members and work with the children for only short periods of time at frequent intervals, 20 minutes twice a week. For older children, ages 8–12, a 30- to 45-minute session is practical. To function effectively, eight should be the maximum number of children in a group.

Fleming (1985; Fleming & Balmer, 1991, 1996) reports that initially he sought to differentiate between the death of a parent and the death of a sibling in his groups, based on the uniqueness of each relationship. He found, however, that children often share similar feelings about type of death and the tasks of grieving are the same. In general, the kind of death experienced does not appear to be a barrier to a cohesive group for children. Programs that are well established may have sufficient members to provide separate groups for each kind of loss. Survivors of suicide may encounter greater degrees of guilt, blame, denial, and anger than survivors of other types of death. It may be difficult to live with the social stigma of suicide, and a conspiracy of silence may emerge. Groups help work through the anguish, guilt, anger, shame, and perplexity and, as Lucas and Seiden (1987) suggest, "It's time to end the silence" (p. 210).

FORMAT

The common experience of loss creates a bond between members that leads to feelings of acceptance and unity despite the groups' varied and changing membership (Roy & Sumpter, 1983). Some groups are open ended; that is, members can join at any point in the life of the group and may terminate at any point. Schwab (1990) cites the advantages of an open format that allows members to come to the group several times without having to make an ongoing commitment. The group remains a safe and supportive resource, and a member has the option of returning to the group during especially difficult times, such as holidays or anniversaries. However, the lack of predictability and the erratic nature of the discussions—sometimes disjointed, sometimes intimate or distant—can have an impact on the worker (Corr, Nabe, & Corr, 2000).

More typically children's bereavement groups tend to utilize a closed (i.e., time-limited) format in order to help members cope with their experience of grief and loss and to maximize their current life experience. Such a structure demands an ongoing commitment to the group to foster trust and a stable sense of community (Lahnes & Kalter, 1994). It is necessary to contract with the members to prevent instability and unnecessary loss in a group that has already sustained multiple losses. Trotzer (1977) states that continuity of membership coupled with frequent contacts helps maximize effectiveness by encouraging cohesiveness within the group, thus allowing the children to get to know and depend on each other.

EVALUATION OF GROUP MEETINGS

Bruckner and Thompson (1987) provide a model for evaluating weekly group sessions with elementary school children that could be adapted for use with bereavement groups for children whose parent died of AIDS. These authors developed an instrument containing the following six incomplete statements and two forced-choice items:

1. I think coming to the group room is _____.
2. Some things I have enjoyed talking about in the group room are _____.
3. Some things I would like to talk about that we have not talked about are _____.
4. I think the group leader is _____.
5. The group leader could be better if _____.
6. Some things I have learned from coming to the group are _____.
7. If I had a choice, I (would) (would not) come to the group.
8. Have you ever talked with your parents (guardian) about things that were discussed in the group? (yes) (no)

Some of these items may be used as a needs survey for future group sessions. Two independent persons rate group members responses on a 5-point scale, ranging from 5, for statements showing an outright positive, accepting attitude toward the item, to a rating of 1 for statements showing an outright rejecting, negative attitude toward the item. A rating of 3 is awarded to neutral, ambivalent, or evasive responses. Limited positive and limited negative responses receive ratings of 4 and 2, respectively. Raters should reach 85% levels of agreement and generally experience little difficulty in obtaining agreement on the remaining 15%.

ISSUES FOR GROUP LEADERS

Haasl and Marnocha (1990) identify some particular characteristics as important for bereavement group leaders. These include comfort with and interest in children; comfort with and knowledge of the grief process; empathy, sensitivity, and warmth; a nonjudgmental attitude; and flexibility. In addition, a facilitator needs to be able to tolerate the pain that grieving children and their parents feel and express. The purpose of the group is to help children move toward grief and not away from it. It is necessary, therefore, for facilitators to be able to tolerate the expression of grief, and to encourage participants to express their painful feelings.

Heegard (1990) notes that it is important for facilitators to acknowledge and share their own personal grief issues for them to be most effective in supporting bereaved children. Exploring his/her own history of losses, including ways of coping, can give a leader insight into a child's current feelings. Further, remembering earlier childhood experiences of loss or death helps put a person in touch again with the unique childhood perspective of such experiences (see the "Personal Death History" form in

Tait & Depta, 1993, p. 183). According to Heegaard (1990), the facilitator's role focuses on six basic tasks:

- Teach basic concepts.
- Help children recognize, accept, and express feelings.
- Provide opportunities for risks and problem solving.
- Encourage open communication and opportunities to learn from each other.
- Give support and encouragement.
- Discover unhealthy misconceptions.

Each of these can be addressed through children's activities, sharing times, and the dynamics of group process. Almost all programs acknowledge the importance of cofacilitation of groups. Tait and Depta (1993) propose that the ratio between supportive adults and children be as low as possible. Having at least two facilitators per group allows one person to attend to the needs of a specific child while the other facilitator continues with the group process. Anschuetz (1990) also suggests that cofacilitators together share the intensity of the emotions that such groups express (and evoke). The importance of having another leader to help plan, process, and evaluate the group is self-evident.

Dyer and Vriend (1988) list 20 group leadership skills crucial for group counseling effectiveness:

1. Identifying, labeling, clarifying, and reflecting *feelings*: the facial expressions, body posture, movements, tone of voice, eye activity, and other behavioral indicators that are indicators of feelings.
2. Identifying, labeling, clarifying, and reflecting *behavioral data*: understanding the meaning and cause of behaviors in relation to the group process itself, the interaction of group members, and the individuals' goals.
3. Identifying, labeling, clarifying, and reflecting *cognitive data*: skills necessary to help members change their methods of thinking and communicating in order to be more effective.
4. Questioning, drawing out, and evoking material for *counseling focus*: helping counselees decide what they are willing to work on, to change, or to risk.
5. Confronting: identifying and pointing out discrepancies in how the group member thinks, feels, or acts, while conveying acceptance of the person.
6. Summarizing and reviewing important material: important for correcting distorted perceptions, to provide focus and direction, to assist members to recall important information, and to help members set goals.

7. Interpreting the underlying meaning of a member's statement or experience in order to correct distortions or misperceptions.

8. Restating the essence of a client's statements in a manner that clarifies and eliminates ambiguity. (This skill is especially important in children's groups because of their limited cognitive abilities.)

9. Establishing connections: attending closely in order to see relationships that help the member gain insight.

10. Information giving: appropriately providing "expert" information about group procedures, leader expectations, direction, and other topics important to the group.

11. Initiating: the ability to develop a plan of action in order to introduce appropriate material at a given moment.

12. Reassuring, encouraging, and supporting: to help members through difficult moments.

13. Intervening: interrupting when the group activity is unproductive (when a member speaks for everyone, blames others for his/her problems, or begins to ramble.)

14. Dealing with silence: recognizing when silence can be productive and when it should be dealt with. (Silence seems to be less a problem in children's groups than in adult groups.)

15. Recognizing and explaining nonverbal behaviors: continually observing the nonverbal signals sent by members and using the information at the appropriate time.

16. Using clear, concise, meaningful communications: avoiding lectures, jargon, sarcasm, talking excessively, rambling. (Working with children requires an appropriate developmental level of language to assure that members understand what is being said.)

17. Focusing or staying on task. (Counselors working with children need to be very proficient in this area. Depending on their age, children need more structure in their groups to stay involved and on track.)

18. Restraining, subduing, and avoiding potentially explosive and divisive group happenings: being able to determine when tensions are rising and deal with them constructively.

19. Goal setting: help members to set individual goals that are specific, relevant, achievable, and measurable.

20. Facilitating closure: effectively summarizing and planning for the end of a session or the end of the group experience.

Workers need to utilize these techniques in addressing the process of the group. The techniques can be adapted by the leader to meet the needs of the group members to foster emotional communication and express their thoughts and feelings.

INTERVENTIONS

Group activities are designed to help children experience and come to terms with their thoughts and feelings about the death. Creative arts, ritual, and storytelling engage them in individual as well as small- and large-group activities. When they work alone, they are encouraged to later share their achievements and interpret their work within the group. Group activities can be designed thematically to assist young children to understand the permanence of death and to express their confusion or denial concerning the irreversibility of death.

Within the group, children can work with their memories through storytelling, drawing, and sharing of tangible memory items. When children listen to their peers' "death stories," they have an opportunity to grapple with the reality of death with each new story. Children can decorate treasure boxes to hold their memory items and share photographs of the deceased. Children who lack a clear memory of their loved one can be encouraged to explore feelings associated with the deceased and talk about their "shattered dreams and wishes."

Rituals

Ritual is set apart from the everyday world and can effectively create a safe "container" for intense emotion. The ritual components of the group create a special place where children can safely share their grief. The opening and closing rituals at the beginning and end of each session help to clearly define the nature of the grief group "container." A memorial service can be designed to honor the memory of the deceased. Children can create and participate in a ritual that can involve lighting candles, drawing a picture of the deceased, reading a special biography of the deceased, saying prayers, reading poems, and playing music. At the end of the service, children can blow out their candles and say good-bye to the deceased (Ormand & Charbonneau, 1995).

Games and Exercises

Segal (1984) recommends games and communication exercises to help children express feelings related to losses. He suggests passing out small blank cards and pencils to children in a group, asking them to write down a question about death or dying, and assuring them that the writer's name will not be revealed. The group leader reads the questions, and the children discuss their thoughts about the questions. Alternatively, the group leader may prefer to write the questions on cards ahead of time and ask each child to draw a card, read the question, and answer it with his/her views. Art techniques, including crayon drawings, clay, or hand puppets, may help children portray their conflicts. Children can be asked to sculpt or carve a figure representing someone for whom they have a great deal of love; usually the figure is the person they lost. These drawings, carvings, or hand puppets can express the pain of the loss more easily than the child can verbalize it.

Segal (1984) describes a technique for illustrating feelings with paper and music. The children draw "peaceful" views of death on one side of the paper while listening to soft music; then they draw "harsh" views of death on the other side of the sheet while listening to dissonant music. Phototherapy (having the child respond to different photographs of men, women, or children) may stimulate discussion concerning losses of loved ones. Use of all nonverbal means of communication should be followed with a discussion of their meaning and of coping strategies for the various problems revealed.

Poppen and Thompson (1975) describe group activities that enhance self-concept by focusing on children's strengths. One such activity is to have members of the group share something about themselves, such as their favorite activity and why they enjoy it, and then have group members write all the good points observed about each member on a 3 × 5 card. Another is to have each group member draw something he/she does well and wear the drawing for the rest of the day. Children seldom have their good points recognized, and these exercises create good feelings and serve as a stimulus for group guidance activities. Bowman (1986) describes an interesting idea for facilitating group guidance. In addition to familiar attention-getting techniques such as puppets, art, music books, dramatics, humor, and yoga that are effective in working with children, he suggests magic. His review of the literature showed that magic increases self-concept, eye-hand coordination, patience, attending behavior, and interpersonal skills; stimulates creative thinking and increases children's curiosity; and reinforces lessons on safety.

CASE EXAMPLE: THE MEMORY LANE BEREAVEMENT GROUP

Grief is a natural and normal response to loss. Sometimes children are denied access to this process due to feelings of shame and social stigma, which frequently accompanies deaths related to AIDS (Doka, 1989). Children often feel embarrassed and remain silent out of fear of being rejected or ridiculed. Oftentimes they feel lonely and isolated. Groups can provide bereaved children a safe supportive context in which they can express feelings that are kept secret in their family. Further they can receive support from both their peers and the group leader and co-leader. The Memory Lane Bereavement Group was developed to meet the needs of children whose parents died of AIDS and who are presently living with their guardians. Both the children and their guardians were members of a church group. The group was offered since many of the parishioners have had an adult child die of AIDS, and many of the surviving families are raising nieces, nephews and grandchildren. The group model, with some modifications, was based on a treatment protocol (Kazdin, 1988) that includes weekly themes and activities.

An abbreviated weekly outline of the group treatment is as follows:

Week 1: Introduction of leader and co-leader, children, and group; expectations of group; confidentiality; rules; promotion of the idea of expression of feelings.

Week 2: General discussion of child and deceased; discussion of how the deceased died and the child's involvement during the illness and at the time of death.

Week 3: Focus on positive memories of the deceased; discussion of feelings regarding self and the change of self since the death; discuss type of support they have; activities that focus on symbolic thanks to the deceased for positives; games that facilitate questions regarding death in general.

Week 4: Art project that focuses on things the children miss from the deceased; discussion of sadness, anger and fears.

Week 5: Focus on unfairness of death and feelings of anger through discussion and tai chi project.

Week 6: Focus on possible reasons for feeling guilty; guided imagery exercise in forgiving self; discussing unfinished business through storytelling.

Week 7: Symbolic good-bye scenario to deceased; ritual to memorialize the impact of the deceased on their lives.

Week 8: Discussion of importance of a support system and good-byes to the deceased and group members.

Family Information

Prior to the group, the children's guardians were interviewed. Ten grandmothers responded to the announcement at the church and the flyers that were posted, advertising a group for bereaved latency-age children, ages 7–11. Each grandmother was interviewed, and questions were asked to assess the child's emotions, thoughts, behaviors, and physical symptoms during the parent's illness and after the death. Queries were made about demographics, the parent's history of AIDS, the disclosure process, the grandmother's reactions to the child after the death, the age of the parent, time of death, funeral services, and the amount of preparation for the parent's anticipated death as well as discussion of postdeath reactions. The proposed Memory Lane Bereavement Group activities were described, and the number of meetings, times, and place were indicated. A consent form was signed. The problem of absenteeism from the group was addressed in advance with the grandmothers (there was a full turnout at all eight meetings). The grandmothers were encouraged to prepare the children for the group and to describe the activities.

After meeting with each grandmother, each child was screened for his/her ability to benefit from the group experience. The proposed activities were described for the 8-week sessions that would take place at 2:00–3:30 after the end of Sunday services. The meeting would be held in the church community room, and refreshments would be served before the group began. The children were spontaneous and open in talking about their parent's death but felt they could not discuss it among their peers, relatives, or friends. Some children said they were called the "AIDS kids" in school. The children had no overt psychiatric problems but had been exposed to a variety of stressors including illness and death in the family, adult drug and alcohol use, and violence in their neighborhood. Seven children were eager to begin the group. Jessica was reluctant to join the group. She had experienced the death of both parents within the last year. They died two months apart. However, she felt she "would give it a try" since her two friends Mol and Keesha were going to attend. The group members were as follows:

Name	Age	Person who died	How long ago
Keesha (sibling of Mol)	8	Mother, sister	2 yr
Beverly	8	Mother, father, brother	2 yr
Jean	8	Mother, two aunts	3 yr
Ronald	9	Mother, uncle, sister	2 yr
Jessica	9	Mother, father	1 yr
Mol (sibling of Keesha)	9	Mother, sister	2 yr
Susan	10	Mother, aunt, uncle	22 mo
Mark (sibling of Jerry)	10	Mother, father	3 yr
Jerry (sibling of Mark)	11	Mother, father	3 yr

All the group members had experienced multiple deaths and their unrelenting feelings of sorrow, loss, and abandonment could be described as "bereavement overload." This occurs when an individual has not completed the bereavement process for one person when another dies. This dynamic adds to the difficulty of coping with the death of a parent (Dane & Levine, 1994). Three of the children indicated that their baby sister and brother died when they were infants. Mark, Jerry, and Jean's parents had contracted HIV through injecting drugs and lived for 2 years in a homeless shelter. Each couple returned to live with their relatives before they died.

Presently, all the group members were active with their grandmothers in the church. The church has been, and continues to be, the original self-help institution and a safe place for emotional release for African Americans (Boyd-Franklin, Steiner, & Boland, 1995). Attitudes among religious individuals toward homosexuality and drug use vary widely. Initially, in the AIDS epidemic the disapproval of the church in African American communities was particularly crucial, since it has historically constituted a major social support, primarily in times of grief and bereavement. However, in recent years ethnic churches have become actively involved and are supportive and helpful to families and individuals who have survived their loved one's death from AIDS (Dane & Miller, 1992). In 1998, the view of death from AIDS in the black community is reflected in statements like "What a waste! What went wrong?" and "Whose fault is it?" (Lynch & Hanson, 1998).

There are social, ethnic, cultural, and religious variations in the expression of emotions. Traditionally, ritual has been an important element of the leave-taking process, and funeral customs are a primary source of this ritual. As clinicians we must be knowledgeable about acceptable practices in helping survivors receive comfort from their religious and cultural beliefs. The power of rituals comes not from magic but from the faith the individual has in his/her ability to provide meaning (Dane & Miller, 1992). All the group members were African American and lived with their mothers, fathers, and other family members through their illness and death. All the children were aware of the parents' death due to AIDS. All but one child attended the funerals of all their family members. The presence of children at different points in time since the death of their parents provided the group with a broad perspective and hope about the bereavement process. Children in this group knew each other within the church context. Confidentiality was discussed with Jessica, Mol, and Keesha, and their feelings about being in the same group were explored since their presence could either help or hurt the process.

Presenting Problem

The bereaved youngsters were referred to the program by their grandmothers, who themselves had sustained multiple losses of family members. The criteria for membership in the group were as follows:

- The death of a parent
- The child's age between 8 and 11 years

- The child's ability to tolerate a group setting with a ratio of two leaders and seven other children
- The child's demeanor and resiliency and ability to tolerate group interaction

The following were the specific goals of the group:

1. To provide a safe place for children to experience and rework emotionally painful aspects of the death
2. To clarify death and AIDS-related issues that present confusion and fear
3. To normalize children's reactions to and experiences of the death of parents, siblings, and relatives
4. To develop coping strategies to deal with their grief
5. To help children maintain an emotional connection to their parents

First Contact with Children

Session 1: Getting Acquainted

The first session is very important in setting the atmosphere for the remaining group meetings. It establishes the tone for the children to connect to the group and allows them to feel safe and secure. As each child enters the room, they are greeted by the leader and co-leader and invited to participate in refreshments of juice and cookies. After 10 minutes, the children are invited to an adjoining room where they sit around a big table. The leader first explains the purpose of the group, including that we will be meeting for 8 weeks. The leader reviews the "rules." The rules are crucial. Confidentiality, not leaving the group space, and allowing "one person to talk at a time" is discussed. The children are invited to suggest other rules. Beverly and Jean shake their heads, saying, "These are enough."

The leader begins by stating that everyone here has experienced the death of a parent and some children have experienced the death of a sister, brother, aunt, uncle, grandparent, and other relatives and friends: "We are here to help each other." An important aspect of the first session is to provide the opportunity to "tell your story." For most children, this may be the first time they have been invited to discuss their family's death. Each child, in turn, is offered the opportunity to introduce him/herself and relate the details of his/her loss. We bring out 12 puppets to bring humor and balance to what can be an overwhelming experience. We ask members to tell us about themselves through the puppet. We have the children each choose a puppet and give it their name. We encourage them to participate to the extent that they feel comfortable. The group leader reminds the members to listen carefully to each other's feelings and thoughts, and to help each other explore possible solutions to a problem. The leaders demonstrate both empathy and listening skills by using a puppet to respond or pass a tissue box or "check-in" with a child. The co-leader, through the puppet, invites the children to take a turn to respond to another member's "story."

The invitation to tell one's story is viewed as an integral beginning in the healing process (Parkes & Weiss, 1983). It also has an additional therapeutic impact. Invariably, as the circumstances of the dying and death unfold, some children possess more information than others do. It is not uncommon for those who lack details or have unanswered questions to seek this missing information from their relatives. Throughout the session, the leader and co-leader empathize and help to label the feelings that emerge. The members show great enthusiasm and an eagerness to tell their story. For children who are bereaved survivors, puncturing the "conspiracy of silence" begins to strengthen their ego to cope with the fantasies about the deceased parent or sibling that are an integral part of grief work.

Session 2: Relationship to the Deceased— before and after Death

Prior to the session the children spend 10 minutes having cookies and juice, and then go to the group room. A ritual of feeding the children before the therapy sessions is beginning, and each session will commence in this way. Therapists who conduct children' groups often structure the group activities to include a snack (Madonna & Caswell, 1991). Davis (1989) found that a snack served as a symbolic manifestation of the children's concerns about trusting adults.

Content of Session	*Analysis and Feelings*
LEADER: Today, we are going to draw *two* pictures. Choose a person that has died in your family. Close your eyes and make a mental picture of that person.	The choice of what the child draws often reveals potentially problematic thought/ feelings that may hinder grief resolution.
THEY RESPOND: I see my mother . . . my father . . . my brother . . . I remember my mother.	
L: Okay, lets take those pictures and draw a scene on one page of that person, when he or she was sick. On the other page, draw a picture of what	

happened on the day of the person's death and funeral.

MOL: That was 2 years ago. My mother's picture is not that sharp!

Painful feelings are emerging that may be suppressed

KEESHA: You can look at my picture, Mol. I remember Mommy.

Group support begins between sibling members.

CO-LEADER: Mol, would you like to sit next to Keesha?

JERRY: This is dumb. *(Looks around and begins to draw a picture of his father.)*

Looks for support. Leader nods, reassuring him he can do it.

PATRICK: *(Looking at Jerry's pictures.)* What's the other picture we have to do, Barbara?

RONALD: Hold on, I'm not ready with finishing my mother. Pass the magic markers.

Some anxiety begins to emerge.

(The children are finished with the first picture.)

CL: Are you ready to draw the second picture?

EVERYONE: Yes.

MARK: What are we going to do with this picture?

CL: For a moment, let's place them on one side. . . . Now, let's draw a picture of what happened to the person *after* he or she died.

JEAN: I didn't see my mother. The coffin was closed. We went to the cemetery.

Reveals possible conflict.

L: You may want to draw a picture of the cemetery.

KEESHA: Did you all go to the cemetery when your parents died?

Anxiety is emerging.

RONALD: I saw my mother in a coffin. She looked so beautiful.

JESSICA: *(Tears begin to surface.)* I did not go to the funeral. You are all so lucky. I was sick.

SUSAN AND JEAN: *(Both touch Jessica's*

Group support is beginning to

hand.) That's terrible! Do you want to look at our pictures? *(Both tasks are completed.)*

L: Who would like to tell us about their pictures?

KEESHA: This is a picture of my mother, when she was sick. She was very skinny and had air going into her nose. When she died she was buried in this coffin. *(Holds picture up.)* It has two angels that live with her in the cemetery. Grandma said they watch over Mommy, Mol, and me.

SUSAN: My mother and aunt had a coffin like that.

BEVERLY: This makes me sad. All of us don't have a mother. *(Looking at both leaders.)* Do you have a mother?

MOL: *(Interrupting.)* I don't have a mother!

SUSAN: *(Interrupting.)* I don't have a mother!

L: Let's each take a turn and give each person a chance to talk about his or her upset feelings.

CL: My mother died when I was very young, and my friend Barbara's mother is still living.

BEVERLY: I feel sad. I don't have a mother. I did not go to the cemetery. I think my mother is angry at me for not coming. We were close friends. I still did not go to the cemetery. My aunt keeps promising, but no action.

CL: What are the rest of you feeling? *(The children slowly begin to place the puppets on the table and ask questions like: How long was your mother sick? Were you screamed at in school when they found your mother had AIDS?—All expressed a wish that things could go back to the way they were. They also said*

emerge. How encouraging they can be to each other!

Thinking about Beverly's history. How old was she when her mother died?

They are all referring to the present. Everyone had a mother—but some remember her more clearly than others.

Reestablishing the ground rules is important.

Disclosure seem to help and normalize the groups feelings

The leaders are very attuned to their sadness. She is angry, and is feeling deprived.

Raw pain is felt by both the children and the leaders. Silence is pervasive to contain the pain.

how they screamed and banged on
chairs, tables, and walls the day their
mother died.)

Toward the end of the session both leaders reflected on the children's affective and sad emotions that came up when they talked about the painful illness and death of their loved ones. This helps minimize the leaders' defense against the terror of death and one's own immortality. Each week, the leaders assessed what is appropriate, helpful, or necessary to raise in the context of a bereavement group and how to bind the normative anxiety that emerges. Leaders can only allow the group to develop, grow, express, and relieve their pain when they feel safe with the discussion. Group members can collude with the worker to avoid dangerous, painful, and self-revealing discussion. Reflecting on both the group process and the leaders' feelings helps contain the powerlessness and stresses that one experiences in a bereavement group.

Session 3: How Things Have Changed

The leader began: "Today we are going to begin by making a circle and creating a story of an imaginary family where the parents were living with AIDS and were very sick. Our story can reflect a day or two in their lives before their death." Common themes that emerged during the "go-round" were caring for the sick parent, self-blame for the death (not getting aspirins for the mother), not enough time to play with friends, fear of going to sleep at night, anger that the parent got AIDS and died, and worry that someone (particularly grandmother) would get sick and die. Several children and one grandmother in the imaginary family repeatedly said things like "Stop doing drugs. You see what happens when you inject that stuff."

This activity allowed group members to explore selective parts of who they were and provided an experiential outlet to release their feelings of anxiety, anger, and sadness. The leaders universalized statements around anger, fear, and confusion. This displacement technique helped the children to address taboo feelings more directly. The children used this time to reminisce with each other about their deceased family members, providing a strong supportive experience.

During the second part of the session, the children worked in two groups. The group leaders helped the children develop a family and then sculpt how the family changed after the death of the person they loved. The children projected the characters, setting, and situations from this family. A few children responded critically to the family picture, which created a dilemma since it was difficult to agree initially on the "new family." The catalyst for change comes as alternative and compromise are worked through:

Content of Session	Analysis and Feelings
LEADER: Who would like the part of the parents?	Testing: Death is a frightening possibility—even in play.
SUSAN: Do we have to die in the play?	
BEVERLY: No, silly, just be very sick.	
CO-LEADER: What would happen if someone played that part, Susan?	Wonder if she has worried about that?
SUSAN: We would know what they were thinking, before they died.	

This intervention helps identify their emotional feelings and the sculpting becomes a portrait of their lives. The first half of the session children process the rupture in their lives created by death. This helps them navigate the pain of loss and rewrite the way things are now, which promotes healing and growth. The leaders help by validating their feelings and accepting their frustrations with their losses and adapting to their new family structure. This activity allows group members to explore selective parts of who they are and provides an expressive outlet to release their feelings of anxiety, anger, and sadness while piecing together a family through active imagination.

Sessions 4 and 5: Missing the Parents/Unfairness of Death—Weather Chart and Tai Chi Animals

These sessions were intended to provide continued opportunities to grieve the loss of the parent. Exercises were created based on tai chi so the children could be spontaneous and continue to find a safe and helpful place to talk about their experience of death.

As early as 190 A.D. Hau T'o, founder of Chinese surgery, wrote about a system of exercises called the frolics of five animals, the tiger, deer, bear, monkey, and bird. Using deep breathing methods, he invented a form of circular movements intended to bring the person to his/her full potential and achieve a longevity of about a hundred years. The exercise directs the breath into the upper, middle, and lower abdomen through focused concentration of the mind and the banishing of all wandering thoughts (Kit, 1993).

We began session 4 by asking the children if they ever saw Bruce Lee's punches. After an overwhelming "yes," we read a story of the animals and demonstrated movements with the body. Immediately they began mimicking the strokes. We had them draw pictures of the animal they would like to be and helped them make a mask. No child wanted to be a bird. We again demonstrated with the masks the breathing and the sounds of each animal.

Each child took a turn being an animal. Throughout this session, we elicited feelings from the children and encouraged each of them to relate these feelings to their parent's death. The leaders talked about common themes that emerged which created a community of support while decreasing levels of anxiety and distress. It highlighted the children's need to release painful feelings and memories of the deceased parent.

In session 5 we asked the children to draw two pictures: one picture was what the weather was like on the day of the funeral; the other was the temperature (inner) they felt today.

Creating a picture is a first step in getting out some of those thoughts and feelings that are building up "inside" (Furth, 1998)—a first step in regaining a feeling of control at a time when so many things can seem out of control if they are put "outside." Once feelings are expressed on paper, group members can show it to other people and talk about it.

A large piece of paper is placed on the floor, a piece large enough for all group members to have a space to draw both their pictures. The children interpret their pictures to the group. Much of the initial anger is gone for most of the children. However, some are still engulfed in the intense pain of grief. The purpose of this session is to allow the children to compare notes as they describe the changes they are struggling with and the coping strategies they employ to survive.

Session 6: Story and Guided Imagery

In session 6 we read a storybook, *Thank You, Jackie Robinson*, about a slowly deepening friendship between 12-year-old Sam Greene and the elderly black cook, Davy, in Mrs. Greene's restaurant. After they have together followed the career of their "main man"—Jackie Robinson—Sam is bereft when Davy suffers a fatal heart attack. The book helped avoid direct anxiety-provoking confrontations by using symbolic language. The therapeutic goals of storytelling are (1) gaining wisdom that comes from a story that specifically educes an understanding of oneself, and (2) directing the child "more to the encouragement and reinforcement of strengths than to the diagnosis of problem areas" (Hynes & Hynes-Berry, 1986, p. 17). These goals promote the belief that the locus of control is from within and that children can access inner strengths from problem solving and self-healing. We process the story through imagery. McAdams (1993) suggests that children "make the image do what they want it to do, even in ways that seem strange and illogical to adults" (p. 55).

Spirituality is as much a part of the human search for fulfillment as any other aspect of humanity. Canda (1989) has emphasized that suffering and alienation are part of human life, so spirituality "involves confronting these courageously and faithfully while developing a sense of meaning and fulfillment that enables coping and transcendence" (p. 43). Guided imagery used to say good-bye helps the children to find meaning. Here is an example:

"Close your eyes and breathe in and out five times. You are in the middle of the deep woods smelling the pine trees and watching the sun glisten through the forest. You are with your immediate family chanting songs for your parent(s) who died. The chants become very loud and strong. There are vigil candles and fresh flowers surrounding you. One by one each family member steps forward and nods his head and says good-bye. It is now your turn. Feel your heart. Surround yourself with the peace, the inner calm and light that is yours. Feel all the love and spiritual strength you have at this moment. Stay connected to that spiritual love. Again, keep connected to your breathing. When you are ready, open your eyes and come back to the room."

Then, for about 15 minutes, we debrief the children about their experiences of feeling relaxed, light, body tingling, wanting to return to the forest, and wondering if they could repeat the image. We encourage the children to do this at home and create their own healing images.

For our session on rituals next week, we ask the children to bring in photos or other objects of attachment to their deceased parent.

Session 7: Rituals; Sharing Photos; Good-bye to Parents

In every culture throughout history mourning rituals have developed to help people accept the deaths of those close to them. In ancient Mesopotamia, tear vials, similar to bud vases, were found buried with the deceased in tombs. This simple act acknowledged the emotional significance of loss, the value of grieving, and—in burying those tears with the deceased—the importance of moving on with life (Walsh & McGoldrick, 1988, 1991).

In this session, the children brought in pictures of their deceased parents or other family members. Some brought other mementos of the person. These were their cherished possessions. The room was lit with candles and a large table with a cloth was in the center of the room. The children sat on the chairs in a semicircle. We first talked about rituals in our everyday lives like brushing our teeth, eating, waking up, and going to school. They added to the list of rituals. Today's ritual is to memorialize the deceased person's memory.

One by one each child brought a picture, doll, handkerchief, and/or ring of the deceased person, and laid it on the table. We encouraged them to tell a story about the object and also the person we were memorializing. Themes of sadness, loss, and good memories were evidenced in the following:

JESSICA: This poem is about my mother.

Mother

I am so glad you were my mother. Remember the time we went to beach and I got
lost. You were so worried. I don't go to the beach anymore.

Miss you, Mother.

Good-bye, Mom.

IN UNISON: Good-bye, Jessica's mother.

JESSICA: I brought a picture of my mother in her casket. Remember, I told you I was sick and could not go to the funeral. *(Holds up her picture.)*

MOL: *(A wooden Santa Claus is placed on the table.)* Mommy, what I miss most is baking the cookies for Santa and leaving them on the table. I always knew you and Uncle Pete ate them when I went to bed. It's two years since you died. I still can't be happy on Christmas.

STEPHEN: Dad this is a picture I drew of what you look like now. Picture shows a tombstone and people crying. Angel overhead says, "Your Dad is OK." I dreamed this one month ago and felt good drawing it and bringing it here today.

PATRICK: This is a letter I wrote to my mom. Picture of mother is posted to the letter.

MOM:

I miss you very much. Sometimes I think I see you on the street or in the subway. I look real hard and know it's not you. I am trying to go on with my life.

Each week grandma, Barbara and Rhonda say its ok to have fun and "go on with life". I know you are watching me and keeping me safe.

Mom, I love you and miss you.

Your son,

Patrick

This session helped the children to hold on the memory of the deceased parent(s) and, through expressions of longing and sadness, go on with their present life. The leaders often reminded the children that their parents would be happy to know that they are enjoying their life and growing up and this does not mean they are disloyal.

Session 8: Good-Bye to the Loved One and to Group

The last session was a good-bye to the deceased loved ones and to the group. Kites were bought for every child and brought to the group.

Content of Session	Analysis and Feelings
Each child selected a kite and two had to negotiate with the co-leader's help on selecting a color that was not their favorite.	Anxiety regarding ending and wanting to delay the process through a distraction.

We suggested they write a letter of good-bye or another wish to the parent. We then taped the letter to the kite. Assembling in the churchyard, we marched about 10 times in a circle with the kites flying in the air. The song "Amazing Grace" was sung. We then released the kites while clapping and throwing kisses.

Once back in the group room we had cookies and juice and took turns saying what we liked and what was helpful and what they would suggest not to repeat. It was hard to choose one activity, and all seemed to be well received. No child could verbalize what he/she would not like repeated. We took group pictures and distributed them so they could have a memory of the Memory Lane group.

CONCLUDING COMMENTS

This chapter described a support group for children, ages 8–11, whose parent(s), siblings, family members, and friends in their immediate communities lived with and died from AIDS. Immediate and timely professional interventions for children mourning these deaths can mitigate some of the negative lifelong responses to this overwhelming trauma. The group gave support to the children while providing a forum of safety to express their feelings and concerns about surviving in the aftermath of AIDS. A therapeutic atmosphere was established through a myriad of planned play activities, which expanded and identified coping skills while validating and supporting their concerns and fears. The leaders demonstrated empathic understanding, genuineness, and respect for group members.

Some reflection for therapists planning a children's bereavement group are proposed in the following topics: the function of food; the use of ritual and storytelling and sharing; number of sessions; mutual support of the leader and the co-leader; siblings; termination; and evaluation.

Function of Food. The group provides opportunities for curative factors described by Yalom (1985). Food serves as a vehicle whereby the therapists can align themselves with the members in a therapeutic partnership. Food can represent love, power, and rapport, serving as a tool to elicit clues as to where there are psychic conflicts related to nurturing.

Rituals and Storytelling/Sharing. Stories offer a natural language for children and adults. Stories that heal often exude optimism and hope, providing nourishment and encouragement about the possibility of change. It is best to avoid all verbal analysis or attempts to promote the children's conscious awareness of the underlying meaning of the stories. Children possess resilience and healing, despite their emotional and spiritual pain related to death. Rituals provide a way to master cycles of disruption while remembering, integrating, and transforming the loss.

Number of Sessions. A time-limited group was adapted from a widely used and systematically researched model of parentally bereaved children (Seigel et al., 1990; Masterman & Reams, 1988; Zambelli & DeRosa, 1992). It was intended to help children cope with difficult feelings, stigma, and their newly reconstituted family following AIDS bereavement. Our announcing in advance that there would be only eight sessions may have helped the children quickly cohere and interact with the leaders and other group members. The techniques of activity and directed leadership may have contributed to the solid cohesiveness of the group, as well as members' shared association as members of the church group.

Mutual Support of the Leader and the Co-Leader. The facilitators were aware of their own history of loss and immediate death experiences. Weekly debriefing following the group session enables the leaders to connect with their personal pain that is evoked when leading bereavement groups and needs to be addressed. Normalizing some of the children's potentially distressing and problematic fantasies and symptoms allows the facilitators an opportunity to discuss how they might intervene during the group sessions when these emotions surface. Comfort with one's feelings and reactions requires the leaders to recognize their limitations as well as their countertransferential feelings of avoidance, overprotectiveness, and personal history of "parentification."

Siblings. Careful assessment needs to be made before the group begins as regards the acceptance of siblings in the same group. The presence of a sibling can either hurt or help the process. In the group described above, two sets of siblings were members. In neither set did one sibling attempt to dominate the other; each showed respect and was able to hear his/her sibling's views, concerns, and fears. This might not happen in all instances. Age and personality differences should be carefully considered.

Termination. This may have warranted more attention than it was given, inasmuch as this particular set of group members experienced multiple losses. Although balanced, thoughtful group selection is generally important, that did not happen in this group, which was self-selected. We did not, however, have children with acting-out and conduct disorders. These children were naturally inclined to verbalize and participate in group activities, thus making the termination a smooth transition.

Evaluation. To address the unmet needs of bereaved children, an evaluation component with a pretest and posttest will need to be built in so that a systematic research model can be developed. A weakness in our group format was not having a follow-up meeting with the grandmothers to share information about any changes that they may have observed over the 8 weeks. Positive reports were received informally from both the grandmothers and members of the church community. To assess the effectiveness of the group for bereaved children we plan to offer this group again, adding a component for evaluation.

*   *   *

Clinical social workers can enhance the grief journey of a child whose parents died of HIV/AIDS through the mutual healing that takes place in a group. When a parent dies, children are often left to mourn alone. Groups fill a void and provide support and a message that each member can enjoy life again.

Children whose world has been darkened by the death of those they loved become less anxious by being exposed to group members who have suffered similar losses and are on the path of developing new insights and strengths as they grieve. Group treatment for latency-age children from families with HIV/AIDS can legitimize their feelings of grief, stigma, shame, and isolation, and so further the healing process.

DISCUSSION QUESTIONS

1. Comment on the first step in achieving confidentiality with children affected by HIV/AIDS. How can the leader respond to the group members when there is a breach of confidentiality?

2. How can leaders respond to their own feelings of sadness/anger and loss during the group session? When is self-disclosure appropriate and/or helpful to both group members and the leaders?

3. If it becomes apparent to the leaders that a child in the group is seriously depressed/withdrawn, how should this be handled? If a child proves to be inappropriate and unresponsive in the group, how do the leaders intervene (with the child, the group, the caretakers)?

REFERENCES

Anschuetz, B. L. (1990). *Bereavement counseling group for adolescents: Training manual.* Ontario, Canada: Author.

Bonkowski, S., Bequette, S., & Boomhower, S. (1984). A group designed to help children adjust to parental divorce. *Social Casework, 65,* 131–137.

Bowman, R. (1986). The magic counselor: Using magic tricks or tools to teach children guidance lessons. *Elementary School Guidance and Counseling, 21,* 128–136.

Boyd-Franklin, N., Steiner, G. L., & Boland, M. G. (Eds.). (1995). *Children, families, and HIV/AIDS: Psychosocial and therapeutic issues.* New York: Guilford Press.

Brazdziunas, D. M., Roizan, N. J. M., Kohrman, A. F., & Smith, D. K. (1994). Children of HIV-positive parents: Implications for intervention. *Psychosocial Rehabilitation Journal, 17,* 145–149.

Bruckner, S., & Thompson, C. (1987). Guidance program evaluation: An example. *Elementary School Guidance and Counseling, 21,* 193–196.

Call, D. A. (1990). School-based groups: A valuable support for children of cancer patients. *Journal of Psychosocial Oncology, 8*(1), 97–118.

Canda, E. (1989). Religious content in social work education: A comparative approach. *Journal of Social Work Education, 25,* 36–45.

Christ, G. H., Siegel, K., Freund, B., Langosch, D., Henderson, S., Sperber, D., & Weinstein, L. (1994). Impact on parental terminal cancer on latency-age children. *American Journal of Orthopsychiatry, 63,* 417–425.

Corr, C. A., Nabe, C. M., & Corr, D. M. (2000). *Death and dying, life and living* (3rd ed.). Belmont, CA: Wadsworth.

Dane, B. O. (1996). Children, HIV infection, and AIDS. In C. A. Corr & D. M. Corr (Eds.), *Handbook of childhood death and bereavement* (pp. 51–70). New York: Springer.

Dane, B. O., & Levine, C. (Eds.). (1994). *AIDS and the new orphans: Coping with death.* Westport, CT: Auburn House.

Dane, B. O., & Miller, S. (1992). *AIDS: Intervening with hidden grievers.* Westport, CT: Auburn House.

Davis, C. B. (1989). The use of art therapy and group process with grieving children. *Special issue: The death of a child, III. Issues in Comprehensive Pediatric Nursing, 12,* 268–280.

Dohrenwend, B. S., & Dohrenwend, B. P. (Eds.). (1981). *Stressful life events and their contexts.* New York: Prodist.

Doka, K. (Ed.). (1989). *Disenfranchised grief: Recognizing hidden sorrow*. New York: Free Press.

Dyer, W., & Vriend, J. (1988). *Group counseling for personal mastery*. New York: Sovereign.

Epstein, Y., & Borduin, C. (1985). Could this happen?: A game for children of divorce. *Psychotherapy, 22*, 770–773.

Fleming, S. J. (1985). Children's grief: Individual and family dynamics. In C. A. Corr & D. M. Corr (Eds.), *Hospice approaches to pediatric care* (pp. 197–218). New York: Springer.

Fleming, S. J., & Balmer, L. (1991). Group intervention with bereaved children. In D. Papadatou & C. Papadatos (Eds.), *Children and death* (pp. 105–124). Washington, DC: Hemisphere.

Fleming, S. J., & Balmer, L. (1996). Bereavement in adolescence. In C. A. Corr & D. E. Balk (Eds.), *Handbook of adolescent death and bereavement* (pp. 139–154). New York: Springer.

Furman, E. (Ed.). (1974). *A child's parent dies: Studies in childhood bereavement*. New Haven, CT: Yale University Press.

Furth, G. M. (1988). *The secret world of drawings: Healing through art*. Boston: Sigo.

Groves, B. M., Zuckerman, B., Marans, S., & Cohen, D. J. (1993). Silent victims: Children who witness violence. *Journal of the American Medical Association, 269*, 262–264.

Haasl, B., & Marnocha, J. (1990). *Bereavement support group program for children*. Muncie, IN: Accelerated Development.

Healy-Romanello, M. A. (1993). The invisible griever: Support groups for bereaved children. *Special Services in the Schools, 8*(1), 67–89.

Heegard, M. E. (1990). *Coping with death and grief*. Minneapolis, MN: Lerner.

Hickey, L. O. (1993). Death of a counselor: A bereavement group for junior high school students. In N. B. Webb (Ed.), *Helping bereaved children: A handbook for practitioners* (pp. 239–266). New York: Guilford Press.

Hynes, A. M., & Hynes-Berry, M. (1986). *Bibliotherapy—the interactive process: A handbook*. Boulder, CO: Westview Press.

Johnson, J., & Johnson, M. (1978). *Tell me, Papa: A family book for children's questions about death and funerals*. Omaha, NE: Centering Corporation.

Kazdin, A. E. (1988). *Child psychotherapy: Developing and identifying effective treatments*. Elmsford, NY: Pergamon Press.

Kit, W. K. (1993). *The art of chi kung: Making the most of your vital energy*. Rockport, MA: Element Press.

Lahnes, K., & Kalter, N. (1994). Preventive intervention groups for parentally bereaved children. *American Journal of Orthopsychiatry, 58*, 562–570.

Lewis, M. (1995). The special case of the uninfected child in the HIV-affected family: Normal developmental tasks and the child's concerns about illness and death. In S. Geballe, J. Greundel, & W. Andiman (Eds.), *Forgotten children of the AIDS epidemic* (pp. 50–63). New Haven, CT: Yale University Press.

Lucas, C., & Seiden, H. (1987). *Silent grief: Living in the wake of suicide*. New York: Scribner.

Lynch, E., & Hanson, M. (1998). *Developing cross-cultural competence* (2nd ed.). Baltimore: Brookes.

Madonna, J. M., & Casewell, P. (1991). The utilization of flexible techniques in group therapy with delinquent adolescent boys. *Journal of Child and Adolescent Group Therapy, 1,* 147–157.

Masterman, S. H., & Reams, R. (1988). Support groups for bereaved pre-school and school-age children. *American Journal of Orthopsychiatry, 58,* 562–570.

McAdams, D. P. (1993). *Stories we live by.* New York: Morrow.

Moody, R. A. & Moody, C. P. (1991). A family perspective: Helping children acknowledge and express grief following the death of a parent. *Death Studies, 15,* 587–602.

Nisivoccia, D., & Lynn, M. (1999). Helping forgotten victims: Using activity groups with children who witness violence. In N. B. Webb (Ed.), *Play therapy with children in crisis* (2nd ed.): *Individual, group, and family treatment* (pp. 74–103). New York: Guilford Press.

Opie, N. D., Goodwin, T., Finke, L. M., Beattey, J. M., Lee, B., & Van Epps, J. (1992). The effects of a bereavement group experience on bereaved children's and adolescents' affective and somatic distress. *Journal of Child and Adolescent Psychiatric and Mental Health Nursing, 5*(1), 20–26.

Ormand, E., & Charbonneau, H. (1995). Grief responses and group treatment interventions for five- to eight-year-old children. In D. Adams & E. Deveau (Eds.), *Beyond the innocence of childhood* (Vol. 3, pp. 181–202). Amityville, NY: Baywood.

Ormont, L. (1992). *The group therapy experience: From theory to practice.* New York: St. Martin's Press.

Parkes, C. M., & Weiss, R. (1983). *Recovery from bereavement.* New York: Basic Books.

Pelcovitz, D. (1999). Betrayed by a trusted adult: Structured time-limited group therapy with elementary school children abused by a school employee. In N. B. Webb (Ed.), *Play therapy with children in crisis* (2nd ed.): *Individual, group, and family treatment* (pp. 183–199). New York: Guilford Press.

Poppen, W., & Thompson, C. (1975). *School counseling: Theories and concepts.* Lincoln, NE: Professional Educators.

Roy, P., & Sumpter, H. (1983). Family support and a child's adjustment to death. *Family Relations, 32,* 43–49.

Rutter, M. (1987). Psychosocial resilience and protective mechanisms. *American Journal of Orthopsychiatry, 57,* 57–72, 316–331.

Saler, L., & Skolnik, N. (1992). Childhood parental death and depression in adulthood: Roles of surviving parent and family environment. *American Journal of Orthopsychiatry, 62*(4), 504–516.

Schilling, R. F., Kohn, Abramovitz, R., & Gilbert, L. (1992). Bereavement groups for inner-city children. *Research on Social Work Practice, 2*(3), 405–419.

Schwab, R. (1990). Paternal and maternal coping with the death of a child. *Death Studies, 14,* 407–422.

Segal, R. (1984). Helping children express grief through symbolic communication. *Social Casework, 65,* 590–599.

Siegel, K., Mesagno, F., & Christ, G. (1990). A prevention program for bereaved children. *American Journal of Orthopsychiatry, 60,* 168–175.

Tait, D. C., & Depta, J.-L. (1993). Play therapy group for bereaved children. In N. B.

Webb (Ed.), *Helping bereaved children: A handbook for practitioners* (pp. 169–185). New York: Guilford Press.

Tonkins, S., & Lambert, M. (1996). A treatment outcome study of bereavement groups for children. *Child and Adolescent Social Work Journal, 13*(1), 3–21.

Trotzer, J. P. (1977). *The counselor and the group: Integrating theory, training, and practice.* Monterey, CA: Brooks/Cole.

Vastola, J., Nierenberg, A., & Graham, E. H. (1986). The lost and found group: Group work with bereaved children. In A. Gitterman & L. Shulman (Eds.), *Mutual aid groups and the life cycle* (pp. 75–90). Itasca, IL: Peacock.

Walsh, F., & McGoldrick, M. (1988). Loss and the family life cycle. In C. J. Falicov (Ed.), *Family transitions: Continuity and change over the life cycle* (pp. 311–336). New York: Guilford Press.

Walsh, F., & McGoldrick, M. (Eds.). (1991). *Living beyond love: Death in the family.* New York: Norton.

Warmbrod, M. E. (1986, June). Counseling bereaved children: Stages in the process. *Journal of Contemporary Social Work,* 351–358.

Webb, N. B. (Ed.). (1999). *Play therapy with children in crisis* (2nd ed.): *Individual, group, and family treatment.* New York: Guilford Press.

Witte, S., & de Ridder, N. (1999). "Positive feelings": Group support for children of HIV-infected mothers. *Child and Adolescent Social Work Journal, 16*(1), 5–16.

Worden, J. W. (1982). *Grief counseling and grief therapy: A handbook for the mental health practitioner.* New York: Springer.

Yalom, I. D. (1995). *The theory and practice of psychotherapy.* New York: Basic Books.

Zambelli, G. C., & DeRosa, A. P. (1992). Bereavement support groups for school-age children: Theory, intervention, and case example. *American Journal of Orthopsychiatry, 62*(4), 484–493.

Zayas, L., & Romano, K. (1994). Adolescents and parental death from AIDS. In B. O. Dane & C. Levine (Eds.), *AIDS and the new orphans* (pp. 59–76). Westport, CT: Auburn House.

13

Art as a Component of Grief Work with Children

ROBIN F. GOODMAN

Childhood is the kingdom where nobody dies.
—MILLAY (1934/1969, p. 203)

Over 2 million children in the United States, or slightly more than 3%, endure the death of a parent before age 18 (U.S. Bureau of the Census, 1990); death clearly *does* invade a child's world. Given this fact, talking to children about death should not be taboo. However, most adults steer clear of the topic with children. An adult's need to maintain an idealized, magically untarnished view of childhood serves perhaps to preserve a fantasy of immortality for him/herself. Children, on the other hand, do not have this need to avoid death. In fact, it becomes a subject of curiosity, as with many events in a child's life. After experiencing death, children often embrace opportunities to communicate their feelings about it despite being confused or upset. But children are not miniature adults, and they don't necessarily have or express their strong feelings in a watered down, diminutive form. We must respect children's unique understanding, manner of displaying, confronting, and mastering their grief. For many children art offers a valuable vehicle for meeting the challenge of bereavement.

This chapter focuses on integrating art therapy into other techniques to help children communicate, understand, and cope with their grief. The

297

case of a 14-year-old boy with recurrent abdominal pain following his father's suicide highlights the value of a nonverbal therapeutic intervention. Art was particularly well suited to the boy due to his shy personality, learning disability, interest in art, and age.

RESEARCH ON CHILD AND ADOLESCENT GRIEF

Research on child and adolescent grief reactions is sparse. Conclusions from existing studies are mixed, yet refer to potential disequilibrium and/or clinical symptomatology for children in the beginning months after a death. Bereaved children and teens may meet criteria for a major depressive episode but overall, they have fewer symptoms than children hospitalized for depression. They differ from normal (nonbereaved) children with respect to school behavior, interest in school, peer involvement, peer enjoyment and self-esteem (Fristad, Jedel, Weller, & Weller, 1993; Weller, Weller, Fristad, & Bowes, 1991). Although less likely to develop an anxiety disorder immediately following a death, children who exhibited the most anxiety were more likely to have a depressive disorder (Sanchez, Fristad, Weller, Weller, & Moye, 1994).

Dysphoria, loss of interest, appetite disturbance, sleep disturbance, psychomotor agitation or retardation, declining school performance, withdrawal, guilt/worthlessness, morbid/suicidal ideation, headaches, and gastrointestinal tract disturbances are the most commonly reported symptoms in bereaved children (Sood, Weller, Weller, Fristad, & Bowes, 1992; Van Eerdewegh, Clayton, & Van Eerdewegh, 1985; Weller et al., 1991). When bereaved and depressed children were compared, symptoms of guilt/worthlessness and fatigue were identified *more* in the bereaved and were the best means of discriminating between the two groups (Weller et al., 1991). Similar to adults, not all bereaved children exhibit these symptoms, and evidence of morbid or suicidal thoughts does not necessarily indicate suicidality. The longing to be reunited with the deceased parent rather than a wish to be dead is the more likely basis for suicidal thinking (Weller et al., 1991). Preexisting child and family mental illness, the gender of the surviving parent, socioeconomic status, and the child's age are some of the compounding variables that influence a child's or teen's reaction and adjustment (Van Eerdewegh et al., 1985; Weller et al., 1991). Inconsistencies between the symptoms reported by the parents and children in many studies indicate the necessity for directly assessing children and teens in addition to interviewing parents in order to obtain a thorough evaluation.

BEREAVEMENT IN ADOLESCENCE

By age 10, most children have acquired a mature understanding of death—an understanding that it is irreversible, final, and inevitable, and an understanding of how it is caused (Goodman, 1999). But the emotional response of any individual child or adolescent depends on pertinent developmental issues. As a teen traverses the path from childhood to adulthood he contends with profound physical, emotional, and social changes. Teenagers must begin a new stage of separation from their family as they are propelled toward independence, are occupied with forming an identity, and are establishing a social network. When a parent dies, the bereaved teen can feel protective of the surviving parent, feel pressure to assume a parental role, and experience a sense of detachment from peers. Bereaved adolescents face special challenges related to their being reluctant to show strong emotions, discomfort talking to parents about feelings, lacking a model or acceptance for strong displays of emotion, and feeling different from and misunderstood by peers at a time when affiliation is important.

Bravado, denial, anger, and sadness can exist separately, coexist, or alternate for teenagers coping with such a loss. They may escape into the world of activities and friends. They may push their emotions underground, and adults may accept their behavior as resistance to accepting help. Adolescents' pain can be difficult to access, and their narcissism can make them difficult to reach. Engaging teens can become a thorny proposition when confronted with the combination of normal adolescent issues and grief. Using a nonverbal and less intimidating intervention can be helpful for the teen who is self-conscious about revealing his/her feelings yet interested in art. Upon remembering what happened when his mother died at age 15, an 18-year-old remarked:

> When my mom died, I thought my heart would break. Yet, I couldn't cry. My friends and family said, "Be strong, you can take it." You just have to face it and get on with your life. . . . Everyone said my mom would have wanted me to go to college. What was interesting about this is that no one would talk about what my mom's death meant to me, but they sure would use her to get me enrolled in the right college. I needed to talk about my mom, but they wanted to talk about college. (in Wolfelt, 1990, pp. 60–61)

CHILDREN, ART, AND BEREAVEMENT

Direct access to a child's world is often achieved by way of his/her imagination, where thoughts, ideas, and feelings interact freely with facts. Therapists can capitalize on this, finding that therapeutic communication can be easier or more direct through the use of symbols or images rather than through the complex world of spoken language. Image making can be powerful for the child and significant for the therapist. Talking and making art are very different activities, even involving different spheres of the brain. Words offer a credible yet often incomplete re-creation of experiences. For example, words can be inadequate when describing the aroma of fresh-baked cookies or a beautiful sunset. The kinesthetic qualities of the recollection are difficult to capture in language unless that language is imagistic. Thus, our deepest, strongest, and most difficult feelings are likely associated closely with nonverbal representations. Visual artists achieve greatness by re-creating an experience for the audience via evocative and poignant images.

Therapy relies on the transfer of private sometimes vague, unpleasant, and confusing feelings, such as those associated with a significant person's death, into something shared. Images have the capacity to capture and confront such abstract, unformed, difficult feelings: "Art has the ability to revive the enshrouded past of a trauma through a dialogue in the present. In creating a holding witnessing 'other' that confirms the reality of the traumatic event, the artist can provide a structure or presence that counteracts the loss of the internal other, and thus can bestow form on chaos " (Laub & Podell, 1995, p. 993). "In narrating about past traumas, the person changes his or her relationship to them and what they mean to him or her in the present" (Mishara, 1995, p. 184). Research on the therapeutic value of writing for Holocaust survivors informs us about the art-making process for those suffering a loss (Pennebaker, Hughes, & O'Heeron, 1987). Individuals who wrote about traumatic experiences "showed significant improvements in immune responsiveness, physical health, and remission from other psychosomatic symptoms" (Mishara, 1995, p. 182). Similarly in art, when a child depicts his/her feelings on paper the therapist then can help the child observe, react, change, correct, and master them.

STRUCTURE AND FORMAT
OF ART THERAPY SESSIONS

Those using art in therapy with children follow one of two different traditions. In general, when using an "art as therapy" approach, the *process and product* are the significant focus for change (Kramer, 1971). In "art psychotherapy," the *thoughts* stimulated by the art making become the focus (Naumburg, 1987). Thus, art making can be used as a valuable tool for symbolic communication without direct reference to a particular topic such as death (art as therapy), or the art may be used to stimulate direct discussion about an issue (art psychotherapy). In either approach, talking and creating can occur simultaneously, where one enhances or clarifies the other. The process of externalizing significant memories in the art becomes a bridge for discussing unarticulated thoughts and feelings about death in the case discussed in this chapter.

The structure of art therapy sessions with bereaved children and adolescents varies. Clients may be seen individually, in families, or in groups, for unspecified ongoing periods of time or for a previously determined amount of time, depending upon the particular case formulation (Junge, 1985; McIntyre, 1990; Zambelli, Clark, & Heegaard, 1989). Within the session, therapists also employ different techniques. A nondirective style allows for a more open-ended unfolding of issues. A more direct presentation of particular themes and activities, based on a core curriculum, is often the method of choice in time-limited sessions and in groups (e.g., Zambelli, Clark, Barile, & de Jong, 1988). Art based therapeutic bereavement groups for children usually occur with companion parent groups (Zambelli et al., 1988). The art therapy literature presents variations on these formats, and on the focus, be it stimulation of feelings, problem solving, or improved family functioning (Zambelli et al., 1989).

Age is a prime consideration when a therapist is determining the form of treatment. Younger children may benefit from more targeted interventions, or gentle suggestions from the therapist, in order to focus on bereavement issues. Older children, on the other hand, may become involved in elaborate projects that encompass complex issues requiring in-depth execution, carry-over for more than one session, and considerable discussion. Thus, I structure sessions with children according to their age, their interest in and skill with particular materials, and their psychological needs. For example, I made symbolic Play Doh memory pills with a 4-year-old whose father had died. She pretended to swallow them in order to guarantee that memories of her father would be locked inside forever. We also decorated a "memory box" filled with styrofoam creations—one object representing past memories with her father, and one unnamed object representative of future memories without him. I encouraged an 8-year-old who endured her younger sister's unsuccessful year-long battle with cancer to draw pictures, in consecutive sessions, of her life before and after her sister died to provide a framework for our understanding the changes in her life.

GENERAL GUIDELINES FOR BEREAVEMENT WORK WITH CHILDREN AND ADOLESCENTS

Assessment of the bereaved child and subsequent verbal or nonverbal intervention involves understanding the child's (Christ, 1999; Liotta, 1996;

Webb, 1996, see also Webb's, *tripartite assessment of the bereaved child*, Chapter 2, this volume):

- Personal thoughts and beliefs about death
- Relationship with the person who has died
- Memories of the person who has died
- Relationship with the surviving family members
- Current feelings and functioning
- Personality
- Family and social environment and supports
- Adaptation to life changes resulting from the death

The *therapist's tasks* include the following (Christ, 1999; Liotta, 1996):

- Assessing bereavement related symptoms, thoughts, and feelings
- Normalizing the grief process
- Allowing nonverbal and verbal content to be revealed at the child's own pace
- Encouraging trust
- Respecting existing feelings
- Aiding adjustment to changed family relationships
- Supporting mastery of the events and emotions
- Promoting continued age appropriate development and reengagement and reinvestment in activities and peers

The *main goals* of the treatment include having the child (Adams-Greenly, 1984; Goodman, Williams, Agell, & Gantt, 1998):

- Establish a trusting relationship
- Express feelings in a safe environment
- Awaken and explore memories of the deceased person
- Understand and adjust to life that has changed

In general, as Hemmings (1995) explains:

The aim or resolution of mourning is not to create an emotionally safe distance between the living and the dead, but a different and new closeness. This closeness should not inhibit or interfere with the bereaved person's ability to form or maintain attachments to others. . . . As the child matures, so her ability to appreciate the significance and personal meaning of this life-event alters. . . . It is . . . wholly inappropriate to expect children to "get over" or "through" early childhood loss because, to a lesser or greater extent, it is part of who they are and is not affected by irrelevant time limits. (p. 21)

The following case highlights the therapeutic tasks and goals as they were addressed through art.

CASE OF RICHARD SULLIVAN, AGE 14

Richard, a 14-year-old fraternal twin, was referred following the suicide of his father.

Family Information

Mother, Joan Sullivan, age 42, bookstore manager
Maternal grandfather, Walter Paterson, died 20 years previously from a heart attack
Maternal grandmother, Judith Paterson, died 10 years previously of lung cancer and with a long history of severe depression
Fraternal twin brother, Philip Sullivan, age 14
Richard Sullivan, age 14, the client
Father, Tom Sullivan, suicide at age 45, 9 months prior to initial contact; diagnosed with schizophrenia at age 31, 3 years after being married
Paternal grandmother, Suzanne Sullivan, died 3 years previously from a stroke at age 69

The paternal grandfather is unknown.

Presenting Problem

Approximately 7 months after Richard's father committed suicide, Richard, his twin brother, Philip, and his mother all had a stomach virus. However, Richard continued to have loose bowels and severe cramps. He was evaluated by his pediatrician and gastroenterologist for various ailments, such as parasites, and treated for various conditions, including lactose intolerance. Due to his significant discomfort Richard stayed home from school for 3 weeks, after which time his pediatrician put him on home school instruction with a tutor. Following a thorough medical workup ruling out any physiological cause for his physical distress, Richard's pediatric gastroenterologist referred him for psychotherapy. Mrs. Sullivan, Richard's mother, also suffered from various stress-related abdominal symptoms (e.g. nausea, upset stomach) following the death of her husband, but she felt the problems were under control when Richard began treatment.

Immediately following the father's death, prior to Richard beginning individual therapy with this therapist, the family went for counseling together for 3 months, and his mother continued in individual treatment for an additional 8 months with the therapist.

Background Information

The family was at home together one spring afternoon when Mr. Sullivan jumped out the window of their fifth-floor apartment. Richard's brother ran to the bedroom on hearing the window open and witnessed his father jumping out. Richard ran downstairs to find his father, still alive, on the ground.

Mr. Sullivan had suffered various mishaps in his life, such as being mugged (leaving him almost blind in one eye) and experiences with law enforcement due to his intermittent delusional behavior. He was on disability secondary to his mental illness and he was inconsistent and noncompliant with his use of psychotropic medications. In addition to the waxing and waning of the symptoms of his schizophrenia, he had a variety of other ailments for which he was receiving pain medication.

Throughout Richard's life Mr. Sullivan had been in various treatment facilities and lived alternately with the family and his own mother. Following the death of Mr. Sullivan's mother 3 years earlier, he moved back with his family full-time.

Richard was currently in special education and had been treated for attention-deficit/hyperactivity disorder from ages 5 until 8. He never needed medication but recalled positive experiences with therapists who taught him how to focus his attention. His brother was diagnosed with dyslexia but was maintained in a regular classroom setting. At the start of treatment, the boys were attending the same school for the first time, in the year following the suicide. They were quite close, with Richard somewhat dependent on his brother. In spite of having some common friends, they also had different styles and engaged in different activities.

Initial Contact with the Client's Mother and First Contact with Richard

Approximately 9 months after her husband's death, I met with Richard's mother to obtain background information, assess the appropriateness of the referral, and formulate a working plan. Mrs. Sullivan was quiet and seemingly distant, expressing her concern for Richard more by what she said than by any display of emotions. Mrs. Sullivan provided details about the suicide and her involvement in managing her husband's schizophrenia. She did not volunteer information about her marriage, her own grief, or her adjustment to her husband's death. My initial impression was that she was a caring mother who admirably had met various challenges growing up as well as in her roles as wife and mother. Her reticence to discuss her feelings suggested there was limited family communication about Richard's father's illness while he was alive and about the circumstances of his death.

After meeting Mrs. Sullivan I conferred with Richard's gastroenterologist to review the case and confirm that there was no organic cause or medical treatment for his symptoms. I scheduled a separate session for Richard.

He is a tall, lanky Caucasian boy with straight dark hair falling over his eyes. He came to his session dressed in typical teen garb of blue jeans and a T-shirt. He was polite and quiet, seeming extremely shy, maintaining little eye contact. Most questions were answered in a few words or involved a shrug of the shoulders.

First Session

Content of Session

THERAPIST: I've heard you haven't been feeling well, and Dr. Curran thought I could help. Tell me what's been going on.

RICHARD: I've been having a lot of cramps, and I go to the bathroom a lot.

T: When did it start?

R: A few months ago.

T: When does it happen?

R: Kind of all the time.

T: Are there any times when it's better or worse?

R: (*Shrugs.*)

T: Is there anything that makes it better?

R: (*Shrugs, mumbles.*) Not really, no.

T: What about school?

R: I'm on home instruction.

T: Why is that?

R: Because my stomach bothers me, and I need to go to the bathroom a lot.

Analysis and Feelings

He knew what type of "doctor" I was and that the medical doctor was not able to alleviate his symptoms. Given Richard's age and problem, I decided it was appropriate to let him know I was aware of his problems and ask directly about his immediate symptoms. However, I left the initial questions open ended enough to allow for him to choose the focus: the stomach problems or the death.

His reticence to answer seems more a matter of being ill at ease than of being resistant.

T: Would you like to go back if that was better?

R: Yes

T: I can help you with that.

I want to encourage positive expectations.

T: I heard about your father

R: He died.

T: How did that happen?

R: He jumped out a window.

T: How has that been?

R: (Shrugs.) Okay.

T: Have you ever been to a therapist before?

R: I went with my brother and mother, and we talked about it a little.

Although Richard knew I had previously met with his mother, he was somewhat uneasy talking about all topics and did not volunteer information about his father's mental illness. Therefore I did not pursue this area directly, being unsure exactly what he knew about his father's history.

T: (Asks Richard if he would be interested in doing something or drawing, and he chooses to draw.)

His mother had informed me that he liked to draw.

R: (Readily and quietly draws a detailed picture he identifies as trees in Africa. He does not elaborate on the background or what the picture means.)

Although I wanted more verbal content to help identify and understand what was going on for Richard, I was heartened and encouraged by the fact that he was so comfortable and at ease when drawing.

T: For next week it would be helpful for me if you could do an assignment and keep track of how you are feeling. Rather than hear from other people like your mother or doctor, I want to find out directly from *you* how things are going. You can record your stomach cramps and diarrhea. Then we can understand exactly when it's better or worse. This will help plan for going back to school.

Given his vague answers I needed some detailed information to get a full appreciation of his stomach problems. In addition, his monitoring the problems would tell me about his level of compliance, and the focus on the monitoring itself could generate an improvement. I also wanted to make him feel more in control of the process.

R: Okay

T: (Gives him a chart to record his symptoms at home.)

Preliminary Assessment

Richard seemed genuinely interested in getting help for his problems and was compliant with requests in the session. I was unsure how to interpret his avoidance of eye contact and his sparse answers. Consistent with the literature, Richard was at particular risk for having a complicated bereavement reaction due to his premorbid history. Given his learning disability, attention-deficit/hyperactivity disorder, physical symptoms, and family history of mental illness, I considered the possibility of an underlying depression or anxiety disorder. In addition, his physical symptoms could result from a grief reaction. Gastrointestinal symptoms are not uncommon in bereaved children or those who have experienced stress. Richard's physical discomfort was also understandable as a reflection of the teenage preference for withdrawal, repression, and avoidance of emotions, complicated by his own shy tendencies. The surviving parent's somatization, in this case Richard's mother's stomach ailments, also increased the likelihood of his somatization (Sood et al., 1992).

Given his style and the conclusions from medical tests, I hypothesized that Richard's abdominal distress was the result of internalized stress and anxiety, and unexpressed anger and sadness about his father. I imagined he was also ashamed and embarrassed by his lack of bowel control. In order to keep Richard motivated for therapy, I chose to work directly on the goal of returning to school. The decision was based on the fact that (1) I felt we could succeed in this area, (2) he expressed a desire for this, and (3) it was concrete and thus less threatening or vague than working on his unacknowledged and unconscious grief.

Second Session

Content of Session

(Richard arrived with his mother, and both informed me that he could not stay because his stomach was bothering him and he needed to go to the bathroom frequently. I said he was free to go to the bathroom whenever needed and we should see how things went. Richard then started the session.)

Analysis and Feelings

While I was sympathetic to Richard's plight, I felt it necessary to be optimistic and suggest more positive coping strategies by telling him he was welcome to use the bathroom at any time. Although I knew that improvement would be a slow process, I worried that Richard and his mother would be pessimistic about treatment and prematurely terminate therapy be-

THERAPIST: Did you get to do your chart?

RICHARD: It's not complete.

T: Let's see what it says.

R: Sometimes at night it's very bad and I can't sleep well.

T: How is it when you get to sleep? Do you have any dreams or have things on your mind?

R: No, not really.

T: *(Upon inquiry as to time of day, particular foods, etc., Richard cannot pinpoint any reason why his symptoms have gotten better or worse.)* Why don't we do some more drawing.

R: *(Quietly begins a drawing of a deserted beach with a lone empty chair. I comment on the drawing and he describes the scene.)*

T: It can help sometimes to do some relaxation techniques when your stomach is hurting and making you feel uncomfortable. Why don't I show you how this works.

cause the problem was not immediately fixed.

Although his physical symptoms are important, I don't want to focus exclusively on this for fear of it becoming a distraction to the underlying grief issues. He also seemed the most relaxed when drawing rather than talking face to face. I wondered if the reported cramps and bowel problems at bedtime were related to a fear of nightmares or actual bad dreams.

Given his affinity for drawn imagery I decide it's worth trying to use this strategy. Also, since he came to the session complaining of stomach pain, I thought having him experience some immediate relief would keep him motivated to continue treatment.

Next Richard rated his stomach discomfort on a scale of 1–10 prior to my teaching him progressive muscle relaxation. Once Richard was relaxed I introduced a guided imagery story based on the beach scene he just drew and described (Figure 13.1). I instructed him to imagine his cramps being waves that gently rolled out to sea. He admitted to feeling better and agreed to try this at home. He was to do the exercises nightly, when going to bed, and at any other time during the day he felt it might help. "Following a major relationship loss, a child may see himself as helpless and vulnerable. It is possible that this image of being frighteningly small and helpless is the most disruptive and disorganizing view of the self that can emerge subsequent to parental death" (Osterweis, Solomon, & Green, 1984). After the session I realized that his picture of the uninhabited

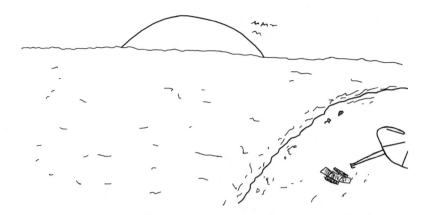

FIGURE 13.1. Pencil sketch of a beach.

beach with a lone empty beach chair might refer to his absent father or his own loneliness. The remote-looking scene mirrored his distant demeanor. It provided an image of solitude that was disquieting rather than soothing. Yet, for Richard the drawing also seemed to suggest calm; while working he seemed comforted by the self-contained activity. I was also struck by his skills of observation and ability to draw evocative scenery. The art allowed his feelings to emerge, and the relaxation exercise allowed him to reclaim and experience some control.

Contrary to his forecast, Richard stayed the entire session without leaving for the bathroom. The following week he came to session on his own, feeling better, and although he forgot to bring his chart, he reported using the relaxation techniques and thinking they helped. I reviewed the technique with him, finding him to be quite accurate and faithful implementing the strategy. Although he would intermittently and abruptly cancel sessions over the next weeks, it seemed clear he was interested in seeing his treatment through.

We established a routine of drawing in each session, periodically preceded by a review of his self-monitoring chart and progress with self-directed relaxation. Occasionally I educated Richard about the connection between his mind and his body—his head and his stomach. I let him know that sometimes his sad or worried thoughts could cause his stomach upset. Therefore, by using the relaxation technique to calm his thoughts he could also calm his stomach. Realizing that the nonverbal avenue of drawing was well suited to his interests and style of interaction, I suggested making a pictorial autobiography. I envisioned it as a way to understand him better, see relationships within his family, avoid a direct focus on his father's death, allow for remembrances, and help him put his grief in perspective. This idea was readily appealing, and he began drawing a picture of himself and his brother in a baby carriage. Over the next 2 weeks he added scenes depicting different events in his life. He included a scene of himself at the beach and told stories about his father picking up sharks and eels and going fishing. Richard easily initiated conversations laced with fond memories of his father, based on his drawings.

Fourth Session

Richard canceled his session, when it was scheduled to start, due to stomach problems. We rescheduled it for the following day. When we started, I reviewed procedures for canceling and encouraged him to attend despite his stomach ailments. I also introduced the idea of returning to school. The discussion centered on two main issues—his being caught up with his academic work and having a plan for using the bathroom. I kept his return to school a priority as a way to actively and concretely work toward increasing normalization and resumption of outside activities. I used his experience of cramps during session as an *in vivo* situation to desensitize him to his anxiety and physical symptoms. Improved coping within the session was used to reinforce his coping ability outside the session.

Content of Session	Analysis and Feelings
RICHARD: *(He continues working on his pictorial autobiography and easily returns to the rhythm of the drawing and talking. He starts the picture at the beginning—with a drawing of himself and his brother in a baby carriage. He now begins adding another scene of himself at an inner-tube playground in the winter.)*	
THERAPIST: Tell me about this scene.	I am surprised and glad that Richard is able to be so honest and open about his father.
RICHARD: My father used to take us to this playground sometimes.	
T: I'd like to hear more about your father and what he was like.	At times Richard would be holding back tears whenever he talked about his father. When this happened, I commented that it was normal and acceptable to be sad, miss his father, and even be upset or mad. I had to monitor my
R: He was a lot of fun.	
T: I know he also had some problems too.	
R: He had schizophrenia. One time he had a reaction to his medication and	

had to go the hospital. He would hear voices.

T: What do you know about schizophrenia?

R: I know it's a disease and that you can't catch it.

T: You're right. How was it to see him like that?

R: *(Shrugs.)*

T: I know it can be hard sometimes to live with someone who has that.

own discomfort and concern, weighing whether the discussion was making him too uncomfortable and embarrassed or whether it was necessary for him to talk about his feelings about the death and hear my comments in a safe environment. I was left to guess that this was the right thing to pursue, even if gingerly, by the fact that he continued to attend, draw, and respond.

Figure 13.2 depicts an interesting sequence of scenes representing a process of separation: from Richard and his twin together as infants to Richard as an independent, lone participant. Richard had said he liked having a twin who "looks like me" and "is always there even though it's annoying sometimes." He felt his brother understands him but they "think differently and have different feelings about our dad." Although others

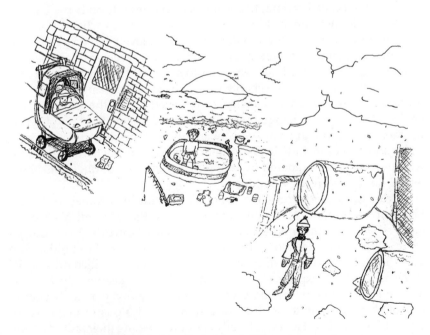

FIGURE 13.2. Pencil sketch of different memories.

were included when describing events, it was clear that the experiences, memories of his father, and the grief belonged to Richard alone. His inclusion of containing structures (baby carriage, pool, tubes, walls, fences) informed me of his need for protection and guardedness, yet his attention to external details suggested a potential for internal self-reflection.

Coordination with Other Professionals

I was fortunate to make an alliance with Richard's school counselor. She was eager to make whatever arrangements were necessary to ease Richard's transition back to school. Over the course of a month, we discussed her notifying teachers of his return, talking to them about integrating the work he had done at home with their own requirements for graduation from middle school, and alerting them about his bathroom needs. We discussed the timing and logistics of Richard's return: meeting with the counselor and his teachers for a shortened first day, then returning for a full day. Although we had to contend with spring vacation, leaving only approximately 1 month of school remaining, I felt strongly that he should return before the end of the year.

The risk of increased avoidance of school was high. With a prolonged absence I feared Richard might become too comfortable on home instruction—lose momentum and his motivation to return to school. With the start of high school a few months away, I believed he was better off reconnecting with peers before the summer. Each week we discussed his feelings and any fears about returning to school. Much of his expressed anxiety was focused on his schoolwork. Richard had the option of switching to his brother's homeroom when he returned to ease the transition, but he decided against a change. Asked what peers knew about his absence, Richard indicated that some were aware of his stomach and bowel problems, and some, including his brother, teased him. Richard believed it was all in jest. We prepared by role-playing answers to questions about where he had been for 4 months.

With Richard's permission I met alone with his brother to discuss his return to school. Although fraternal twins, Richard and his brother have strikingly similar looks and mannerisms. However his brother's more extroverted and calm nature was readily apparent. His brother also gave limited answers to questions yet did not convey Richard's social awkwardness. He expressed concern about Richard keeping up with the academics when he returned to school, and he seemed genuinely protective of Richard in spite of also being somewhat jealous of his more indulged status of late. He spoke briefly about witnessing their father's death when asked, but denied having any untoward symptoms or feelings.

I had made contact with Mrs. Sullivan's therapist, who had previously seen Richard in family therapy. His isolation and withdrawal had been of concern to her, but she had not seen him in 6 months. I also arranged a psychiatric consultation to further evaluate Richard's symptoms of anxiety and depression. The psychiatrist diagnosed him as having irritable bowel syndrome, exacerbated by anxiety, and recommended an antianxiety medication. Richard tried the medication for a couple of weeks and thought it helped. However, he soon used it inconsistently, and within 2 months stopped using it completely and cancelled follow-up appointments with the psychiatrist. Without the benefit of the art as a nonthreatening arena in which Richard could talk, others had difficulty assessing and understanding him. After the first month of our treatment, due to the significant improvement in Richard's relatedness and commitment to change, I was no longer concerned about his having psychiatric symptoms and therefore did not pursue the medication issue further.

Richard returned to school for a few hours the day before spring vacation and continued full-time following vacation. He reported that his friends were glad to see him again and that the schoolwork was manageable. I began gingerly but directly approaching the issue of extracurricular activities—going out with friends and doing sports. In session, he began working on a picture of a visit to a theme park. This had been a happy occasion with his brother, mother, and father.

Content of Session	*Analysis and Feelings*
(Richard canceled his appointment right before his session because he didn't feel well. We rescheduled it for the next day.)	I was both frustrated and concerned about Richard's cancellation. Richard knew that it was not always possible to reschedule sessions and that he was responsible for keeping up with his appointments. However, I was concerned that I keep a close watch on any increase in symptoms of anxiety or stomach problems, now that he was back at school. I wanted his return to be a success, thus preventing a more difficult case of school refusal.
THERAPIST: How are things going in school?	
RICHARD: Things are fine.	
T: How's the work?	
R: OK, not so bad.	
T: What about friends?	
R: It's good to see them.	
T: How has your stomach been?	
R: So-so, still bothers me sometimes.	
(We discuss how he is doing with the classwork and getting to a bathroom when needed.)	

T: It sounds like you're doing a good job. It seems as if what we talked about is true, that things aren't as bad as you think and your mind can makes things seem worse than they are.

R: Yeah.

At times I referred back to the cognitive-behavioral strategies he had learned.

T: Do you want to get back to work on your drawing?

R: Yeah. *(Continues to work on the drawing of rides at the theme park.)*

T: So what ride is that?

R: The bumper cars.

T: How was that?

R: We kept hitting each other.

T: It must have been fun. I like hearing stories about when you were younger. You must miss your dad.

R: Yeah. *(Talked more than usual about his father and, although sad, seemed more comfortable talking about his death.)*

T: Some kids think or wish they could've done something.

R: I could've grabbed him.

T: Then what would have happened?

R: I would've gone out the window too.

T: It's hard to think about what you could've done to stop it.

R: My aunt realized he mentioned his plans but didn't know what it meant until afterward. One time my father had a bad reaction to his medication and the police were called.

This is the most open Richard has been about his father's death and the thoughts that have probably been plaguing him for months. Although he seems aware of and understanding of his father's mental illness, he struggles with a not uncommon guilt over not saving his father.

T: What did you think?

R: It was bad, but he needed his medication.

T: I like hearing about your father. I know you miss him, and it's good to talk about him so your thoughts don't stay stuck inside and upset your stomach.

His understanding of his father's need for medication to manage his schizophrenia may have influenced his noncompliance with his own psychiatrically prescribed medication—fearing he was or would become like his father.

The scene of bumper cars in Figure 13.3 is quite a departure from the earlier desolate beach scene. It corresponds to Richard's current increased activity and involvement outside the house, albeit a reference to his awkward, somewhat stilted interpersonal interactions. Although a possible metaphor for Richard's earlier and current feelings bumping into each other and finally being revealed, it is also hopeful for its suggestion of a reengagement in life and social relationships. Not unlike the anchor for the cars, I felt the need to be a tether for Richard.

Fortunately the return to school was a positive experience. Richard felt confident in being caught up with his work yet became worried about impending end-of-the-year tests. He was more conversant about his life—past, present and future. He told me about his learning disability and attention-deficit/hyperactivity disorder, and about the therapist who taught him how to stay in control. It was worthy of note that he reported feeling better than when he was young and did not currently exhibit the signs of hyperactivity he said were part of his past. I capitalized on his ability to discuss his father in the context of his drawing and pursued upcoming issues related to the future, particularly his summer plans and transfer to a new high school in the fall.

Richard did not show up for his next session; when I called, I found him home sick with a cold. (Given typical teenage behavior, such a call to follow up can be an exasperating experience when phone lines are

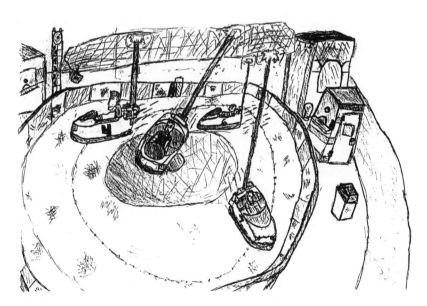

FIGURE 13.3. Pencil sketch of bumper car rides.

continually busy due to Internet use and the like.) I was aware of the approaching anniversary of his father's death, so I was particularly concerned about maintaining contact with Richard and his mother. Once he returned to our sessions I reiterated the need to attend even when feeling under the weather, associating this to not letting his stomach problems interfere with his life.

Wondering if his canceled sessions corresponded to feeling he revealed too much in the previous session, I acknowledged that it might be difficult to talk about his father. He continued to do relaxation exercises as needed. He was excited about his upcoming graduation from middle school and end-of-the-year trip to a theme park, the same one he had drawn and visited as a child. Given his inconsistent attendance and the upcoming anniversary, I decided to increase the structure between sessions again by having him rate and time his stomach problems. In addition, I made him a diary and suggested he write down any thoughts he had about his father. I wanted to relieve any pressure he felt about telling me things that made him uncomfortable, and doing this at home might decrease any ruminations.

Content of Session	Analysis and Feelings
(*Session following his class trip.*)	I was encouraged by Richard's engaging in a social activity away from home and his high level of functioning despite still having symptoms
THERAPIST: How was the trip?	
RICHARD: I had a good time, it was fun. (*Told me about the rides and how it was different from when he went as a child.*)	
T: How was your stomach?	
R: It's better, I didn't do the chart, but it's between 4 and 6 (on a 10-point scale of discomfort) and only about four times a day. (*Continues to work on a picture he started of a Little League baseball game, talking about his father watching as he played on the team.*)	
R: I saw a TV program on schizophrenia using virtual reality—that's what my father had. It showed how you could see and hear things and not be able to get them out of your mind.	
T: I guess you could see what it was like for your dad.	
R: My father was good when he was on his medications, but he didn't always take them.	Richard's successful reintegration into school seems to have increased his confidence and

T: Do you think you should've done something to make him take them?

R: *(Shrugged.)*

T: You might feel it was your job, but it wasn't, you couldn't control that for your father. But I understand you wish it were different. *(Continues working and also tells me about having to make different 4th of July holiday plans because the aunt had died who used to have them over.)*

ability to withstand exploration of more difficult issues related to his father.

Richard seems to have experienced an unusual number of family deaths in a relatively short time, adding to a loss of a sense of stability.

Even with intermittent lapses in his attendance, Richard continued to progress; he was excited about ending school and, for the first time he could remember, he did not need summer school.

My encouraging Richard to make summer plans was met with passivity. Although he had played on Little League baseball teams in past summers, this summer he made little effort to do so again. Most of my suggestions or inquiries prompted excuses or a rationale for why it could not happen. I also spoke to his guidance counselor to get ideas for outside involvement and passed along names and numbers for various programs to Richard's mother. While making positive strides in other areas, he was able to discuss still being sad about his father. For example, he missed his father when he watched baseball games on television because they used to do it together. As the summer progressed, Richard showed marked improvement in many areas. His affect was more open and relaxed, his eye contact was better, and his activity level outside of sessions increased. He reported going out with friends and had plans for starting karate classes. He also was diligent about using his symptom chart, which showed a decrease in the severity and frequency of attacks. Although I never asked to see the results, he reported having used his diary to record thoughts about his father. I reinforced all this by noting that things were going well and that he was taking control of making himself better. He began drawing a baseball stadium, talking about the different times he went to baseball games with his brother and parents.

Content of Session

THERAPIST: You really remember a lot about the stadium—you have a lot of details.

RICHARD: I went to three different games. My father came to one. He used to come to a lot of my Little League

Analysis and Feelings

Although Richard told me he enjoyed playing baseball in

games. I didn't play well last summer after my dad died. I can't really
play baseball good anymore.

T: Why is that?

R: He used to always be there to cheer
me on, but he wouldn't be there
now.

R: Is that why you didn't go out for baseball this summer?

R: Yeah.

T: Maybe you didn't play so well last
year because you were sad about
your dad and didn't quite feel like
yourself. It's takes time to get over
something like your dad dying, and
it doesn't mean you could never
play as well again.

R: I know. . . . (A pause as he draws.)

R: You can see the game from these buildings. And there are people outside
selling tickets. One time there was a
guy in my neighborhood selling
World Series tickets, but we didn't
get them because my mother had to
work.

past summers, he was uncoop-
erative about pursuing it this
summer. I was never able to
quite understand the source of
the resistance or change. It
now became clear that he was
anticipating that it would be
painful without his father. I
also thought it would help to
reframe the meaning of his father's death and help him to
see that feelings and behaviors can be multiply determined.

Richard contends that he likes
the top-down perspective because it allows him to draw
more details; however, it is an
"outsider view," and it made
me think of his looking down
upon his father after he
jumped or his father now looking down on him. I have
found other children to be relieved and comforted by having a concrete concept of the
person who has died being
physically above, in heaven,
with a guarding watchful vantage point.

As was his usual pattern, Richard attended our sessions in spurts
throughout the summer. Whenever in session he was engaged and talk-
ative and clearly happier than at the start of treatment. He continued to
elaborate on his baseball stadium picture, laboriously adding more details,
as if it was a metaphor for his expanding life (Figure 13.4).

While drawing, Richard was also able to talk more directly about
the day his father died. He recounted that he, his brother, and mother
were in the same part of the apartment when his father jumped out the

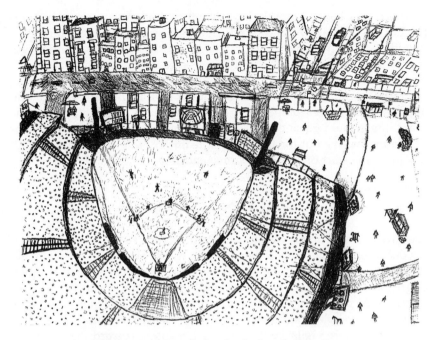

FIGURE 13.4. Pencil sketch of a baseball stadium.

window. His brother ran to the bedroom and saw the window open from where his father jumped, but Richard ran downstairs. Richard saw his father breathing and gagging with a bloodied arm. Looking up he could see a gate on which his father hurt his arm and the snapped wires and cords that had entangled his father. A neighbor was at the scene and later at the wake described to the family what she had seen when the father was falling. Firemen from a station down the block and paramedics immediately arrived. His father was still alive the last time Richard saw him. Richard returned to the apartment when his father was taken to the hospital. When the family arrived at the hospital they were told his father had died in the ambulance.

Comment

Both the beach scene and the baseball stadium offer a bird's-eye (overhead) view, hinting at Richard's seeing his father down on the ground or, conversely, being watched over by his father. It is also conforms to Richard's tendency to be more of an observer than a participant in life. But the contrast and progression from a scene empty of people (Figure

13.1) to one he began 4 months later, in which thousands are in attendance (Figure 13.4), speaks volumes for Richard's new outlook. He commented that his "stomach is fine," having only occasional loose stools, which was confirmed by his mother. Richard also reported not using his diary much nor being as sad about his father anymore. I remarked that not feeling sad didn't mean he stopped caring about or missing his father. In talking about back-to-school preparation for fall, Richard was quite optimistic that things would go smoothly, and he spontaneously informed me that he planned to try out for the baseball team. True to his prediction, and our plan, the start of school was uneventful and successful.

CONCLUDING COMMENTS

Richard was well on his way to reclaiming control of his life and moving beyond the trauma of his father's death. In the beginning of treatment, his resistance to coming and to talking seemed associated with the pain of grief and shame about his symptoms. Richard's later inconsistent attendance seemed more positive, as a sign of teenage rebellion and hence improved psychological functioning. Given the passive family style, I had to maintain more vigilance than with other cases. Toward the middle of treatment, I recognized that I had not fully appreciated the extent of Richard's learning problems. For example, coexisting with his intense focus on details and his drawing skill was an inability to remember dates or even accurately sequence the months of the year. Thus his forgetting the actual anniversary of his father's death and appointment times was not a result of psychological defensiveness. Hence, I gave him reminder cards at the end of each session. It was also important to avoid asking about his brother and comparing Richard's functioning and ability to those of his twin. Although I investigated his twin's ability to be supportive and encouraged their sibling bond, I capitalized on the individuation Richard had established and portrayed in his early drawings.

Art making allowed for the re-creation and restoration of memories for Richard (Zambelli et al., 1989). Drawing the specific enabled him to articulate the unformed—his feelings. Discussing the content of the art also provided the opportunity for clarification of concepts—as when we talked about Richard's father's mental illness and the impossibility of Richard's preventing the suicide; as when I gave encouragement to his problem solving; or as when we worked through Richard's future participation in baseball. "Symbols restore a sense of unity by integrating and connecting emotions, perceptions, and thoughts not previously brought into juxtaposition and, in so doing, create a complex subjective experience that is deeply moving and cathartic" (Lewis & Langer, 1994, p. 232).

DISCUSSION QUESTIONS

1. How did Richard's being a twin influence his reactions and coping with his father's death?
2. Do you think the whole family could or should have been integrated into the treatment differently?
3. What would be the pros and cons of having Richard draw the actual scene he saw when his father died?

REFERENCES

Adams-Greenly, M. (1984). Helping children communicate about serious illness and death. *Journal of Psychosocial Oncology, 2*(2), 61–72.

Christ, G. H. (1999). *Healing children's grief.* New York: Oxford University Press.

Fristad, M. A., Jedel, F., Weller, R. A., & Weller, E. B. (1993). Psychosocial functioning in children after the death of a parent. *American Journal of Psychiatry, 150*(3), 511–513.

Goodman, R. (1999). Childhood cancer and the family: Case of Tim, age 6, and follow-up at age 15. In N. B. Webb (Ed.), *Play therapy with children in crisis* (2nd ed.). *Individual, group, and family treatment* (pp. 380–404). New York: Guilford Press.

Goodman, R., Williams, K., Agell, G., & Gantt, L. (1998). Talk, talk, talk, when do we draw? *American Journal of Art Therapy, 37,* 39–65.

Hemmings, P. (1995). Communicating with children through play. In S. C. Smith & M. Pennells (Eds.), *Interventions with bereaved children* (pp. 9–23). London & Bristol, PA: Kingsley.

Junge, M. (1985, March). The book about Daddy dying: A preventive art therapy technique to help families deal with the death of a family member. *Art Therapy, 2,* 4–10.

Kramer, E. (1971). *Art as therapy with children.* New York: Brunner/Mazel.

Laub, D., & Podell, D. (1995). Art and trauma. *International Journal of Psychoanalysis, 76,* 991–1005.

Lewis, L., & Langer, K. C. (1994). Symbolization in psychotherapy with patients who are disabled. *Journal of Psychotherapy, 48*(2), 231–239.

Liotta, E. J. (1996). *When students grieve.* Alexandria, PA: LRP Publications.

McIntyre, B. B. (1990). Art therapy with bereaved youth. *Journal of Palliative Care, 6*(1), 16–23.

Millay, E. St. V. (1969). Childhood is the kingdom where nobody dies. In *Edna St. Vincent Millay collected lyrics* (p. 208). New York: Harper & Row. (Original work published 1934)

Mishara, A. I. (1995). Narrative and psychotherapy: The phenomenology of healing. *American Journal of Psychotherapy, 49*(2), 180–195.

Naumburg, M. (1987). *Dynamically oriented art therapy: Its principles and practice.* Chicago, IL: Magnolia Street Publishing.

Osterweis, M., Solomon, F., & Green, M. (Eds.). (1984). *Bereavement: Reactions, consequences and care.* Washington, DC: Institute of Medicine—National Academy Press.

Pennebaker, J. W., Hughes, C. F., & O'Heeron, R. C. (1987). The psychophysiology of confession: Linking inhibitory and psychosomatic processes. *Journal of Personality and Social Psychology, 52*(4), 781–793.

Sanchez, L., Fristad, M., Weller, R. A., Weller, E. B., & Moye, J. (1994). Anxiety in acutely bereaved prepubertal children. *Journal of Clinical Psychiatry, 6*(1), 39–43.

Sood, B., Weller, E. B., Weller, R. A., Fristad, M. A., & Bowes, J. M. (1992). Somatic complaints in grieving children. *Comprehensive Mental Health Care, 2*(1), 17–25.

U.S. Bureau of the Census. (1990). *Statistical abstract of the United States: 1990* (119th ed.). Washington, DC: U.S. Government Printing Office.

Van Eerdewegh, M. W., Clayton, P. J., & Van Eerdewegh, P. (1985). The bereaved child: Variables influencing early psychopathology. *British Journal of Psychiatry, 147*, 188–194.

Webb, N. B. (1996). *Social work practice with children.* New York: Guilford Press.

Weller, R. A., Weller, E. B., Fristad, M. A., & Bowes, J. M. (1991). Depression in recently bereaved prepubertal children. *American Journal of Psychiatry, 148*(11), 1536–1540.

Wolfelt, A. D. (1990, February). *Bereavement Magazine,* pp. 60–61.

Zambelli, G. C., Clark, E. J., Barile, L., & de Jong, A. F. (1988). An interdisciplinary approach to clinical intervention for childhood bereavement. *Death Studies, 12*, 41–50.

Zambelli, G. C., Clark, E. J., & Heegaard, M. (1989). Art therapy for bereaved children. In H. Wadeson, J. Durkin, & D. Perach (Eds.), *Advances in art therapy* (pp. 60–80). New York: Wiley.

14

✿

Storytelling with Bereaved Children

DONNA O'TOOLE

Stories are not merely a nice or fun decoration added to the real stuff of mental development. They are in many respects, the real stuff of mental development. . . . Through stories children construct a self and communicate that self to others.
—ENGEL (1995, p. 206)

Each time a story is told it also becomes a text and, therefore, an object that you can reflect on.
—ENGEL (1995, p. 188)

FINDING OUR WAY THROUGH STORIES: A TRANSGENERATIONAL JOURNEY

Storytelling is as ancient as human civilization. Yet, with the rise of analytical psychology the value of storytelling receded, was discounted, and held suspicious. Today, the tidal wave has again reversed. Our interest in finding family roots through tales, legends, and myths from around the world and in understanding the meaning of life through stories has regained credibility. The imaginative story adventures of an orphaned boy named Harry Potter have captured audiences of all ages, making J. K. Rowling's books (1998, 1999, 2000a, 2000b) phenomenal overnight bestsellers. In the professional arena, postmodern psychology has incorporated storymaking and storytelling through its constructionist or narrative approach to define and guide therapeutic practice.

My work with stories extends the boundaries of psychological theory by embracing the story as a valuable and practical art form of the people. As such, stories hold the wisdom of the ages. Human beings who are inherently meaning makers resonate to stories as a natural way through which we can navigate and understand our world. Stories can imprint solutions, guide our quests, and emerge as beacons of light in times of darkness and despair.

Such has been my own experience with stories. The story *Aarvy Aardvark Finds Hope* (O'Toole, 1988) came to me 6 months after the death of my 21-year-old son, Matthew Schmidt. I can still remember the contrast of the light streaming through the windows on that late November afternoon and the darkness of the sadness I was feeling. During the previous several weeks I had been experiencing the pain of intense longing for my son. Then, while I was at work writing a graduate thesis on the value of using creative expression in times of grief, the story of a bereaved animal, an Aardvark, who named himself Aarvy Aardvark, came to me. I did not consciously think this story into being. Rather, the story came to me, unbidden, persistent, and image filled. It was more an experience of something moving through my body than through my head.

So intense was the story that I could not block it from awareness. Thus, Aarvy's story simply unfolded before my eyes. When finally I picked up a pad of paper and a pen the words of the story, without effort or thought, flowed onto the pages. This was a new kind of knowing for me, an experience of words, yet an experience that our language is inept to describe. The story, which at first I kept hidden from others, was eventually shared and much later published as *Aarvy Aardvark Finds Hope*.

Gradually, as I read, reread, and shared the Aarvy story with others, I discovered the deeper meanings embedded in the story, for others as well as for myself. I found many intergenerational factors of my own life history in Aarvy's story. Here were situations that spoke to my own early childhood as much as to my experiences with my son, Matt. As I turned the story around in my mind, shadows of my own childhood losses emerged into light. Miraculously, it seemed, I was restorying my own self with these poignant memories and newly discovered meanings.

Over time, and through the feedback of many others who came to know and appreciate *Aarvy Aardvark Finds Hope*, I have come to value Aarvy's story as timeless and universal. Aarvy's story demonstrates the possibility that grief which is realized, expressed, validated, guided, attended to, and witnessed can be a natural healing process.

Mama Mockingbird's Story

Mama Mockingbird (Wood, 1998) is another modern-day folk story that demonstrates how stories can emerge from sorrow, transforming sadness and quickening hope. Shattered by the sudden death of her grown son, Scot Kenneth Wood, in 1982, and at times doubting whether her "pieces" would ever get back together again, Saunie Wood was walking the hills near her home when the story of *Mama Mockingbird* came to her, as she says, "through the wind." Like the Mama Mockingbird in her story, Saunie was in search of the lost vitality and joy of the way she had known life when her son was living. In the story Mama Mockingbird's son dies. Mama Mockingbird and her family cry and cry. They cry so long and so hard that they forget how to sing. Later, as Mama Mockingbird sets out on a journey to find her song, she says to her family, "I have lost my son, but I do not think I was meant to lose my song."

Like myself, Saunie was at first startled by the power of the story that came to her. For a long time she hid her story and told it to no one, as had I. One day a counseling friend gave Saunie a copy of *Aarvy Aardvark Finds Hope*. She so resonated to Aarvy's story that, as a gift, Saunie sent me a taped version of her story, *Mama Mockingbird*, and gave me permission to share and tell the story as I saw fit. Although Saunie is a gifted storyteller herself, *Mamma Mockingbird* was then too painfully personal a story for her to tell.

Gradually Saunie's pain was lifting. The story that was given to her, as she said, "through the wind" was heard by others through my telling, was recognized for its depth and beauty, and was published. The *Mama Mockingbird* story is a beautiful story that uses the natural world as a metaphor for the nature and naturalness of the healing process of grief. Once again a healing story offered comfort and meaning long before the author had a cognitive understanding of her experience.

Adults are not the only ones who have used stories to quicken hope and to guide them toward understanding and an amelioriation of suffering. My son, Matthew Schmidt, as a 19-year-old, and 5-year-old Joeri Breebaart, further demonstrate how even the very young can find their way through loss with storymaking and storytelling.

Matthew's Story

Although he was pale, thin, and often seriously ill, Matthew wrote about himself in a different and powerful way—as "Super Cystic" (Schmidt, 1981). Matt was born with cystic fibrosis, a hereditary disease that adversely affects the internal secreting functions of the body. To help himself and others dealing with the boredom, homesickness, and fear that young children feel when they enter a hospital for treatment, he developed a coloring book of characters who faced up to and outwitted the challenges of their disease.

Super Cystic had many powerful friends and cohorts (see Figure 14.1). There was an inventive nurse named Fabulous Fran Fibrosis, as well as IV Man, Bob the Breather, Carol Capsule, Polly Pounder, Ralph Respiratory, and Erving Enzyme. Together Super Cystic and his mighty and wise companions battled the powerful bad guys—the bugs—Boris Bacteria and Nasty Pneumonia.

Although often hospitalized and ill, Matt lived with integrity, imagination, and humor to age 21. His brief life challenged and inspired me and many others to live life creatively and fully. A year after his death, Matt's coloring book was posthumously published by a pharmaceutical company (Schmidt, 1981), which made it available so that other youngsters with cystic fibrosis might have a greater understanding of the nature of their illness, thereby fostering hope and personal enpowerment in these young patients.

Joeri's Story

But, we might ask, can even very young children make use of story as a part of their healing process? The true story of Joeri Breebaart and his father, Piet Breebaart, gives insight. From the foreword of their book, *When I Die, Will I Get Better?* (Breebaart & Breebaart, 1993), Piet tells in his own words what happened after his son Remi died suddenly of meningitis when Remi was 2 years and 8 months old; At the time Joeri, who shared a bedroom and had been very close to his brother, was 5:

> In the weeks after the funeral, Joeri was not only sad, but also very withdrawn and often angry. He was confused and disturbed by the loss of Remi and the concept of death and dying. He couldn't really talk about Remi's illness and death, and we had a hard time trying to reach Joeri and understand his feelings. We looked for children's books on death but there wasn't much that appealed to us.
>
> About six weeks after Remi's death, Joeri and I came to talk about Joe Rabbit. Joe was an invented character about whom we used to tell stories to Remi at bedtime. For Joeri, Joe Rabbit stood for Remi. Joeri himself was Fred Rabbit, Joe's brother. Joeri said it was impossible to make up stories about Joe Rabbit now, since Remi was dead. I then suggested making up a story in which Joe would die. That was fine with Joeri.
>
> Joeri created the story himself and always told me what he wanted

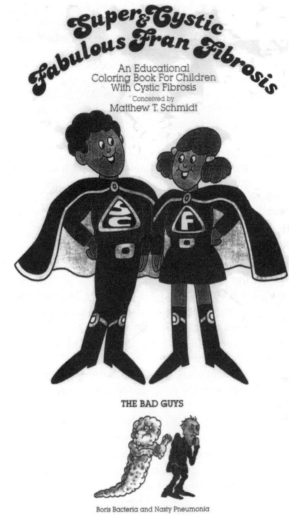

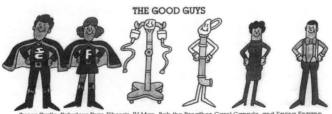

FIGURE 14.1. Illustrations of Super Cystic and cohorts. From Schmidt (1981). Reprinted by permission of Organon Inc.

me to draw for the next illustration. I then wrote down the story and made the drawing, sometimes the same day, sometimes a few days later. It was important to Joeri that I followed his indications. When for example, I had made a fox for a doctor, he didn't agree, for the fox would eat the rabbits. No, the doctor ought to be an owl. There were also days, when Joeri didn't want to talk about it.

The story describes Joeri's own experience. We entitled the story, *When I Die, Will I Get Better?* It tells how Remi got ill, how he died, the funeral, the loss, the coming to terms with the sadness. For us it meant a possibility to talk about it all with Joeri. It wasn't threatening this way. Joeri talked about the rabbits, and about us.

This healing process took about four weeks, and Joeri was very proud of the result. He told his teacher he had made a book about rabbits. Later he could tell her it was about his brother. He took the book to school and his teacher read it out loud in class. This meant a great deal to Joeri. (Breebaart & Breebaart, 1993, p. 2)

It meant a great deal to Joeri's father as well. Healing stories reach across the generations. Just as I found comfort in witnessing my son's creative capacity for restorying hope by helping himself and others imagine strength and wholeness in the midst of illness and disease, so too was Piet comforted. As he watched and listened, and as he illustrated the words that Joeri told him to depict the death of his brother, he was bonded to his sons in a process that moved from the pain of unbearable silence to that of a new type of presence, one of remembering. Storymaking and storytelling allow the essence of a life to be savored, honored, known, and remembered.

Stories that carry themes of resilience and wholeness can assist healing during times of loss and grief (Taylor, 1996; Dwivedi, 1997). Stories weave or reweave lives together. A healing story can clarify and validate, as well as provide new information and insight. A story theme can resonate across races, ages, and circumstances, illuminating connections and lessening isolation and uncertainty (Taylor, 1996).

Those of us wishing to help bereaved children grieve and grow can enhance our abilities to coach and validate these children by expanding our storytelling, storymaking, and storysharing abilities. We can use stories to address unique circumstances and needs, and to encourage insight, imagination, and understanding. Through such stories we can break down isolation, quicken hope, and normalize the many intense ups and downs of the grief process. Although stories will not keep children from hurting, they may keep them from hurting for the wrong reasons, and from feeling strange and alone. We can help children restore (restory) hope for a more meaningful, happier tomorrow.

THE ROLE OF RESILIENCY AND HARDINESS IN RESTORYING

Resiliency and hardiness research provides a scaffold by which we can elicit and stimulate healing stories. The research on hardiness and resilience (O'Connell Higgins, 1994; Flach, 1988; Walsh, 1998; Kobasa, 1985) can strengthen our confidence in helping children through story forms. This research documents how children and adults positively transform loss and adversity into life-enhancing ways of being. Resilient persons are those who have weathered great gales and storms in life, emerging from these trials as optimistic people. They become hope-based rather than fear-based individuals (Schneider, 2000). Rather than being diminished by their losses, they are made stronger. They feel somehow enhanced by these rough circumstances, having endured and become integrated into the tapestry of life.

As the Skin Horse in the story *The Velveteen Rabbit* tells us, this restorying—this integration of the chapters of a life—doesn't happen as an event but as a process: "It doesn't happen all at once. You become. It takes a long time. That's why it doesn't happen to people who break easily, or have sharp edges, or who have to be carefully kept. . . . [But] once you are *Real* you can't be ugly, except to people who don't understand" (Williams, 1958; emphasis added).

Helpers, or interaction agents (a term I prefer), who desire to assist bereaved children, need to know what can go right (resiliency, positive reformulation and transformation), as well as what may go wrong (complicated grief and pathology). We must differentiate grief experiences that may naturally reoccur across the life span from complicated grief that is currently often overdiagnosed as depression (Schneider, 2000). For all professionals working with bereaved children, I recommend a thorough review of the work of Therese Rando (1993) and John Schneider (2000), as well as perusal of the current developmental literature.

In choosing stories to tell and share as potentially healing stories for children and their families, I look for tales that exhibit the following elements which I have extrapolated from the literature as key traits of those who possess hope-based resilient personalities:

- Examples of hopefulness—characters that find or maintain an enduring belief in the possibility of fervent wishes. In challenges of uncertainity and fear these characters face (rather than avoid) the unknown. They proceed through grief not without fear and uncertainity but with the help of some small inner hopeful voice. They are moved by determination rather than held back by mistrust or resignation.

- Characters and story elements that display personal nonjudgmental awareness and acceptance of needs, emotions, values, and mental and physical states.
- Characters with intact personal boundaries.
- Characters that express their needs and feelings assertively as a hallmark of personal choice rather than coercion, manipulation, or judgment.
- Characters that display congeniality—the ability to engage and be engaged.
- Stories that demonstrate remembrance and commemoration in ordinary life or through recognized rituals. These stories tangibly or symbolically recognize and make real the loss, its value, and meaning.
- Some story element that honors or demonstrates affinity, a connection or kinship to something greater and/or beyond the self.
- Elements that demonstrate and encourage active imagination—the willingness and capacity to dream and to conceive of ideas and possibilities and mystery, all of which offer the possibility of an unfolding, ongoing, and changing story rather than a certain absolute end or solution.
- Stories that favor forgiveness and awareness over blame and shame. Forgiveness here implies the ability to accommodate to the imperfection of oneself and of others.

Annotated lists of storybooks for children and adolescents facing loss and bereavement can be found in the *Compassion Books Catalog* (O'Toole, 2002) and in Corr (2000), Corr, Nabe, & Corr (2000), and O'Toole (1995).

GRIEVING AS A LIFE SKILL

From the cradle to the grave, loss and grief is a part of life. Young people need to understand various responses to loss across the life span. By understanding how grief manifests itself through thought, emotion, behavior, and spiritual questioning and meaning making, children can learn to build awareness, acceptance, and competency.

Grieving can be thought of as a life skill that can be taught and learned (O'Toole, 1989). Adults can use teachable moments of grief in many ways: to normalize the experience of grief (e.g., for the death of a pet); to witness, to validate, and to label a child's feelings of loss (e.g., a move to a new home) without judging those feelings; and to model and guide ways of externalizing feelings that avoid harm to the child or to others.

Adults who have themselves navigated loss have an important and crucial role in modeling and holding hope for bereaved children (Jevne & Miller, 1999). It *is* possible for children to overcome great adversity and grievous losses and thrive. Maintaining hope and being able to imagine a meaningful future lies at the foundation of positive outcomes from a grievous loss (Schneider, 2000).

THE NATURE OF NARRATIVE: A MEANING-MAKING PROCESS

A storytelling or narrative view of life recognizes that grief can be a lifetime process—a spiral of feedback loops rather than a single event that follows a prescribed path. A metaphor, a theory, or stage model of grief, extrapolated from the experiences of many, may present a road map of grief but is unlikely to show the specific terrain any individual child or adult will travel as each experiences his/her own grief process.

Narrative, as a topic of inquiry, presents an enormous playing field (I use narrative and story interchangeably). For both the storyteller and story listener narrative approaches involve all aspects of self (mind, body, spiritual, and social), often simultaneously. Therefore, story approaches are inherently holistic in nature and difficult to analyze by separating elements. They emerge at the intersection of experience, emotion, and language as a meaning-making process.

Western culture, preoccupied with immediate outcomes that can be manipulated, measured, and defined, is uncomfortable and even suspicious of both narrative practices and grief, which may appear unproductive. However, from a *spiritual* perspective, one in which meaning making and personal spiritual development are included and valued, both story and grief provide a cornucopia of lifelong opportunity. As we process our losses across the life span through experience and selective attention, and as we alter and elaborate on stories that unfold, we are creating the "true" story—the meaning of our life. Moreover, the key to transforming losses into something positive lies in embracing our memory. In this way we remember ourselves (Harvey, 1996)—or, in story terms, we restory (and restore) ourselves.

Narrative approaches are highly child or client centered. From a narrative point of view a person whose intention is to be part of a healing process for a grieving child (or family) plays the role of interaction agent rather than expert. Using their current awareness and intuitive insights, the children and adults play with story possibilities to explore and co-create connections, change, and healing.

Additionally, using storytelling as a way of processing a loss experience calls for a leveled playing field. Storytelling is an interaction process between the teller and the listener. This process evolves over time with flow and mystery rather than through fixed, stable expectations that are certain and provable. Story approaches imply a collaborative, rather than a hierarchical, process. Both the listener and the teller are affected by the telling. Both are changed by the process. Since possibilities are offered but not prescribed, choice abounds. The locus of control is shared and internal. In this approach, authority is often based on intuition and personal experience rather than objective formulas or power.

Naming an event, designating it as a specific vignette, a story, or a chapter of life, gives it importance. By naming, writing, and telling our stories, we lay claim to their rightful place in our memory. Matt and Joeris's stories as told, written, and titled remind us that those we care about give life quality and meaning long after they are gone from our sight.

Stories can also cause us to explore our personal histories. From the story of Aarvy Aardvark, who loses his entire family at a very young age, I can explore memories of abandonment which I felt as a young child when my father left our family. By working with Aarvy's story I have been able to realizing ways that I and my entire family were forever changed by this loss.

My mother is no longer living, but from the vantage point of Aarvy, a profoundly bereaved creature, I can explore my relationship with my mother. Why did she grow to mistrust imagination and guide me to value facts rather than fiction? As I remember my mother, I also remember my sister, Sharon, 5 years older than I, who was tireless in reading fairy tales to me and who told me made-up stories with great enthusiam. Now, as a storyteller I feel deeply connected to my sister. I wonder who her story heroes are now and who were they as a child. Together we can wonder about the different themes we created as children in a family going through the many profound losses of the Great Depression and World War II. Whether recognized or not, storytelling and storysharing are intergenerational processes of continuity with a cast of thousands—those known and those unknown to us.

> We tell stories because we hope to find or create significant
> connections between things. Stories link past, present, and
> future in a way that tells us where we have been (even before
> we were born), where we are, and where we are going.
> —TAYLOR (1996, p. 1)

THE ROLE OF STORY ALTERATION
AND STORY CHOICE

The selection of a story for telling or reading to bereaved children can be both science and art. Selecting a story takes awareness, knowledge, and a sensitivity to the individual needs and developmental aptitudes of your audience. However, once you are familiar with various materials and stories it is likely to take only a short time to determine if a particular book is appropriate and satisfactory. You may even experience yourself capable of making up stories on the spot to match particular situations. Doris Brett's book, *Annie Stories* (1988), is an excellent resource that shows how brief but poignant made-up stories can help children cope with a variety of real or anticipated loss situations.

Often a story will need some alteration of words, location, or character to fit an particular child or audience. A favorite folk tale of mine was placed into written form by storyteller David Novak (1994). The story, named *The Three Dolls*, was told to David by a musician from northern India named Mr. Dasgupta. Later, Novak recast the story from an oral to a written presentation. As a storyteller I look for guidance and permission to be true to my own experiences. This ancient story not only creatively solved a perplexing problem, it also instructed me—showing me that I could alter stories so that their content matches their audiences.

Story choosing and story alteration is a necessary skill in the use of stories with bereaved children or with adults. *A word of caution here*: When altering stories which are not in the public domain but are under copyright, one must first consult the story's author (and/or copyright holder) to obtain his/her permission for a literal retelling. It is helpful to understand that copyright does not protect an idea, only the fixed form of expression of an idea. A more in-depth discussion of copyright issues related to storytelling is found in *The Storyteller's Guide* (Mooney & Holt, 1996).

As already noted, storytelling is an interaction between the listener and teller. When you are telling a story in a way that makes use of all aspects of the self (mind, body, spirit) to engage and convey the story, you, the storyteller, will be changed by the reception of the listener(s). This is often true even in writing.

For instance, as I interact here with the imagined ear of you, the listener, someone I wish to connect with in a meaningful way, I imagine the story in the context of this book. I think about what the story might mean to you, am challenged by how I can describe what it means to me, and am curious as to what it might mean to the editor of this book, whom I appreciate and admire. I am informed by my belief that effective storytellers do more than tell a tale, they embody it (Stotter, 1994). I ask myself, "What should I add or take from my story experience that will bring you, the reader, with me into the written story? How can I create an environment of words and spirit that will help this story sing?—That will encourage you to discover your own stories and to use stories in your work with children?"

In my experience one thing seems certain: Stories that heal will offer kinesthetic and emotional possibilities and memories as well as intellectual ones; stories that have the greatest potential for healing are those that create shifts in awareness, understanding, and well-being. This emotional resonance may replace or surpass cognitive understanding.

The Crucial Role of Imagination

Following a loss, the ability to imagine new possibilities and the ability to reformulate old experiences are essential components for finding our way or growing through grief. This imaginative capacity is needed by children and adults alike. It allows us to re-create or reconstruct meaning and hope for a life that may be new or altered but still holds value and promise. The imaginative capacity also serves as a foundation for building resilient, purposeful, and unique human beings.

RECOGNIZING THERAPEUTIC STORIES

In choosing and developing stories for therapeutic value, I rely heavily on two sources as guidelines: First, I count on my understanding of practices and attributes derived from the literature and research on resiliency, heartiness, and transformation and growth through loss and trauma, some of which I have previously listed. Secondly, I have gained greatly from workshops and study with various professional storytellers, especially Donald Davis (1993), Robin Moore (1991), David Holt & Bill Mooney (1994, 1996), Jim Mays (1996), and Kendall Haven (1999). I often return to their teachings when searching for stories or when writing or telling my own. All of these storytellers have published works with August House Publishers in Little Rock, Arkansas.

Finding and Telling Stories
That Resonate Wholeness

There is a "Family Circle" cartoon in which a little boy is distraught after hearing the nursery rhyme *Humpty Dumpty*. He looks up seriously at his father and says, "Maybe they didn't try hard enough."

Story is the natural language of children. At an early age children know what is and what isn't a satisfying story (McAdams, 1993) and are able to manipulate story images to obtain more satisfactory outcomes. In the case of the Humpty Dumpty cartoon, the child hearing the story knows that something is wrong with its ending.

At a week-long training I attended with storyteller Donald Davis, he presented a three-part formula for determining if a story is whole or complete. Davis sees this formula as a means to measure a story's ability to both entertain and to be known by the listerner as a wholesome life experience. From his point of view a whole story begins as the listener feels at home and in place in the world of the story.

This is done first by providing the story with descriptions that identify the time, location, and people of the narrative in the normal routine of the characters' daily life and allow the listener to experience them. This first phase of the telling is the story foundation, or story setting, and often takes the most words and time to construct and deliver.

Secondly, with the world now known to the listener, a crisis or some trouble begins to surface in the narrative and is worked through. Davis defines a crisis as anything that takes a piece of the world we are comfortable with and turns it upside down so that we have to make adjustments to go forward. The grievous losses of children certainly fit this criterion. The crisis may be sudden and dramatic or subtle and drawn out. A crisis can be chosen or involuntary, positive or negative. Davis describes this story phase by saying, "trouble's coming . . . trouble's coming . . . trouble's coming . . . trouble comes." Davis points out that a whole story gives much more attention and time to setting the stage and to presenting the "trouble's coming" component than to the part of the story in which the trouble or crisis actually happens and is worked through. But, in a whole story, a healing story, a working through, some solution must be realized. The boy in the cartoon (discussed above) had a valid point. He knew that the problem of Humpty Dumpty was not resolved. As he saw the story, nothing was learned or discovered. So while Humpty Dumpty may be useful as a rhyme presenting the notion of loss as permanent and irreplaceable, it does little as a story to teach the concepts of resilience or connection, both of which are known to foster hope and well-being for children experiencing a loss (Klass, Silverman, & Nickman, 1996). For these purposes we look to whole stories containing the three elements suggested by Davis.

The third part of a whole story is its briefest component. This is the learning that is achieved and/or discovery that is made. Here Davis warns us not to get caught up in long prescriptive teachings. Children love to learn, but like adults rarely love to be taught. *Let them discover.* Therefore, while the discovery or learning from a story is an important component, it needs only a short amount of narrative time.

In *The Healing Power of Stories*, Daniel Taylor (1996, pp. 85–86) gives three parallel requirements of stories with the potential for healing losses and fostering resiliency. Taylor says that first the story must explain the experience, externally or internally. Secondly, these stories must have explanations that are satisfactory. They need to create a world in which we find it possible—even desirable—to live. Thirdly, like Davis, Taylor tells us that healing stories must assure us that life is worth the pain, that meaning is not an illusion, that others share and value our experience.

Here, then, is an example of a different ending for the Humpty Dumpty story, one that honors connection and memory:

> So while all the King's horses and all the king's men couldn't put Humpty Dumpty together again, they could none the less care for him and remember him. And this they did. Some of the King's men carefully gathered up every last piece of Humpty Dumpty's shell, some called Humpty Dumpty's family and friends. Some gathered round in silence, listening while others told stories about what he was like before he fell and cracked into so many pieces. Those who had loved Humpty still felt their love for him. That hadn't changed, although now their love had a great sadness as well. When all the work was done they held hands and remembered Humpty Dumpty by singing this song: "Humpty Dumpty sat on a wall, Humpty Dumpty had a great fall, all the King's horses and all the King's men would always remember him as their special neighbor and friend."

REASONS FOR USING STORIES WITH BEREAVED CHILDREN AND FAMILIES

Stories with children who are bereaved can be used in many ways. When choosing a story for a therapeutic use, keep in mind the particular need the story embodies, remembering that the most useful stories often *describe* rather than *prescribe*. These stories may suggest or describe change, but they do not demand it through pedantic persuasion.

Stories that assist healing have spiritual elements as well as intellectual and emotional content. They allow the teller and the listener to enter into the mystery of what is known and what is not known. They present possibilities rather than dispense solutions.

Stories can provide information, provide distractions from the burden of sorrow, encourage curiosity and imagination, give validation, and present alternatives. Stories may give a sudden burst of insight or may provide a gradual, indirect entry into awareness.

Stories can give new or additional information to correct faulty assumptions and can be used to normalize the grief process. Through story we can remember the past, validate what a child holds important, commemorate and honor what has been lost, and build bridges of hope for future development (Gersie, 1991). By diminishing isolation, quickening hope, and making a child's world more familiar and safe, stories also aid his/her spiritual development. (Coles, 1991).

STORY FORMS AND PRACTICES

With the rising interest and current research into narrative as a therapeutic practice, many story forms have promise. These include poetry reading and writing, journal keeping, story circles, read-aloud storysharing, and collaboratively written poems, plays, and stories.

Enhanced stories—those that can be enacted through puppetry, play, music, video, and theater—are beyond the scope of this chapter but are worth mentioning. To help grieving children, Steve Dawson and Laura Harris (1997, 1999) have developed an intriguing process called Grief Dramatics. Their work offers a 9-week children's bereavement group curriculum as well as scripts and activity pages. GriefDramatics can be used in individual or group settings, or in bereavement camps for school-age children.

The *Aarvy Aardvark Finds Hope* story discussed earlier provides another look at enacted story. Because his family has all been taken away, young Aarvy Aardvark is all alone. He feels so sad and devoid of hope that he even wishes he were dead. Thanks to a wise rabbit that befriends Aarvy through sharing his own experiences and witnessing Aarvy's pain, Arvy gradually finds his own inner strength and begins to imagine a future. Through a slow and gradual awareness that culminates in a ritual of remembrance, Aarvy discovers the courage to grieve his losses. After the ritual, a time when Aarvy honors the memory of his mother, he can once again remember the beauty of rainbows of every color.

Aarvy's story, adapted as a live puppet show, is regularly performed by trained volunteers in two urban North Carolina school systems. Hundreds of performances of the Aarvy story are given each year to fourth-grade students. The shows help teachers and school counselors identify bereaved children. Other young students not currently suffering a loss learn to recognize the universality of loss and the feelings and behaviors of grief as natural and normal. Other schools use the *Aarvy Aardvark Finds Hope* puppet video program (O'Toole, 1998) for the same purposes.

Bereavement counselors can learn to use stories in four distinct categories: (1) spoken stories, (2) written stories and bookmaking, (3) story books—story readings, and (4) sharing personal stories and story listening.

Spoken Stories

For therapeutic value, storytelling is perhaps the most compelling medium of all the story forms. I have had many opportunities to present stories about loss and grief, and death and dying, to individuals and to audiences large and small, young and old. These are stories I have either composed or have chosen and adapted from folk literature. During and after the storytelling I have witnessed the depth and breadth of learning as people respond, resonate, and extract what they need. People can and do enter into stories to create and discover their own meaning.

Telling Home-Made Individualized Stories

Doris Brett, an Australian psychologist and practitioner of therapeutic storytelling, has effectively constructed stories to help children deal with fear, pain, hospitalization, and death (Brett, 1988, 1992). She began her use of stories with her daughter, Annie, as together they faced various developmental hurdles and challenging life events. Later she fashioned her stories using materials and circumstances being faced by troubled youngsters who were her clients. Brett gives the following outline for making up your own therapeutic stories:

1. *Model the story character after the child.* This assists the child in using the story through identifying with the character.
2. *Make the problems and conflicts echo those of the child.* The narrative tone of the story should match how the child sees the conflict, not how you see it. This assists identification with the story character. The idea is to have the child think, "Yes, that's exactly how I feel." After the child has identified with the character, you introduce the way the story character comes to shift its thinking as it struggles with and then resolves its concern.
3. *Keep things simple.* Use concepts and language the child can understand. Tailor the length of the story to the child's attention span.
4. *Have the story honestly portray real conflict, uncertainty, and struggle.* Children have internal experiences of these feelings that need to be matched by the story characters if the story is to be believable.
5. *Remember to identify the strengths of the child and weave them into the story.* This helps the child recognize these traits in him/herself and to increase the individual sense of worth and potency.

6. *Use humor whenever possible.* It, too, allows for psychic shifts to take place and helps to release tension.
7. *When the child is tense, use your voice as an instrument to encourage relaxation.*
8. *As you tell the story, watch the child's body language for cues.* If the child is engaged, you are on target. If the child is disinterested, you might be on the wrong track or the content may be something he/she is not ready to hear.
9. *If you're unsure of where to go next, ask the child,* "What do you think Tommy did then?" Encourage responses through such a guessing game until you have enough direction to continue.
10. *Give the child hope by ending in a way that brings relief to the story character's distress.* Brett suggests these positive endings be honest and possible, something the child can use.

Mutual Storytelling

Brett's guidelines apply when creating a story for a specific situation. Another method of creating stories for therapeutic use is the mutual storytelling technique developed by Richard Gardner (1993). His work is thorough and instructive and provides considerable insight, especially into ways the mutual storytelling technique can be effectively used in clearly identified therapy situations. His work, based on the psychodynamic interpretation of the child's story themes, may seem challenging to persons who offer supportive rather than therapeutic bereavement counseling.

The work of Joyce Mills and Richard Crowley (1986) shifts the focus from psychodynamic analysis to the beharioral subtleties they observe and extrapolate in their work with children. Using metaphors and stories, Mills and Crowley found greater success when they paralleled a child's situation with metaphors that the child did not overtly identify with as personally applicable. Their clinical success with metaphors and simple stories is a tribute to the healing power of the interactive story, especially when the content is carefully and sensitively chosen and is altered by a child's verbal and nonverbal responses. Their approach favors the story process, one in which the child co-creates the story, over the story content. Mills and Crowley believe a story can bring about positive internal shifts and gains even when the child is unable to articulate that change through cognitive recognition or articulation.

Written Stories and Bookmaking

In recent years there has been an increase in popularity of personal stories for adults as well as for children. The *Chicken Soup for the Soul* (Canfield & Hansen, 1993) books tell short personal stories of inspiration that have enjoyed many months on best-seller lists. National publishing houses publish hundreds of personal stories each year, and many authors—unable to negotiate contracts with publishers—have self-published their memoirs. In the latest edition of the *Compassion Books Catalog* (O'Toole, 2002), issued by a mail-order company in Burnsville, North Carolina, specializing in materials that can help people of all ages grow through grief, many of the more than 400 books carried are personal experience stories written by children and adults.

Bookmaking can be used by parents and professionals alike, as demonstrated in the father–son publication, *When I Die, Will I Get Better?* (Breehaart & Breehaart, 1993). The technique of bookmaking as a therapeutic process is carefully outlined for parents and practitioners in *Homemade Books to Help Kids Cope*, by Robert Ziegler (1992). Another example of bookmaking is the *Pain Getting Better Book* created as a metaphorical tool to help children cope with physical pain (Mills & Crowley, 1986).

Story Books—Story Readings

Many of us remember a particular book, poem, song, or story that came to us at just the right time. We remember how we were given some glimpse of hope or some insight to face some challenge. A story, *The Little Engine That Could* (Piper, 1990), evokes many such remembrances. In that story a train faces a big hurdle in taking its load of toys across a great hill to waiting children. It seems an impossible task. But the Little Engine, empowered with resilient traits, turns boldly to the task. Although the going is steep and difficult, the Little Engine never loses hope: "I think I can, I think I can" is its constant refrain.

Many stories have been told of how *The Little Engine That Could* has been used by children and adults to help them complete tasks that appeared impossible. One of these stories reports how an elementary school child pulled his mother, who was injured and unable to walk, from a wrecked car and up an incline to safety. The mother remembers hearing her son's repetitive refrain, "I think I can, I think I can," as he cajoled her to move while he dragged and pulled her away from danger.

A less dramatic but none-the-less evocative reenactment of the power of *The Little Engine That Could* is a personal experience I had at the age of 41 while biking 28 hilly miles around Lake Willowby in northern Vermont. I quickly learned that that beautiful route far exceeded my physical conditioning. All alone, trailing at least a mile behind others and barely able to peddle up a long steep grade, I was feeling very discouraged. As I slowly pedaled, my head looking mostly down at the pavement, I realized a song had begun to sing itself to me. The song seemed to be coming from somewhere deep inside my body. I was too out of breath and too despondent to sing that song out loud, but still I benefited from its helpful determination. As I listened to the song, my legs became more steady and confident. The words I was hearing, and they came to me in the musical tone of my remembered sister's voice, were "I think I can, I think I can, I think I have a plan. And I can do most anything if I just think I can." Happily I caught up with the other bikers and completed the trip with great exhilaration.

As the author of *Aarvy Aardvark Finds Hope*, I have also experienced the power of a tale to heal. I have been privileged to receive many poignant phone calls and letters from adults and children whom I would otherwise not have known. They have told me how they used Aarvy's story and Ralphy's imaginary presence to hold onto hope during periods of despair and loneliness.

One such woman was a single parent whom I doubt that I will ever meet but cannot imagine I will ever forget. On the phone she told me how her only child had been killed in a car crash. She told me how desperately she had herself wished to die. This she said was the only way she could imagine being reunited with her daughter. For months she had reached out to touch the copy of *Aarvy Aardvark Finds Hope* that a friend had given her. She kept the book on her bedside table, beside a night light, which she kept on. She said that on the many nights when she could not sleep she would reach out and touch the book cover. As she did so, she would hope that, like Aarvy, she too might find the will to live, that she might someday, like him, be able to imagine a rainbow of every color. Then she told me how one day while she was walking from the grocery store to her car, she saw a brilliant rainbow that arched across the city. She immediately felt a momentary burst of hope and joy. She said in that instant she felt reconnected to her daughter, to everything, everywhere. For her it marked a turning point. She had a long way to go, she told me, but she knew now that she was not alone, that she belonged, and that somehow she would find her way.

I am convinced there is more at work here than the story itself. For me there is experience, co-creation, and no small amount of what I can only call divine mystery. Through the stories we tell, especially those with which we resonate and so retell ourselves, we not only construct ourselves (Engel, 1995) but we are also held in the arms of mystery and love. In this way storytelling does indeed push back isolation, as well as help us know ourselves and broaden our community.

Sharing Personal Stories and Story Listening

As a person who has experienced healing and growth through many different story forms, I would be remiss if I did not speak of the inherent value of personal dialogue and listening in various settings. Whether in individual encounters, in dyads, in storysharing circles, or in other group settings, storysharing enables us to see and reformulate our world. Through the transparency of self we can externalize beliefs, validate what gives meaning to our lives, and release internalized or repressed feelings. Sharing like this allows our own words to be mirrors in which we can see ourselves from the inside out.

Thus, in listening to our own words, we are better able to decide whether to appreciate and maintain the story as it stands or to take steps to alter it through present experience, knowledge, and awareness.

Similiarly, we benefit from listening to the stories of others. Listening stimulates opportunities for new insights as we learn about the many and varied ways individuals experience similiar circumstances. Listening as a benevolent, nonjudgmental presence can greatly enrich our ability to understand ourselves and others. As Rumi, the great and wise poet, so wonderfully reminds us, "[stories of] grief can be a garden of compassion."

OUR CHALLENGE: TO FOSTER NARRATIVE DEVELOPMENT IN CHILDREN

If we are to nurture resilient children, we will do well to nurture children in the telling of stories. Susan Engel (1995) suggests that we can enhance the natural abilities of children to tell stories by listening attentively, responding substantively, and using collaboration to clarify and expand the tales. She also recommends a multiplicity of voices and genres for story expression, encouraging the use of a wide range of forms and permitting, even encouraging, stories about things that matter to the individual child.

As adults desiring to prepare children for the vicissitudes of life, we are called to encourage, reformulate, hold and witness the stories of those we cherish. Together, as we make the transgenerational journey, we can find our way with the help of such stories. For healing stories are more than fiction—they can be our means of recognition, insight, and liberation. Stories are how we can connect with our children, how we can connect with ourselves. Stories can make us *real*.

> So now the story has made camp in your heads.
> The story will hunt for you
> and at night its campfires will keep you alive.
> —DIANE GLANCY (in Taylor, 1996)

DISCUSSION QUESTIONS

1. Imagine that you are a school social worker who has been asked to provide a consultation to a third-grade classroom teacher regarding the death in a car accident of one of the students in her class. The teacher has asked you to give her the names of some books she can read to the class. How would you prepare for this consultation? Discuss both in terms of possible resources for the teacher and with regard to suggested activities for the children to help them grieve their loss.

2. Using animal characters, create a story about the death of a parent. After selecting the age and abilities of the child with whom the story will be developed, indicate how you might help the child incorporate Donald Davis's three-part formula for an effective story. Role-play this process with someone who will play the part of the child.

3. Review three stories from folk literature or books mentioned in this chapter, such as *When I Die, Will I Get Better?* and *Aarvy Aardvark Finds Hope*, to identify factors that contributed to the resiliency of the story characters. Write these factors down. Then find someone else to read the books and to also identify what assisted their healing. Discuss and collaborate on your findings as to what factors and qualities enhanced healing.

4. Do you think that everyone can learn to use storytelling with bereaved children? What might interfere with a counselor's willingness or ability to use this modality, and how could he/she become more comfortable using this method?

5. Discuss some of the pros and cons of reading a story to a bereaved child, compared to telling the story in your own words or creating one together with the child. What would be some of the advantages of using a video such as *Aarvy Aardvark Finds Hope* in a bereavement group like those conducted by some hospice programs. How could the facilitator stimulate group discussion following viewing of the video?

REFERENCES

Breebaart, J., & Breebaart, P. (1993). *When I die, will I get better?* New York: Bedrick Books.

Brett, D. (1988). *Annie stories*. New York: Workman.

Brett, D. (1992). *More Annie stories*. Washington, DC: Magination Press—American Psychological Association.

Canfield, J., & Hansen, M. (1993). *Chicken soup for the soul*. Deerfield Beach, FL: Health Communications.

Coles, R. (1991). *The spiritual life of children*. New York: Houghton Mifflin.

Corr, C. A. (2000). Using books to help children and adolescents cope with death:

Guidelines and bibliography. In K. Doka (Ed.), *Living with grief: Children, adolescents, and loss* (pp. 295–314). Washington, DC: Hospice Foundation of America.

Corr, C. A., Nabe, C. M., & Corr, D. M. (2000). *Death and dying, life and living* (3rd ed.). Belmont, CA: Wadsworth.

Davis, D. (1993). *Telling your own stories*. Little Rock, AR: August House.

Dawson, S., & Harris, L. (1997). *Adventures in the land of grief*. Wilmore, KY: Words on the Wind.

Dawson, S., & Harris, L. (1999). *Death of a forest queen*. Wilmore, KY: Words on the Wind.

Dwivedi, K. N. (1997). *The therapeutic use of stories*. New York: Routledge.

Engel, S. (1995). *The stories children tell*. New York: Freeman.

Flach, F. (1988). *Resilience: Discovering a new strength at times of stress*. New York: Ballantine Books.

Gardner, R. (1993). *Storytelling in psychotherapy with children*. Northvale, NJ: Aronson.

Gersie, A. (1991). *Storymaking in bereavement*. London: Kingsley.

Harris, L., & Dawson, S. (1999). *Death of the forest queen*. Wilmore, KY: Words on the Wind.

Harvey, J. (1996). *Embracing their memory: Loss and the social psychology of storytelling*. Needham Heights, MA: Allyn & Bacon (Simon & Shuster).

Haven, K. (1999). *Write, right: Creative writing using storytelling techniques*: Little Rock, AR: August House.

Holt, D., & Mooney, B. (Eds.). (1994). *Ready-to-tell tales*. Little Rock, AR: August House.

Holt, D., & Mooney, B. (1996). *The storyteller's guide*. Little Rock, AR: August House.

Jevne, R., & Miller, J. (1999). *Finding hope*. Fort Wayne, IN: Willowgreen.

Klass, D., Silverman, P., & Nickman, S. (1996). *Contuining bonds*. Washington, DC: Taylor & Francis.

Kobosa, S. (1985). Stressful life events, personality, and health: An inquiry into hardiness. In A. Monat & R. S. Lazarus (Eds.), *Stress and coping* (2nd ed.). New York: Columbia University Press.

Mays, J. (1989). *The farm on Nippersink Creek*. Little Rock, AR: August House.

McAdams, D. (1993). *Stories we live by*. New York: Morrow.

Mills, J., & Crowley, R. (1986). *Therapeutic metaphors for children and the child within*. New York: Brunner/Mazel.

Mooney, B., & Holt, D. (1996). *The storyteller's guide* (pp. 183–199). Little Rock, AR: August House.

Moore, R. (1991). *Awakening the hidden storyteller*. Boston: Shambhala.

Novak, D. (1994). The three dolls. In D. Holt & B. Mooney (Eds.), *Ready-to-tell tales* (pp. 13–15). Little Rock, AR: August House.

O'Connell Higgins, G. (1994). *Resilient adults*. San Franciso: Jossey-Bass.

O'Toole, D. (1988). *Aarvy aardvark finds hope* [Book]. Burnsville, NC: Compassion Press.

O'Toole, D. (1989). *Growing through grief: A K–12 curriculum to help young people through all kinds of loss*. Burnsville, NC: Compassion Press.

O'Toole, D. (1995). Using story to help children cope with dying, death and bereavement issues: An annotated resource. In D. W. Adams & E. J. Deveau (Eds.), *Beyond the innocence of childhood* (Vol. 2, pp. 335–346). Amityville, NY: Baywood.

O'Toole, D. (1998). *Aarvy aardvark finds hope* [Video]. Burnsville, NC: Compassion Press.

O'Toole, D. (2002), *The compassion books catalog*. Burnsville, NC: Compassion Books, Inc. Available on-line from *www.compassionbooks.com*

Piper, W. (1990). *The little engine that could*. New York: Platt & Munk.

Rando, T. (1993). *Treatment of complicated mourning,*. Champaign, IL: Research Press.

Rowling, J. K. (1998). *Harry Potter and the sorcerer's stone*. New York: Scholastic.

Rowling, J. K. (1999). *Harry Potter and the prisoner of Azkaban*. New York: Scholastic.

Rowling, J. K. (2000a). *Harry Potter and the chamber of secrets*. New York: Scholastic.

Rowling, J. K. (2000b). *Harry Potter and the goblet of fire*. New York: Scholastic.

Schmidt, M. (1981). *Super cystic fibrosis and fabulous Fran fibrosis*. West Orange, NJ: Organon Inc.

Schneider, J. (2000). *The overdiagnosis of depression: Recognizing grief and its transformative potential*. Traverse City, MI: Season's Press.

Stotter, R. (1994). *About story*. Stinson Beach, CA: Stotter Press.

Taylor, D. (1996). *The healing power of stories*. New York: Bantam Doubleday Dell.

Walsh, F. (1998). *Strengthening family resilience*. New York: Guilford Press.

Williams, M. (1958). *The velveteen rabbit*. New York: Doubleday.

Wood, S. (1998). *Mama mockingbird*. Omaha, NE: Centering Corporation.

Ziegler, R. (1992). *Homemade books to help kids cope*. New York: Brunner/Mazel.

15

✄

Self-Care for
Bereavement Counselors

SARAH J. GAMBLE

> In much wisdom is much grief, and he that increaseth
> knowledge increaseth sorrow.
> —ECCLESIASTES (1:18)

> Listening to my patient's lives made the world darker for me. I
> became more cognizant of the damage people can do to each
> other, and more protective against others' behavior toward me
> and my loved ones. I became more aware of how hard it is to
> repair the damage that . . . people sustain, and of human frailty
> under massive assault. At the same time, it helped me to
> understand my own life by seeing my experience mirrored back
> to me in my patients.
> —S. D. PERLMAN (1999, pp. 128–129)

On the day I first sat down to work on this chapter a "self-care" catalog
arrived in the mail. Within its glossy pages were specialized gadgets for
personal hygiene, expensive antiaging potions, and a very pricey weight
loss system that seemed to consist of eating nothing but dehydrated soup.
As I flipped through the catalog I reflected on the different meanings of
"self-care" and realized that the self-care I would be writing about concerns one's internal, psychological life rather than one's external appearance or image. As I thought about the sorrow one carries as a bereavement
counselor, that soul weariness and heavyheartedness, the catalog items
seemed ludicrous. Improving one's appearance, pampering oneself, and

indulging in sensory pleasures provide only temporary respite from work that involves sustained empathy with grieving children.

A specialization in grief (or, in my case, trauma) is a lifestyle choice for a counselor. Most of us don't realize that when we enter the field, but ongoing practice brings immersion into the shadows and dark places of other people's lives that gradually colors one's perception of the world. Many of these changes are positive: we have the satisfaction of doing meaningful work; we see clients reclaim themselves and their lives; we gain wisdom; and we have endless opportunities to learn about the deeper recesses of the human heart, our own included. Many of us become especially sensitive to the fleeting nature and preciousness of life, and of how things are always in transition. The insight that change is the norm, that nothing ever stays the same, can enhance our ability to savor the sweet moments in our own lives ("This is wonderful, and it is temporary") as well as to withstand the periods of loss and inner desolation that we inevitably encounter ("This is horrible, and it is also temporary"). This heightened awareness and enlarged perspective accompany one's ongoing development as a psychotherapist.

At the same time that we experience success and satisfaction in our work, however, some of the ways our work affects us can be deeply disturbing. This chapter is about some of those disturbing effects and what counselors can do in response. Examining the negative effects of one's work may seem disconcerting or even distressing, but it also makes room for greater self-empathy. One is not "unprofessional" if haunted or preoccupied by the pain of one's clients. The work of grief therapy places great strain on professionals' emotional and spiritual resources. In the long run, understanding the real emotional costs of one's work is a healthier strategy than numbly insisting that such costs don't exist. As one of my favorite authors writes, "When we are numb, we are not available for joy or hope" (Lewin, 1996).

In this chapter I provide a framework (the concept of *vicarious traumatization*) for understanding the negative effects of trauma and bereavement work, offer questions for self-reflection and assessment, and make some suggestions on how to address the specific disruptions of self that may occur. I write from my perspective and experience as a psychologist working primarily with adult trauma survivors. Many of my clients are survivors of traumatic losses, and the work we do can rightly be called "grief therapy." Although I do not work with children, I have presented on vicarious traumatization to a wide variety of counselors, including those who work with grieving children. I have found that vicarious traumatization is a concept that resonates with most mental health clinicians. While our clients may be of different ages and stages, the impact of our work as counselors on our selves and how we perceive the world is very much alike.

I hope readers use this chapter as a springboard for discussion with colleagues, classmates, supervisors, students, and supervisees. As we so often remind our clients, talking *does* help.

CASE EXAMPLES

Anna struggled to write her clinical notes after she finished her session with Miguel, a 10-year-old who had witnessed his mother's murder a year ago. She felt as if every nerve in her body was exposed. Her mind swam with gory images—predominantly her own imagination, she realized—since Miguel was mostly mute and withdrawn and Anna had purposefully tried to shield herself from any details about the crime when it was reported in the news. Miguel's play was repetitive and joyless: Pokémon figures endlessly attacking each other. He was surely clinically depressed. Anna knew she would have nightmares again tonight. "He's affecting *me* more than I'm getting through to him," she thought, as her mind sped on to fears about her teenage daughter's safety. "Why did I think it was okay for her to go over to Shirley's? Where is my judgment? Didn't Shirley's family live over in that section of town where residents had complained about gangs?"

Jeff, a practicum student, was in session with his 7-year-old client, Heather. "Do you think my sister is watching us?" Heather asked as she colored the stick figure drawing of her sister in heaven. Jeff looked at the drawing and responded, "Your drawing shows her looking down from the clouds. Is that how you think of her?" "Mmmhhmm," Heather replied. "My mom says she's an angel and that means she's flying around in the sky." Jeff felt a pang of envy and thought, "What I wouldn't give for that kind of optimistic certainty." Had he been that sunny and unshaken at one point in his life? Heck, he hardly knew *what* he believed anymore. He hadn't gone to church in ages but was afraid that if he did he'd hear more platitudes about a loving God. Just the thought of that made him angry. When he had mentioned some of these feelings in his last supervision session he had felt shamed by his supervisor's response: "It sounds like you've got a lot of work to do on your adolescent issues and perhaps you also need some medication. I can make some recommendations about who to see—or do you prefer to go through your insurance?"

Marion packed her briefcase at the end of her long day and tidied up the toys she had used in the last session. As she walked the carpeted hallway of the mental health center, she caught sight of her colleague, Sheila, and pretended not to notice the look that Sheila had that said, "Help! I need some on-the-fly supervision!" "Not tonight, Sheila," Marion thought, and kept her gaze straight ahead as she left the building. "Hey, we all have tough cases—you just deal with it," she thought defensively. As she drove home she remembered her partner's complaints last night that she was shut down and tuned out. Maybe a jolt of strong coffee on her way home could do the trick. "Marion, you've changed" had been the exact words. "You're not responsive. It seems like you don't let anything or anyone in anymore. What's going on?" Marion began to tear up as she thought about how she could no longer use the excuse of "It was a bad day." In fact, today had been a relatively good day. The "Good Grief" group she ran for kids was off and running. In fact, she had been asked to expand the program into the school system.

Anna, Jeff, and Marion are skilled, caring, and ethical counselors who work with grieving children. They are also each suffering from a process my colleagues and I refer to as *vicarious traumatization* (McCann & Pearlman, 1990a; Neumann & Gamble, 1995; L. A. Pearlman & Saakvitne, 1995).

Anna is besieged with affect and imagery related to her client's traumatic experiences. She has disruptions in her ability to trust others and also questions her own judgment. Her beliefs about the safety of her loved ones have shifted in a pessimistic way. She has extra sensitivity to media accounts of violence and tries to protect herself by avoiding newspapers and news broadcasts.

Jeff, the counselor-in-training, is struggling with his spiritual beliefs. He is highly anxious and is having trouble soothing himself. His ability to tolerate his own strong affect is compromised. His supervisors' off-target response to Jeff's efforts to communicate his distress and seek support has pathologized his thoughts and feelings, thus increasing Jeff's sense of shame and isolation.

Marion's intimate behavior and her interpersonal relationships in general have been seriously changed by her work. While her professional career has taken off, internally her experience parallels someone with posttraumatic stress disorder (PTSD) who so fears flooding she has become numb. She has stopped doing things she used to enjoy and she experiences others' interactions with her as unwelcome burdens. She has lost much of her idealism and zest. Previously known by her partner and friends as a warm and generous person—Marion's changed behavior alarms and frustrates her social network.

DEFINITION OF VICARIOUS TRAUMATIZATION

Vicarious traumatization (VT) refers to the deleterious effects of trauma work on the self of the therapist. We define VT as *the negative transformation in a helper's inner experience that takes place as the result of deep empathic engagement with traumatized clients coupled with a sense of professional responsibility to help* (Saakvitne, Gamble, Pearlman, & Tabor Lev, 2000). VT is not a tangible thing or a single experience; rather, it is an inner *process* that happens over time as helpers sustain their connection with human beings grappling with worlds shattered by loss or other trauma. All counselors who work with trauma survivors (and certainly this includes those who work with grieving children) need to be informed about VT because it is an unavoidable, inescapable, occupational hazard.

Like grief, VT won't go away through denial, minimization, or medication. Like grief, VT has at its core the pain of caring and attachment to one's clients. VT develops because of deep concern for clients. We cannot be effective healers without being vulnerable to VT; the only way to become invulnerable to this painful aspect of our work would be to avoid empathizing with our clients, and then, of course, we would be unable to help them.

Addressing our VT requires treating our own pain as seriously as we regard the pain of our clients. This process entails developing self-compassion. Recognizing and working through our painful responses to clinical work will benefit clients as well as ourselves. Our healing and our clients' healing are interconnected; what helps us to open our hearts will also serve our clients. Mohandas K. Gandhi taught that treating ourselves with compassion and mercy makes us more available to aid in the healing of others (Muller, 1992). In like manner, Pema Chodron (1997) writes, "As we learn to have compassion for ourselves, the circle of compassion for others—what and whom we can work with, and how—becomes wider" (p. 85).

VICARIOUS TRAUMATIZATION AS DISTINCT FROM OTHER CONCEPTIONS OF WORK STRESS

The negative effects of human service work have long been recognized and were described by Maslach and Jackson (1986) as *burnout*—a construct which encompasses the three components of emotional exhaustion, depersonalization, and reduced feelings of personal accomplishment. Others have written about "secondary traumatization," "traumatic countertransference," and "compassion fatigue" (Munroe et al., 1995; Herman, 1992; Figley, 1995). These constructs share a certain amount of overlap with burnout and VT but place most of the emphasis on symptoms (i.e., how therapists may experience somatic symptoms that parallel those of their traumatized clients).

In contrast to a symptom-focused approach, the concept of VT is grounded in constructivist self-development theory (CSDT). CSDT is a comprehensive model of human adaptation to extreme stress developed by my colleagues at the Traumatic Stress Institute (McCann & Pearlman, 1990b; L. A. Pearlman & Saakvitne, 1995). CSDT provides both a framework for assessing and treating trauma survivors, as well as a map for exploring the inner changes helpers may experience as a result of their work. A major emphasis of the theory is how people subjectively interpret and make meaning of their experiences: What is distressing and disruptive to one helper will be different from what is most impactful to another. Thus, the most important distinction between VT and other constructs is the emphasis on meaning, subjectivity, and the uniqueness of helpers' responses to their engagement with traumatized clients.

VICARIOUS TRAUMATIZATION IN THE REALM OF FRAME OF REFERENCE

A person's *frame of reference* is his/her characteristic way of making meaning out of his/her experiences. Like a pair of prescription eyeglasses, it selectively perceives the ongoing stream of experience so that his/her basic beliefs about self, others, and the world tend to be repeatedly confirmed. The frame of reference allows that individual to organize and interpret incoming data. Psychologically, the frame of reference includes his/her *worldview* (the person's conception of causality, why things happen as they do), his/her sense of *identity*, and his/her *spirituality* (sense of connection to something larger than the self).

A hallmark of trauma is disruption in the survivor's frame of reference. In an acute situation, this change is sudden and shattering. In an ongoing, chronically traumatizing environment, the person's frame of reference evolves toward pessimism, passivity, and randomness. In a parallel but clearly less intense way, therapists who work with trauma survivors can experience dramatic as well as subtle and insidious shifts in their frames of reference.

Worldview

Traumatized people ask, "Why me?" and "Why did this happen?" Their view of the world is inalterably changed—nothing seems to be the way it was originally: "I thought there was always a way to make sense out of things, but now that's gone." When a person's worldview is punctured, tremendous anxiety rushes in; many survivors experience panic and fear that they are losing their minds.

Counselors who experience VT in the realm of worldview sometimes describe a "deskilling" phenomenon in which all their training and theoretical grounding falls away or seems insufficient in light of the enormity of crises and needs in their caseloads. They may have trouble prioritizing tasks and attending to the incoming information from clients. Some counselors notice worldview disruption in their overall sense of being dislocated and overwhelmed. Similar to traumatized clients, therapists can be flooded with anxiety as they struggle to make sense of their experiences.

Working with bereaved and traumatized children may call into question cherished beliefs about the sanctity of childhood, namely, that childhood is a carefree, idyllic time in which parents can protect their children from suffering. Counselors may notice that their view of the world has become tragic—that they see loss everywhere and find it hard to believe that anyone grows to a ripe old age or dies a good death. When a senseless loss shatters a child's world (e.g., losing a sibling in a drive-by shooting), all adults struggle to comfort and provide explanations for the unexplainable. Parents, teachers, clergy, and counselors alike don't have "answers" to grieving childrens' universal question, "Why did it have to happen?"

Identity

"This can't be me," "I no longer know who I am," and "I feel like I've lost who I was" are identity themes encountered repeatedly in work with survivors of traumatic losses. As therapists, our sense of identity usually rests heavily on our ability to be helpful, nonjudgmental, "tuned in," and emotionally steady. We like to take complicated, messy situations and find ways to understand and intervene.

At times, however, our clinical work disturbs our sense of ourselves. We feel the feelings our blocked clients struggle to avoid, and our own equilibrium can be threatened. Sometimes a client's grief is massively complicated and protracted. We may feel frustrated, angry, and impatient in response. We may find ourselves internally labeling a difficult child as "manipulative" or "bratty" or some other pejorative, as if that could let us off the hook from the uncomfortable feelings of judgment and disdain we may be experiencing.

Grieving children can be very angry and may express their rage toward their therapists. Despite knowledge that contextualizes anger as part of the grief process, counselors can understandably feel hurt when they are targets of clients' anger or outright hatred. Children may see us in unflattering ways and criticize us in just the way that triggers our worst images of ourselves. A family may drop out of treatment with no explanation, a parent may vent despair on the counselor ("Nothing can help, and bringing my child here to play just makes her feel worse!"), and clients who had been doing beautifully can have setbacks. Such experiences challenge one's identity as a caring and sensitive therapist. On a deeper level the strain of one's work can invade a counselor's capacity to hang on to a sense of self that is "good enough."

Spirituality

In the wake of loss and other trauma, spiritual concerns are common. Some survivors question their long-cherished religious beliefs—"How could I believe in a God who let this happen?"—a searingly painful loss. Others, perhaps for the first time in their lives, begin to mull over the existential "big questions" about the ultimate meaning and purpose of life, what happens after death, and whether it makes sense to hold hope in a world so full of despair.

Our clients' struggles with spiritual and existential issues can be provocative and highly challenging for us. A precocious preteen whose mother had died of breast cancer angrily demanded of her therapist, "Tell me the meaning of life!" Her therapist felt on the spot, nailed as an "emperor with no clothes." As exemplified in the previous example of Jeff, a helper can be thrust into an existential crisis even when his/her clients' own spiritual views are tidily in place.

NEEDS AND BELIEFS

CSDT describes five basic need areas (and beliefs related to those needs) that are most sensitive to disruption by traumatic events: *safety, trust, esteem, intimacy,* and *control*. For helpers, these same needs are sensitive to vicarious traumatization. Sometimes a counselor's changed attitudes are readily recognized. One therapist realized her sense of control had been disrupted when she found herself jumping to the conclusion that her daughter's bruised leg indicated leukemia. At other times, a friend points out the changes: "You've become such a worrywart! You see accidents waiting to happen everywhere!"

Again and again in workshops on VT clinicians have described their changed needs and beliefs:

"I had an alarm system installed in my house. I never used to be so vigilant, but now I think about crime all the time." (safety)

"I can't stand having my son in day care. I worry constantly—what if someone hurts him? I can't stand it that I have to hand him over to someone else who does things differently from me. I worry that

I'm going to get a terminal disease and he's going to be stuck with this huge hole of grief." (safety, trust, control)

"My opinions of others have changed. I'm so much more critical—seeing people as frivolous and wasting their time here on this planet. Don't they realize life is a gift, we're all going to die sometime, and every day is precious?" (esteem for others)

"I'm more inward. I go through such intense experiences in my work but can't talk about it with my husband or my friends. It's not just the confidentiality, it's also this sense that I'm living on this different, heavier level." (intimacy)

VICARIOUS TRAUMATIZATION SELF-ASSESSMENT

All counselors need to recognize VT as an occupational hazard so that they can develop strategies to safeguard their hope and well-being. As part of this recognition, it is important to assess the level of one's VT regularly. Table 15.1 offers questions to help counselors in this effort. Other, more detailed assessment tools are available in *Transforming the Pain: A Workbook of Vicarious Traumatization* (Saakvitne, Pearlman, et al., 1996). As you look over your answers, what themes stand out? Which need areas are most salient for you at this time? How is this related to

TABLE 15.1. Self-Assessment: Vicarioius Traumatization

Frame of reference

• Why am I doing this work? Has this changed over time?
• What do I believe about myself? How is this consistent (or not) with my beliefs in the past?
• What do I believe about the world? Was this true before I did this work?
• What are my spiritual beliefs? Which spiritual issues of my clients are the hardest for me to work with?
• What gives me hope?

Needs and beliefs

• Do I feel reasonably safe? Do I believe my loved ones are safe?
• Am I proud of who I am? Do I generally think well of others?
• Can I trust my own judgment? Can I trust or depend on others?
• How much control do I have over my life? How much can I influence others?
• Am I good company for myself? How much can I allow others to know me?

your work and your own life experiences? What might you do to respond to any negative changes you have noted in yourself? What gets in the way of attending to your needs?

SELF-CARE FOR
VICARIOUS TRAUMATIZATION

My colleagues and I have identified awareness, balance, and connection as the ABC's of addressing vicarious traumatization (Saakvitne et al., 2000).

Awareness

Awareness includes not only becoming aware of VT—specifically, the areas in which you are disrupted—but also becoming mindful of your thoughts and feelings, your yearnings, your physical self, and your relationships. This requires "waking up" to your experience rather than distracting yourself, tuning out, and numbing. It may include some heart-to-heart discussions with colleagues and loved ones about changes they have noticed in you. It may involve cutting down or eliminating the use of alcohol or other substances that artificially alter awareness.

For many professionals awareness can only happen with a concerted effort to slow down, to do less, to stop running. This may be facilitated by meditation practice, prayer, or any form of focused contemplation that allows one a chance to step back and take a "time-out." Therapists who meditate regularly describe the calming aspects of inward reflection as well as increased access to their creative imagination and heightened ability to just "be with" clients without preconceived (and thus limiting) ideas (Fleischman & Fleischman, 1999; Rosenthal, 1990).

Balance

Balance is a philosophy and an ideal. It may be about balancing your work so that you carry only a few difficult trauma or loss cases in your caseload at any one time. It may be about balancing the type of work you do so that you use your professional knowledge and skills in a *variety* of roles in addition to direct clinical work. It may encompass how you schedule your clients so that no one day is "too much." It may be about the emphasis you place on trauma and loss themes as you listen and respond to your clients. A balanced approach to listening includes being open to themes of restoration and growth as well as of loss and decay.

Balance involves setting limits on our availability to clients and keeping realistic boundaries for our therapeutic work. This means that we have to be alert to rescue fantasies which will be regularly triggered in response to our clients' compelling needs. Repeatedly we must remind ourselves about the perils of overextension and examine any of our movements away from an empathic, reflective stance with our clients. We need to keep reminding ourselves that providing a therapeutic space, a relationship, and our best efforts of connected and disciplined attention is in and of itself extremely valuable to our clients.

Balance is also about one's personal priorities and recognizing how these change over the life cycle. In my own life, as I've juggled the competing needs of my young family (which also includes a special-needs child), my work, and myself, I have had to face my personal limits of energy and attention. I have had to accept that as much as I love my work, it is also profoundly draining. The realization that I was giving the best of myself to my clients rather than my children was painful and hugely guilt inducing. Acknowledging that I had "dropped the ball" in important areas of my juggling life led me to look hard at the issue of balance between work, home, and self.

As a result, I have cut down on the number of clients I see, work-related travel, and the number of projects I take on. It has been humbling to realize I can't do it all, or do it well enough to suit my own standards, without doing less. "Less is more" is my new mantra.

Connection

Human relationships are vital in addressing issues of VT. None of us should do loss or trauma work alone. We all need personal and professional anchors to moor us, offer us perspective, and counteract the isolation of our work. Professionally, we need a supportive and nonjudgmental atmosphere in which to explore and discuss our emotional responses to our clients' material. We can use colleagues, supervisors, consultants, or personal therapists—but at a minimum we need at least one caring, safe, and confidential relationship in which to address our responses to our work.

At my workplace we have weekly clinical "feelings" meetings where we talk about our experiences of VT, countertransference, and general stress. At agencies or work settings where needs of practitioners are not sufficiently recognized, staff can lobby administrators for scheduled time to provide "VT peer consultation." Some clinicians with whom we have consulted have arranged informal peer support groups outside of work (Ryan, 1999).

Attending to VT can be seen as a primary prevention effort to maintain staff morale, avoid staff turnover, and protect the integrity of clinical services. When agencies take the needs of counselors seriously, everyone benefits.

In our personal lives we need the opportunity to connect with others in roles other than that of "therapist" or "counselor." We need people with whom we can be spontaneous, sometimes irrational, and hands-on. We need people who will challenge our beliefs and assumptions in a positive direction. We need to be regular, everyday, ordinary folks—not always the expert, the "wise one," or the one on whom others depend. We need to explore and express forms of intimacy other than the intimacy of the therapeutic relationship.

CONCLUDING COMMENTS

Ultimately, caring for ourselves as healers requires spiritual grounding. Whether we identify ourselves as "religious" or not, we need this grounding to help sustain our hope and optimism in the face of the suffering and brokenness we routinely encounter in our offices. Spiritual practices connect us to ourselves, to others, and to that which is larger than we. "Spirituality" in the broadest sense is about being open to an awareness beyond what is tangible or material. It is about being available to joy and beauty, even side by side with cruelty and pain. Spirituality concerns finding that doorway to experiences of awe, to feelings of connectedness to others, and to a sense of wholeness both within ourselves and without.

Spirituality is deeply personal, individualized, and idiosyncratic. It can be hard to put into words with a great degree of specificity. For some of us our spirituality includes some form of theism, whereas for others spirituality is nontheistic. Often, spirituality involves an organized religious community and tradition, but it does not have to.

Sacred depth can be found in many places and practices—in nature, in meditation, in music, in dance, in traditions and rituals, in gardening, in social activism, and in scholarly study, to name but a few. Simpkinson and Simpkinson (1998) define spiritual practice as "the regular use of a method that helps us to step out of everyday consciousness and build a relationship with the Divine" (p. 250).

Bereavement counselors need to build healthy, life-affirming practices into their everyday lives. Such practices aim to see beyond the current (perhaps hopeless) situation without denying the seriousness and reality of pain. With intention, one may pray, contemplate, do yoga, or engage in other attention-based practices which help to clear out the clutter of one's mind. When one can quiet the distracting inner voices, the thoughts and feelings, the lists of what needs doing, the worries about what may happen in the future, one can create a space in which to encounter a larger perspective. With intention, one can seek to simply be still at the center of one's being so that one can make room to hold the dialectics of joy and sorrow, hope and hopelessness, life and death.

In leading VT workshops for mental health professionals, my colleagues and I often use an experiential exercise we developed to engage with the competing poles of hope and despair. The exercise is called "Hope and Despair" and consists of a guided visualization followed by group poetry writing. To give readers a sense of this exercise, I will describe it in detail.

After leading participants through a guided relaxation sequence, we invite them to visualize hope. We give participants sufficient time to fully elaborate their images of hope and then direct them to shift their awareness to an image of despair. We encourage the audience to stay with their despair imagery even though they may find it uncomfortable. We ask them to be curious about their images, to explore them from many angles and vantage points. When enough time has passed, we direct participants to combine their images of hope and despair. Usually, people find this last task very challenging; it is, after all, what we are asked to do as therapists—to contain our clients' despair while also holding hope. In a state of quiet focus and interpersonal support, this exercise guides participants to see hope and despair as two aspects of a whole, as interconnected and overlapping. Last, we reorient participants to wakeful attention and have them form groups of three to five people. With instructions to "be imperfect," each group works quickly on a poem to express their imagery. The exercise closes with a member of each group reading their poem aloud to the group as a whole. This never fails to be profoundly moving and inspirational. Below are two poems from a group of counselors I was privileged to lead several years ago:

> *Hope and Despair (1)*
>
> Hope exceeds all expectations
> Despair prevails despite our efforts
> Despair heard, is hope
>
> Hope is the neighbor of despair
> They live side-by-side
> Day-by-day

> *Hope and Despair (2)*
>
> There's a light at the end of the dark
> Tunnel, a cup in the saucer
> A howling inside the dog
> A closed door can be opened, an open door can be closed.

A paradise in the beyond,
A hope in the present,
Hope grapples with despair
. . . And I reach the end of the tunnel . . . .

The ancient Jewish mystical tradition of Kabbalah, like the Buddhist practice of "mindfulness meditation," encourages spiritual seekers to develop "awareness with intention"—the effort to bring a spiritual perspective to anything and everything one does. Perhaps one of the most useful strategies in addressing VT is to bring to our clinical work the same questions and intentions we bring to our spiritual lives. In each clinical encounter, we can wonder, "What does this client have to teach me?" and "If this client were carrying a message specifically for me, what might it be?"

Seeing one's work from a spiritual perspective does not mean "preaching" or trying to convert clients to any system of belief. Rather, it is about tuning in to what is universal about our client's experience, continually developing our compassion and self-compassion, working with issues of forgiveness as they arise for our clients, staying open to influences that are not "scientific" and rational, and being grateful for signs of hope and healing, even when they are small.

To honor the spiritual depth of our work, we can arrange our offices so that they are sacred spaces—with artifacts and pictures of the beautiful natural world, with reminders of people who have given us wise counsel, with objects that connect us to thoughts of healing, and with books that have given us inspiration. One trauma therapist writes of her office, "Everything in this room gives off an air of gentleness and sends a message that healing is possible." (Collins, 1999). In my own office I have a fountain which reminds me of the healing nature of tears, the life-giving powers of water, and the miraculous cycles of regeneration that are all around us.

John Welwood (2000) writes, "When practiced in a spiritual context, psychotherapy can be a form of soul-work." Increasingly, I am finding this to be true. As I work with my client's suffering, my own pain is stirred. As I work with clients' defenses, I am called to notice where I am blocked and shut down, to notice where my heart has become closed. As my clients wrestle with what makes life worth living, I revisit the question in terms of my own life.

Ongoing contemplation deepens my experience. At times this is painful and I envy the lucky souls I imagine who skim along the surface of life, unencumbered by introspective tendencies. At other times I am more in touch with the gifts of all this "mulling over." I notice that I am becoming more tolerant of not knowing the answers; I am becoming less critical toward myself as well as others; I have become more tolerant and accepting of the messiness of life and human relationships; I am more and more comfortable with not feeling much like an expert.

When I return home to my children, the mounds of laundry, the bills, and the dishes, I often feel grateful to focus on the mundane. The children's squabbles are like a breath of fresh air. The homework struggles, the preschool art projects, and the bedtime rituals are childhood incarnate—early memories in the making that I know from my clients will last a lifetime. That back and forth between everydayness and issues of meaning is something I have come to value more and more.

Tuning in to a spiritual perspective has changed my reading habits. After years of sole focus on trauma, I have moved into reading about healing, finding meaning, optimism, wisdom, and compassion (e.g., Baltes & Staudinger, 2000; Dowrick, 1997; Lewin, 1996; Seligman & Csikszentmihalyi, 2000). Exploring spirituality in its broadest sense, I have gained new language for compassion and "being with" pain rather than working to chase it away. I keep this quote from Pema Chodron (1997) taped to my desk, where I see it as I review clinical notes before beginning a session:

> We think the point is to pass the test or to overcome the problem, but the truth is that things don't really get solved. They come together and they fall apart. Then they come together and they fall apart again. It's just like that. The healing comes from letting there be room for grief, for relief, for misery, for joy. (p. 8)

Chodron's stark words provide wise guidance for all of us in the helping professions. Taking good care of ourselves as grief counselors is very much about "letting there be room" within us for the myriad responses we have to our very compelling clients. This sounds simple but is in fact very challenging. Like successful grieving, it often involves swimming in an ocean of sadness—trusting, having faith, holding some glimmer of hope that there is in fact a tranquil shore somewhere in the distance.

DISCUSSION QUESTIONS

1. Jot down responses to the self-assessment questions in this chapter. What do you notice? Discuss your responses with someone who knows you well.

2. Have you ever experienced despair? What were the circumstances? How is this similar or different from your clients' experiences?

3. What gives you hope? Do you engage in any of the spiritual practices described in the chapter? If not, why? Discuss your answers with a trusted person.

REFERENCES

Baltes, P. B., & Staudinger, U. M. (2000). Wisdom: A metaheuristic (pragmatic) to orchestrate mind and virtue toward excellence. *American Psychologist, 55*(1), 122–135.

Chodron, P. (1997). *When things fall apart.* Boston: Shambhala.

Collins, B. J. (1999). Some thoughts on avoiding vicarious traumatization. *Treating Abuse Today, 9*(2), 40–41.

Dowrick, S. (1997). *Forgiveness and other acts of love.* New York: Norton.

Figley, C. R. (Ed.). (1995). *Compassion fatigue: Coping with secondary traumatic stress disorder in those who treat the traumatized. Psychosocial Stress, No. 23.* New York: Brunner/Mazel.

Fleischman, P. R., & Fleischman, F. D. (1999). *Karma and chaos: New and collected essays on Vipassana meditation.* Seattle, WA: Vipassana Research Publications.

Herman, J. (1992). *Trauma and recovery: The aftermath of violence.* New York: Basic Books.

Lewin, R. A. (1996). *Compassion: The core value that animates psychotherapy.* Northvale, NJ: Aronson.

Maslach, C., & Jackson, S. E. (1986). *Maslach Burnout Inventory* (2nd ed.). Palo Alto, CA: Consulting Psychologists Press.

McCann, I. L., & Pearlman, L. A. (1990a). Vicarious traumatization: A framework for understanding the psychological effects of working with victims. *Journal of Traumatic Stress, 3*(1), 131–149.

McCann, I. L., & Pearlman, L. A. (1990b). *Psychological trauma and the adult survivor: Theory, therapy, and transformation.* New York: Brunner/Mazel.

Muller, W. (1992). *Legacy of the heart.* New York: Simon & Schuster.

Munroe, J. F., Shay, J., Fisher, L., Makary, C., Rapperport, K., & Zimering, R. (1995). Preventing traumatized therapists: A team treatment model. In C. R. Figley (Ed.), *Compassion fatigue: Coping with secondary traumatic stress disorder in those who treat the traumatized. Psychosocial Stress, No. 23,* (pp. 209–231). New York: Brunner/Mazel.

Neumann, D., & Gamble, S. J. (1995). Issues in the professional development of psychotherapists: Countertransference and vicarious traumatization in the new trauma therapist. *Psychotherapy, 32*(2), 341–348.

Pearlman, L. A., & Saakvitne, K. W. (1995). *Trauma and the therapist.* New York: Norton.

Perlman, S. D. (1999). *The therapist's emotional survival: Dealing with the pain of exploring trauma.* Northvale, NJ: Aronson.

Rosenthal, J. (1990). The meditative therapist. *The Family Therapy Networker, 14*(5), 38–41, 70–71.

Ryan, K. (1999). Self-help for the helpers: Preventing vicarious traumatization. In

N. B. Webb (Ed.), *Play therapy with children in crisis* (2nd ed.): *Individual, group, and family treatment* (pp. 471–491). New York: Guilford Press.

Saakvitne, K. W., Gamble, S., Pearlman, L. A., & Tabor Lev, B. (2000). *Risking connection: A training curriculum for working with survivors of childhood abuse.* Lutherville, MD: Sidran Press.

Saakvitne, K. W., Pearlman, L. A., & the staff of the Traumatic Stress Institute (1996). *Transforming the pain: A workbook on vicarious traumatization for helping professionals who work with traumatized clients.* New York: Norton.

Seligman, M. E. P., & Csikszentmihalyi, M. (2000). Positive psychology: An introduction. *American Psychologist, 55*(1), 5–14.

Simpkinson, A. A., & Simpkinson, C. H. (1998). *Soul work.* New York: Harper Perennial.

Welwood, J. (2000). *Toward a psychology of awakening.* Boston: Shambhala.

PART V

❧

Helping Children Bereaved by Terrorism

16

September 11, 2001

NANCY BOYD WEBB

Several thousand children were suddenly bereaved by the terrorist attacks on the United States on September 11, 2001. The *New York Times* (2001a) estimated that possibly 15,000 children lost a father or a mother who, in many cases, was a single parent. The exact number of missing and dead changed daily after the disaster, as body parts were retrieved in the rubble and identified through DNA testing. This was a very slow process, however, and 3 months following September 11 there were still 3,045 persons reported dead or missing at the New York World Trade Center (WTC) and 495 death certificates issued by the medical examiner's office. An additional 1,976 death certificates were issued at the request of families (*New York Times*, 2001c). At the Pentagon, 189 were dead or missing 3 months after September 11. In addition there were 246 passengers and crew who perished on the four hijacked planes and 19 hijackers (*New York Times*, 2001b). Several hundred police, firefighters, and other rescue personnel were also among the victims.

The greatest toll was in New York, where thousands were buried in the rubble of the two multistory WTC towers. Families waited for days and weeks hoping that their missing loved one would be found. Because the reality of the attacks was so difficult to comprehend and accept, many people were unable to face the probability that their relative was dead. Without the evidence of a dead body, family members remained waiting and hopeful. Even after hope had died, some relatives wanted to receive some small bit of evidence from the debris as confirmation of the death and as a token to bury. A few deaths were confirmed with each passing day, but several thousand persons remain undiscovered and unidentified more than 3 months after the attacks. In this state of suspended belief many adults avoided revealing their worst fears to their children. The toll of human life and property destroyed in these attacks was horrendous. Two previous well-publicized terrorist acts in the United States occurred in 1993 and 1995. The truck bombing of the WTC in New York City on February 26, 1993, killed six persons and injured more than 1,000, and the truck bombing of the Alfred P. Murrah Federal Building in Oklahoma City on April 19, 1995, killed 168 people and injured more than 500 others (Kight, 1998). The extent of deaths and destruction of September 11, 2001, was far more numerous and extensive than these earlier attacks, thereby confirming the statement made after the Oklahoma City bombing that "terrorism is now a reality in America" (Krug, Nixon, & Vincent, 1996, p. 105).

TERRORISM

The term *terrorism* refers to "violence or threat of violence, in which civilians or locations habituated by civilians are targets or are frequently involved in the conflict" (Picard, 1993, p.11). This working definition of terrorism makes clear that terrorism operates as a *threat* as well as an actuality, and it usually claims civilians as victims (Kastenbaum, 2001).

The psychological effects of terrorism include an overall weakening of the sense of security, with resultant "changes in the way a society thinks about itself and the rules it enforces" (Kastenbaum, 2001, p. 236). The realization that destruction and deaths occurred as a result of *intentional* actions on September 11 adds to the complicated mixture of emotions experienced by survivors. Kastenbaum (2001, p. 236) states "we should not underestimate the emotional devastation of sudden death on survivors. Research on grief has made it clear that a sudden, unexpected death is much more difficult to bear." Additionally, worry about the possibility of more serious future attacks has compromised any effort to put closure on this traumatic experience of terrorism. Resumption of usual daily activities may be delayed or impossible, particularly since the ongoing retaliatory U.S. air strikes on Afghanistan have emphasized the continuous nature of the "war on terrorism." The anxiety of most Americans has remained high, and many adults have found it hard to reassure children that they are safe. Some children, like adults, have become worried that nuclear, chemical, or biological warfare may ensue. Indeed, the scattered cases of anthrax in the United States in which the biological agents were sent by mail have greatly increased that anxiety.

The section that follows reviews the nature of traumatic bereavement and the special circumstances of "ambiguous loss," in situations where the dead body remains missing. This is presented in the context of "complicated bereavement" for the family and the community, with special implications for children.

TRAUMA, LOSS, AND COMPLICATED BEREAVEMENT

Reactions to Trauma and to Bereavement

Although there are some similar emotional responses following experiences of bereavement and of trauma, important differences between the two relate to the process of reminiscence about the person who died. Bereaved persons typically mourn by remembering a mixture of happy recollections about the person as well as experiences about which they may feel sad or have some regrets. This remembering and talking about the deceased helps the individual gradually come to terms with the fact that the person has died. In normal bereavement, remembering the deceased is a part of the course of adaptation, reorganization, and recovery: "It may engender pleasurable as well as sad thoughts and generates (for children) play that assists the child in working through, accepting, and redefining the relationship with the deceased" (Nader, 1997, p. 21, citing Raphael, 1983).

This acceptance and understanding, however, becomes derailed when the associations are traumatic, terrifying, and overwhelming. Rando (1993, p. 587) states that "traumatic death can leave the individual with an overlay of post-traumatic symptomatology . . . [which is] like a blanket covering the mourning." Thus it makes sense that the stress of the trauma must be addressed first in order to reach the underlying feelings of grief.

When family members of persons lost in the September 11 attacks see and think about the frightening death scene (labeled by the media as "Ground Zero"), terrible images of destruction and horror block out their more intimate personal recollections about their loved one. Preoccupation with the traumatic circumstances of a death occurs whether or not the person actually witnessed the violent death scene or merely heard it described by others. The repeated TV replays of the terrorist attacks on September 11 gave everyone in the United States pictures not only of the airplanes hitting the WTC but also of terrified people running for their lives, including some who were bloody and injured and others who jumped from the windows. Reports of thousands of people trapped in the collapsed towers precipitated anguish and worry about inevitable multiple casualties and deaths, even among citizens who did not have a relative or friend in the doomed buildings. For family members, neighbors, and friends of missing persons the shock of the tragedy and the hunt for their missing loved ones took center stage in their lives. Clearly, *grief* about the loss of a family member cannot begin until there has been some recognition or evidence as to the reality of the death. In these uncertain circumstances children take their cues from the adults around them. Older children may have heard reports from other sources, such as their teachers, their peers, and the media. In this particular case, because the events were so unique and disturbing, the responses of many children probably reflected the pervasive confusion of adults.

In situations of traumatic bereavement people often try to avoid anything that reminds them of the person who died, because they cannot bear the thoughts about the *manner* of the death. This avoidance is one of the criteria for posttraumatic stress disorder (PTSD) (American Psychiatric Association, 2000). Reactions to trauma, therefore, can seriously interfere with and block expressions of grief and make it impossible for the individual to engage fully in bereavement counseling. However, once the individual has reviewed and processed the traumatic event, his/her energies that were previously focused on warding off memories of the trauma can be directed toward memories about the person who died. Examples of dealing with the traumatic elements of loss before addressing bereavement is discussed in this volume in Chapter 8 (Webb), with reference to a child's refusal to go near the home of her friend who died in a fatal car accident, and in Chapter 10 (Nader) with regard to a child whose sister died in a sniper attack on a playground. Nader (1997, p. 39) states that "the complicated nature of traumatic death strongly suggests that an understanding of trauma, grief, and the interaction of the two is essential to [facilitate] recovery."

Complicated Bereavement

This term refers to a distorted or failed mourning process, given the amount of time since the death (Rando, 1993). Circumstances that may predispose any individual to complicated mourning include sudden, un-expected death (especially when the situation involves trauma, violence, mutilation, or randomness) and when the person perceives the death as preventable (Rando, 1993). All of these conditions certainly apply to the terrorist attacks on September 11 and clearly justify referring to the be-reavement of family members, friends, and the community at large as complicated.

Ambiguous Loss

The grief process of families may be frozen and unresolved when they lack any tangible evidence of death, as for the families of the several thousand unrecovered victims of September 11. This lack of verification of a missing person as alive or dead creates a state of what Boss (1999) refers to as "ambiguous loss," which sometimes lasts for years in families waiting for news about soldiers lost in battle or kidnapped children who disappeared without a trace.

The traumatic events of September 11 have been so well documented that families with missing persons who were working in or visiting the affected buildings or their immediate vicinity will not be able to avoid the bitter conclusion that their loved one must have died during or following the attack. However, most still want some evidence to verify the death, and in New York many surviving parents have taken their children to give DNA samples to match with the physical remains that have already been recovered or to place on file for future matching. For some young children this can be very confusing; one child questioned the nurse taking swabs from his mouth as to whether this would help bring his daddy back! As discussed in the next section, a child's age and ability to comprehend the meaning of death clearly affects his/her reactions to the deaths caused by these terrorist attacks.

ONGOING STRESS RELATED TO POSSIBLE FUTURE ATTACKS

Threats of danger constitute a major component of terrorism. Since September 11, the United States has become a country "on alert" for attacks of all types, at unknown times, in unspecified locations. At the time of this writing almost 3 months after the attacks the war continues overseas and on the home front, in laboratories and hospitals identifying and tracking anthrax spores of unknown derivation. Fear of future attacks on bridges and other locations of national importance keep citizens in various states of anxiety, and lacking in the confidence to effectively reassure children about their safety. This is a new type of stress for Americans, and we may need to consult with countries that have a history of ongoing warfare in order to learn how, or if it is possible, to protect children during lengthy periods of continuing anxiety.

Almost 20 years ago, a reporter traveled through locations such as Belfast, Ireland; Israel; Palestine; Cambodia; and Vietnam to try to learn about the experiences of children living in areas that had been at war for the previous 20 years (Rosenblatt, 1984). The writer states that "the children living in these places have known nothing but war in their experience. The elements of war—explosions, noises, fires, death, separation, torture, grief—which ought to be extraordinary and temporary for any life, are for these children normal and constant. Everything they understand, they have learned in an atmosphere of wildness and danger. Everything they feel and sense occurs in a situation where their lives may be ruined at any moment" (Rosenblatt, 1984, pp. 15–16). While these conditions do not apply directly to the United States, the sense of danger and of an uncertain future does prevail for many children, especially for those who were close to the events of September 11.

According to Garbarino and his former colleagues at the Erickson Institute in Chicago, there is a price to pay for living in an environment of chronic danger (Garbarino, Kostelny, & Dubrow, 1991). The resulting accommodations may include "persistent PTSD, alterations of personality, and major changes in patterns of behavior or interpretations of the world that make sense of ongoing danger" (p. 377). They observe further that "there is a growing body of research and clinical observations based on a concern that children and youth caught up in the war and other forms of social crisis will adapt in ways that produce developmental impairment, physical damage, and emotional trauma" (p. 378). Whereas these predictions might not be applicable to the United States in the situation of unease following September 11, they do provide an overview of reactions of children under the chronic stress of war and community violence that could help suggest possible preventive strategies. Several studies (Aisenberg & Mennen, 2000; Berthold, 2000) emphasize the importance of perceived social support and the influence of the child's parents as mediating influences on the effects of violence. Further study and research can inform us further about the risks of chronic stress on children and youth as well about factors that protect them.

ASSESSMENT OF THE TRAUMATICALLY BEREAVED CHILD

Over the past 10 years I have developed several different versions of interactive tripartite assessment models. These include the following: (1) the assessment of the individual in crisis (Webb, 1991, 1999a); (2) the assessment of the bereaved child (Webb, 1993; also Chapter 2, this volume); (3) the assessment of the child in a nontraditional family (Webb, 1996); and (4) the assessment of a child who is placed out of the home (Webb, 1996). All of the assessment models feature three sets of interacting variables with unique factors that apply to different situations. In order to understand the impact of *traumatic* bereavement on a child I have now created a model combining the tripartite crisis assessment and the tripartite assessment of the bereaved child (see Figure 16.1).

In this conceptualization the interaction of three different sets of variables will determine a child's specific responses:

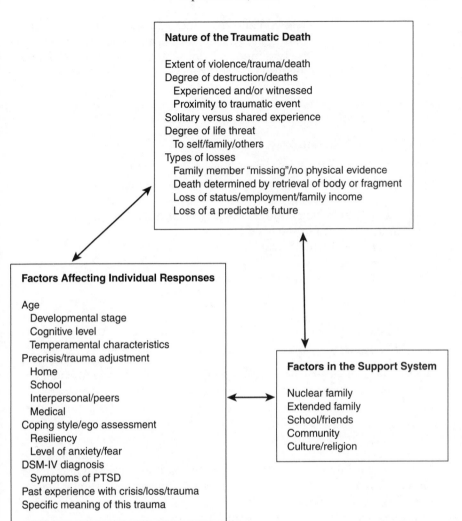

Nature of the Traumatic Death

Extent of violence/trauma/death
Degree of destruction/deaths
  Experienced and/or witnessed
  Proximity to traumatic event
Solitary versus shared experience
Degree of life threat
  To self/family/others
Types of losses
  Family member "missing"/no physical evidence
  Death determined by retrieval of body or fragment
  Loss of status/employment/family income
  Loss of a predictable future

Factors Affecting Individual Responses

Age
  Developmental stage
  Cognitive level
  Temperamental characteristics
Precrisis/trauma adjustment
  Home
  School
  Interpersonal/peers
  Medical
Coping style/ego assessment
  Resiliency
  Level of anxiety/fear
DSM-IV diagnosis
  Symptoms of PTSD
Past experience with crisis/loss/trauma
Specific meaning of this trauma

Factors in the Support System

Nuclear family
Extended family
School/friends
Community
Culture/religion

FIGURE 16.1. Interactive components of the assessment of the traumatically be-reaved child: Webb.

1. The nature of the traumatic death
2. The child's individual characteristics
3. The strengths and weaknesses of the support from family and community

Readers who are familiar with my tripartite conceptualization model for crisis and for bereavement will notice that in the current assessment of the traumatically bereaved child the subcategories "Factors Affecting Individual Responses" and "Factors in the Support System" are very similar from those in the two models from which it was derived. However, the subcategory "Nature of the Traumatic Death" is very different and must be carefully evaluated in order to understand its impact on a particular child.

Nature of the Traumatic Death

Factors that are particularly compelling with regard to traumatically bereaved children following terrorist attacks include the following:

- Extent of violence/trauma/death (including degree of destruction and proximity to the event)
- Degree of the life threat
- Solitary versus shared experience
- Loss of a family member (typically a parent)
- Loss of a predictable future

Extent of Violence/Trauma/Death and Degree of Destruction/Proximity

The tremendous destruction caused by the terrorist attacks of September 11 is without precedent. Children's appreciation of these events increases directly with their age. The older the child, the greater is his/her understanding about the underlying reasons for the attacks and about their possible significance. For example, a 7-year-old asked her mother if the attacks meant we were going to have a war, whereas a 16-year-old boy questioned his father about why he should continue studying and doing homework if we are all going to die anyway. The boy's question suggests that he feels the loss of a predictable future, which (taken with other symptoms) can contribute to posttraumatic stress disorder.

Although an individual's *perception* of a traumatic event is of primary importance in determining its impact, certain objective components of the traumatic situation also contribute to its meaning. For example, the sheer number of dead and missing following September 11 had great significance. Relatives of casualties were so numerous in many communities and schools throughout the metropolitan New York City area that even children who did not suffer a personal loss knew someone who did. Some children even claimed untruthfully that they had a missing parent or other relative, possibly because so much attention was given to classmates who had suffered losses (Goodnough, 2001). Clearly, the reactions of parents and the community, together with the media reports, emphasized the enormous impact of the attacks, which children absorbed and understood depending on their age and general knowledge of world events.

Traumatic deaths are distinct from other deaths and even from crisis events because of the frightening nature of the death. Previous studies (Pynoos & Nader, 1989; Nader, Pynoos, Fairbanks, & Frederick, 1990) have documented that the closer the individual is to the traumatic event, the greater and more serious is her/his response. However, Gurwitch, Sullivan, and Long (1998) point out that exposure may be emotional instead of physical, meaning that some children who have heard about a traumatic event may experience similar symptoms as those of children with direct contact with the trauma.

In New York on September 11 some schoolchildren were firsthand witnesses. A 12-year-old boy who several years before had attended one of the schools in the vicinity of the WTC said to his father, "Dad, I can't imagine what the little kids in Mrs. McCarthy's class must be feeling." Mrs. McCarthy was one of his elementary school teachers. Her classroom overlooks the skyline. "Dad," he said, "those little kids must have seen the whole thing! It's really sick, Dad" (Malekoff, 2001). The serious concerns of this boy reflect both his empathy and his realization that the attacks resulted in many deaths.

Solitary versus Shared Experience

The mental health literature is inconclusive regarding whether children who experience a traumatic event later seek out or avoid other children who endured the same ordeal. Terr (1979, 1991) reports that children who survived the Chowchilla kidnapping subsequently *avoided* contact with one another, almost as if to protect themselves from the anxiety of remembering the trauma. On the other hand, there are scattered anecdotal reports (Webb, 1993; Goodnough, 2001) of children *not* actually bereaved by a tragedy who subsequently claimed (untruthfully) that one of their parents had died. This suggests that those who were not directly affected wanted to be part of the group that was.

We know that children do not like to be different from their peers and that a parent's death may make them very different. However, when several thousand children have lost a parent and received the attention and concern of the community and nation it would be conceivable that other children might envy the attention given to those who were bereaved. In time, researchers will try to learn about the unique strains suffered by children who lost parents in these events as well as about the impact on other children. The magnitude of this trauma has the capacity to affect even children who are not personally bereaved.

Types of Losses

The absence of a dead body to mourn and bury means that families had to decide whether to acknowledge the probable death or whether to continue to wait for positive notification. Some held a "photo wake" followed by a Mass or a memorial service without a body. Even after tissue samples were identified, families were asked to indicate whether they wanted to be notified at a later date if additional samples were located. Children may be very confused about this process. One 6-year-old volunteered to loan a bereaved classmate his own father *until all the parts of the boy's missing father were found and put together again!*

New York City gave each family with a missing and/or dead person an urn containing powdered debris from the WTC at a ceremony held late in October 2001. While this fulfilled the desire of many families to have a tangible remembrance of their loved one, it could reopen wounds for those families who had already had funerals or their own memorial services. Some young children may have wondered if their parent died twice!

In addition to the loss of a loved person, families suffered the loss of income from that person's salary, and they will need to replace this and also to find ways to fill the roles of the one who died. The surviving parent may be depressed and overwhelmed and other family members, neighbors, and friends in the community and church/synagogue will need to offer support and help. It is not known as yet how many children lost both parents in the September 11 tragedy. However, the *New York Times* on September 26 stated that "hundreds of children will eventually need foster care or adoption" (*New York Times* 2001a, p. A18).

Factors Affecting Individual Responses

Any assessment of a child includes an overview of certain basic factors such as the child's age, developmental stage, cognitive level, and temperamental characteristics. In addition, a review of the child's history also must be considered, including the child's adjustment at home, school, and peer relationships, in addition to his/her overall health and coping style.

Factors that are extremely important in the assessment of the *traumatically* bereaved child include the following:

- Level of anxiety/fear
- DSM-IV diagnosis (especially symptoms of PTSD)

- Past experience with loss/crisis/trauma
- Specific meaning of this trauma

Level of Anxiety/Fear

The fear responses of children, like those of adults, depend on their perception of danger. Whereas the preschool child may think it strange that airplanes flew into tall buildings and then the buildings collapsed, many preschoolers did not initially realize that there were people in the buildings and that many of them died trying to get out. In time the children may have learned this, but preschoolers do not have a mature understanding about death (as in the example of the boy who thought that the body of a missing father could be pieced together and returned to his son). Therefore, they might not have become upset about the attacks unless they experienced a personal loss of a family member or unless the caretaking adults around them were unduly anxious. The older the child, the more knowledgeable he/she will tend to be and therefore more subject to anxiety and fear. For example, a 10-year-old child sent the following e-mail to a site for preteen girls: "Every night I think terrorists are going to crash into something and a close relative or even I will die. I don't know what to do. It's not that my parents won't listen to me. It's just that when I want to talk about it I get nervous and cry. What should I do?" (Merrick, 2001). Teen Internet sites have been inundated with similar messages of concern. Adolescents have thus adapted an electronic method as a way of coping with their anxiety about the terrorism.

DSM-IV Diagnosis, Especially PTSD

Gurwitch et al. (1998) state that the most common responses of children to trauma are specific fears, reenactment play and dreams, separation difficulties, and some symptoms of PTSD such as avoidance and arousal. The requirement that symptoms must be present for a month before diagnosis of PTSD is given means that children's early responses of clinging, avoidance, and arousal may be classified initially as acute anxiety disorder (American Psychiatric Association, 2000). However, the literature on disaster characterizes extreme responses to traumatic experiences as "normal responses to abnormal events" (Shalev, 1996, p. 77), thereby normalizing the early symptoms of PTSD that actually may subside over time for many people. An average of 36% of children exposed to traumatic events are actually diagnosed with PTSD; an even greater number (39%) are diagnosed with generalized anxiety, and about 25% are diagnosed with depression (Fletcher, 1994).

Past Experience with Loss/Crisis/Trauma

Logic suggests that individuals who have had histories of exposure to loss, crisis, and/or trauma would become more stressed with repeated experiences. Fletcher (1996) confirms this reasoning in a statement that "considerable evidence has accumulated that a history of stressful life events is associated with higher levels of PTSD in children when they are later exposed to traumatic stressors" (p. 263). Similarly, Gurwitch et al. (1998, p. 27) state "a child's response to trauma and disaster may be affected by prior life events or pre-existing problems that place the child at greater risk for PTSD symptomatology." Later in this chapter I discuss preventive interventions that may be used with children soon after exposure to a traumatic event in order to help reduce their anxiety levels and thereby possibly reduce the later development of PTSD.

Specific Meaning of This Trauma

Fears about other future terrorist attacks or about the spread of biological warfare in the United States weigh on the hearts and souls of many adults, adolescents, and even some young children who have heard about these threats. People are saying that the world will never be the same again, and some are behaving as if there may not be any tomorrow. This erosion of hope and stability will have serious repercussions on children who sense the anxieties and fears of the adults around them and who respond accordingly.

Factors in the Support System

There was an outpouring of support in the United States for the families of the victims of the terrorist attacks. Children in schools across the country sent messages, money, and toys to New York City. Schoolchildren in New York drew pictures with notes on them that later were attached to the food packages given to the rescue workers. Flags continue to fly everywhere as if to assert our national identity and resolve to combat terrorism.

The sheer number of funerals and memorial services reinforced the reality of the multiple losses. Families and children who did not want to admit that a loved one died or think about the manner of the death nonetheless began their own grieving process by attending the wakes and funerals of others. Numerous memorial services and funerals occurred during the months after September 11, sponsored by various municipal and private organizations and professional groups. The victims have been designated as "heroes" with the promise that their memory will be forever honored.

At the same time that leaders urged all citizens to resume their usual lives, many adults have been very fearful about the possible recurrence of similar attacks and/or of biological warfare. This chapter has stressed the impact of adult responses on children, but as we now consider some different helping approaches for children I must emphasize that the effectiveness of these will be greatly diminished unless adults can find a way to reassure children about the restoration of balance and stability in their lives. Practitioners who work with traumatically bereaved children must connect with their parents and offer guidance accordingly. When children have been exposed to trauma, the impact of their parents' responses cannot be overstated. In fact, parents, therapists, teachers, and all adults must learn to take care of themselves to avoid the effects of secondary/vicarious traumatization, both for their own benefit, as well as for the children who depend on them for security. (See Gamble, Chapter 15, this volume, and Pearlman and Saakvitne, 1995, for further discussion).

HELPING INTERVENTIONS FOR TRAUMATIZED CHILDREN

Helping interventions for children following a traumatic event can occur at different periods of time (Pynoos & Nader, 1993; Gurwitch et al., 1998). The timing and typical interventions include the following:

- Immediately after the disaster (psychological first aid in the schools)
- From 1 week to 3 months postdisaster (debriefing and short-term therapy)
- After 3 months postdisaster (long-term therapy)

Immediately Following a Disaster/ Traumatic Event

When large numbers of children have been exposed to a trauma, schools provide the ideal setting for group interventions as soon as possible after the event. Different helping interventions following a traumatic event include "classroom presentations," "debriefing," and "defusing." All these methods emphasize the importance of helping those involved to express their feelings related to the traumatic experience.

Steele (1998) considers *classroom presentations* as the ideal method for reaching the majority of students immediately following an incident. This format provides educational information related to the facts of the event and about appropriate ways to cope. The goal is to normalize the kinds of reactions that typically occur following critical incidents. During the classroom presentation the children whose behavior suggests their possible need for additional help would be identified for later individual assessment to determine the need for further services, including debriefing.

An outline for a classroom presentation, including verbatim suggested commentary, appears in Steele (1998). The recommended presentation includes a *beginning phase* that summarizes what is known so far about the event, and invites students to respond on a personal level. This is followed by a discussion about *"normal" or typical reactions* to the type of trauma under consideration, and a review of *appropriate behavior* to be expected in this type of situation. The presentation ends with a *conclusion* that invites further questions, explains what to do if a student wants help in the next few days, and finishes by mentioning planned activities, such as memorial services. This presentation can last from 25 minutes to an entire class period. Because the classroom presentation consists of primarily *verbal* helping it might be too cognitive for many young children for whom the defusing method described below is more appropriate.

Steele (1998) recommends that the staff of the school who are known to the children conduct the classroom presentations. This might avoid a negative response such as occurred in New York City when a number of students asked to leave the classroom when some counselors unknown to them arrived and attempted to engage them in talking about their feelings about the WTC attacks (Goodnough, 2001).

From 1 Week to 3 Months Postdisaster

Other specialized methods for helping children who appear to be having some difficulties following a traumatic event include *debriefing* (including a particular form called *critical incident stress debriefing*) and *defusing*.

Debriefing is "the process of putting the incident (trauma) and the individual's reactions in perspective" (Petersen & Straub, 1992). It is "a group process designed to mitigate the impact of the event and to accelerate normal recovery" (Mitchell, 1991, CISD Video, quoted in Steele, 1998, p. 1). The debriefing method has been adapted for use in schools by Pynoos and Nader (1993), Petersen and Straub (1992), and Steele (1998) from its origins in a military protocol to help emergency health care workers and rescue personnel. Steele prefers to restrict the provision of debriefing to those who were most affected by the event, namely, individuals who witnessed the trauma or were surviving victims of the incident or were related or a close friend of the victim. Because it is important for each participant to have time to share the details of his/her experience, Steele suggests that debriefing groups consist of no more than 8–10 individuals. Petersen and Straub (1992) and Meichenbaum (1994) also recommend a limited number of participants to facilitate participation in debriefing sessions. Sessions may last from 30 minutes to 2 hours (depending on the age of the participants and the amount of time available).

Another model of intervention, critical incident stress debriefing, has been developed by Mitchell and Everly (1997). They also recommend small groups but would permit a maximum number of 25 participants, which is larger than in most other models. The purpose of critical incident stress debriefing is to reduce symptoms and bring about psychological closure, providing referrals for individual crisis intervention when indicated. Mitchell and Everly (1997) have written extensively and conducted training nationwide on critical incident stress debriefing. However, most of their work is targeted for use with adults rather than children.

Defusing is similar to debriefing, but (in Steele's 1998 model) it is more appropriate for use with younger children since it uses drawing and storytelling to help preschool to 12-year-old children convey the details of their traumatic experience. Petersen and Straub (1992) describe defusing as a process of providing information, promoting ventilation, preparing students and parents for possible reactions, normalization, suggestions for coping, and preparation regarding what to expect in the next few days. This sounds a lot like the content of a classroom presentation, as previously discussed. Still another definition describes defusing as "a 45 minute, structured small group discussion provided within hours of a crisis for the purposes of assessment, triaging, and acute symptom mitigation" (Mitchell & Everly, 1997, p. 7). Although there seems to be a lack of precision and uniformity about terminology among these different models, practitioners are unanimous about the importance of providing children with opportunities to express their feelings about their traumatic experiences.

Because young children do not have well-developed verbal skills, children's books and stuffed animals can be used to tell a story about a traumatic event. One such book dramatizes a situation of a traumatized cat who receives help from another cat (Sheppard, 1998). The story of Bart, a cat who had something "very bad, sad, and scary happen to him," helps traumatized children identify with the cat who appears to have many symptoms of PTSD. In the story, a cat named "Helping Hannah" encourages Bart to draw in her sandbox and later arranges for him to participate in a group with other cats who have had similar experiences. This story helps engage children and encourages them to draw and talk about their own experiences and feelings related to a traumatic event. After the Bart story, the leader in the debriefing group asks the children to draw a picture about what happened to each of them and then tell a story about it. After all the children have told their stories, the leader normalizes all their expressed reactions. The session concludes with some enjoyable activity.

After 3 Months Postdisaster (Long-Term Therapy)

When a child seems to need more help than provided in the classroom presentation, or in a debriefing or a defusing, he/she may be referred for an individual assessment. Drawing and storytelling also may be used in individual assessment sessions to help children depict their traumatic experiences (Nader & Pynoos, 1990; Pynoos & Eth, 1996). When indicated, some children may be referred to a bereavement group (typically 8–10 sessions), and others may require long-term therapy. Usually long-term therapy is indicated when the child had preexisting difficulties and the traumatic event caused an overload of stress, symptoms of PTSD, or depression, or when the child experienced multiple losses and did not have the fortitude and/or support to assist with developmental challenges. Use of the tripartite assessment of the traumatically bereaved child can help identify areas of strain that need to be addressed in therapy.

GUIDELINES FOR HELPING TRAUMATIZED CHILDREN

In earlier publications (Webb, 1996, 1999b) I discussed the use of verbal and play reenactment of crisis/traumatic experiences as a means to prevent the formation of PTSD. Because we do not know which children will develop symptoms following a traumatic event, it is advisable to provide classroom presentations and debriefing and defusing to reach the maximum number of children. The following guidelines would be implemented in these group meetings:

- *Give information about the crisis/trauma.* In the events of September 11 there was a lot of confusion about the extent of the attacks and about who was responsible. In a situation like this the adults should tell children that "Something very bad happened, and we don't know yet exactly what happened and who was to blame." Parents should be told what the children were told, and parents should be given instructions about reassuring children about their safety. An excellent manual for guiding administrators and mental health professionals in helping children and teens cope with traumatic events and death was prepared by the New York University Child Study Center (Goodman, 2001). This 70-page document includes guidelines for mental health staff, teachers, and parents, with selected sections for parents in Spanish.

• *Encourage the children to describe/portray or reenact the trauma, as they think it happened.* Younger children do not have good verbal ability, but many 3-year-olds actually spontaneously played out the scene they had witnessed on T.V. of an airplane colliding into something and knocking it down. Practitioners can explain to parents that this is one way for children to try to understand what happened and get control of their feelings. Older children may find relief by drawing or writing in a journal what they saw and say how they felt. When these drawings or journal excerpts are shared in a group the children have the opportunity to learn that others are sharing similar feelings. Many pictures were drawn by children of scenes of the bombing and events of September 11.

One drawing by an 8-year-old boy in the New York metropolitan area depicts what he saw on televised reports. (See Figure 16.2.) This child's picture shows the twin towers with balls of smoke at the top and several bodies falling from the buildings. Children and adolescents who

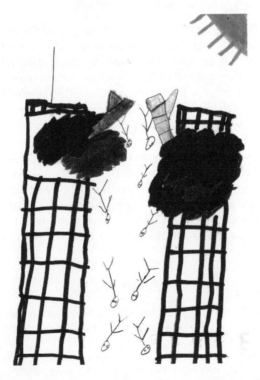

FIGURE 16.2. Drawing by an 8-year-old boy who viewed the attacks on television.

witnessed this scene were puzzled by it; some asked their parents if the people landed on trampolines (Smith, 2001). The process of drawing what they saw helps individuals try to comprehend what happened.

Writing in a journal can serve a similar purpose for older children. The ABC web site (Norris, 2001) reported an assignment for 6th grade students to keep a journal in the days following the attack. The teacher referred to the process of writing as "letting steam off a pot." One child wrote as follows: "This is a nightmare and I'll never forget this and my life will never be the same. So many people died because of this, people jumping off holding hands. It was raining people" (Norris, 2001).

• *Universalize and normalize children's reactions.* Even when personal accounts are not shared, the leader can validate each individual child's drawing or written story.

• *Identify strengths and new coping abilities.* While this may seem to be unrealistic for children mourning the death of a parent, the outpouring of support and attention from so many people might help some children realize that they are not alone in their grief. Children who attend bereavement groups would have the opportunity to bond with other children who were similarly impacted in these attacks.

The effects of September 11 have had many consequences for children, families, and all citizens in the United States. Because this chapter was initially written within 6 weeks following the events, I have discussed the immediate aftermath and the types of interventions that are most appropriate soon after a traumatic event of this magnitude. Only time will reveal the long-term impact on children and others. As already discussed, the continuing fears of many adults regarding our future vulnerability prevents the sense of closure and resumption of stability that traumatized children need to proceed with their development. However, children do find ways to survive, and even thrive, in situations of ongoing stress of terrorism and warfare such as in Israel or Northern Ireland. Most Americans have rediscovered a strong sense of national identity and purpose since September 11. There is thus hope that the children who were bereaved by these attacks will, in time, come to terms with the deaths of their loved ones.

REFERENCES

Aisenberg, E., & Mennen, F. E. (2000). Children exposed to community violence: Issues for assessment and treatment. *Child and Adolescent Social Work Journal*, 17(5), 341–360.

American Psychiatric Association. (2000). *Diagnostic and statistical manual of mental disorders* (4th ed., text rev.). Washington, DC: Author.

Berthold, S. M. (2000). War trauma and community violence: Psychological, behavioral, and academic outcomes among Khmer refugee adolescents. *Journal of Multicultural Social Work, 8*(1), 15–46.

Boss, P. (1999). *Ambiguous loss: Learning to live with unresolved grief.* Cambridge, MA: Harvard University Press.

Fletcher, K. E. (1994). *What we know about children's posttraumatic stress responses: A meta-analysis of the empirical literature.* Unpublished manuscript, University of Massachusetts Medical Center, Worcester.

Fletcher, K. E. (1996). Childhood posttraumatic stress disorder. In E. J. Mash & R. A. Barkley (Eds.), *Child psychopathology* (pp. 242–276). New York: Guilford Press.

Garbarino, J., Kostelny, K., & Dubrow, N. (1991). What children can tell us about living in danger. *American Psychologist, 46*(4), 376–383.

Goodman, R. (2001). *Helping children and teens cope with traumatic events and death: Manual for administrators and mental health professionals* (4th ed.). New York: New York University Child Study Center.

Goodnough, A. (2001, October 3). Schools struggle, delicately, to balance the normal with the surreal. *New York Times,* p. D1.

Gurwitch, R. H., Sullivan, M. A., & Long, P. J. (1998). The impact of trauma and disaster on young children. *Stress in Children, 7*(1), 19–32.

Kastenbaum, R. J. (2001). *Death, society, and human experience* (7th ed.). Boston: Allyn & Bacon.

Kight, M. (Comp.). (1998). *Forever changed: Remembering Oklahoma City, April 19, 1995.* Amherst, NY: Prometheus Books.

Krug, R. S., Nixon, S. J., & Vincent, R. (1996). Psychological response to the Oklahoma City bombing. *Journal of Clinical Psychology, 52*(1), 103–105.

Malekoff, A. (2001, September 20). *Zero degrees of separation.* Address presented to BlueCross/BlueShield, Long Island City, NY.

Meichenbaum, D. (1994). *A clinical handbook/practical therapist manual for assessing and treating adults with post-traumatic stress disorder (PTSD).* Waterloo, Ontario, Canada: Institute Press.

Merrick, A. (2001, October 18). Youths turn to web magazines to unload fears. *Wall Street Journal,* p. B1.

Mitchell, J. T. (1991). *Techniques of debriefing: Critical incident stress debriefing* [video]. Ellicott City, MD: Chevron.

Mitchell, J. T., & Everly, G. S. (1997). *Critical incident stress debriefing: An operations manual for CISD, defusing and other group crisis intervention services* (3rd ed.). Ellicott City, MD: Chevron.

Nader, K. O. (1997). Childhood traumatic loss: The interaction of trauma and grief. In C. R. Figley, B. E. Bride, & N. Mazza (Eds.), *Death and trauma: The traumatology of grieving* (pp. 17–41). Washington, DC: Taylor & Francis.

Nader, K., & Pynoos, R. S. (1990). Drawing and play in the diagnosis and assessment of childhood post-traumatic stress syndromes. In C. Schaeffer (Ed.), *Play, diagnosis and assessment* (pp. 375–389). New York: Wiley.

Nader, K., Pynoos, R. S., Fairbanks, L., & Frederick, C. (1990). Children's PTSD reactions one year after a sniper attack at their school. *American Journal of Psychiatry, 147,* 1526–1530.

New York Times. (2001a, September 26). *Helping the youngest victims.* Editorial, p. A18.

New York Times. (2001b, October 11). Dead and missing, p. B2.

New York Times. (2001c, December 11). Dead and missing, p. B2.

Norris, M. (2001, October 8). Troubled emotions: Children struggle to cope with terror attacks. ABCNEWS.com. http://abcnews.go.com/sections/living/DailyNews/wtc_childrencope010924.html

Pearlman, L. A., & Saakvitne, K. (1995). *Trauma and the therapist.* New York: Norton.

Petersen, S., & Straub, R. (1992). *School crisis survival guide.* New York: Center for Applied Research in Education.

Picard, R. G. (1993). *Media portrayals of terrorism.* Ames: Iowa State University Press.

Pynoos, R. S., & Eth, S. (1996). Witness to violence: The child interview. *Journal of the Academy of Child Psychiatry, 25,* 306–319.

Pynoos, R. S., & Nader, K. O. (1988). Psychological first aid and treatment approach for children exposed to community violence: Research implications. *Journal of Traumatic Stress, 1,* 445–473.

Pynoos, R. S., & Nader, K. O. (1989). Children's memory and proximity to violence. *Journal of the American Academy of Child and Adolescent Psychiatry, 28,* 236–241.

Pynoos, R. S., & Nader, K. (1993). Issues in the treatment of posttraumatic stress in children and adolescents. In J. Wilson & B. Raphael (Eds.), *The international handbook of traumatic stress syndromes* (pp. 535–539). New York: Plenum Press.

Rando, T. A. (1993). *Treatment of complicated mourning.* Champaign, IL: Research Press.

Raphael, B. (1983). *The anatomy of bereavement.* New York: Basic Books.

Rosenblatt, R. (1984). *Children of war.* Garden City, NY: Anchor Press/Doubleday.

Shalev, A. Y. (1996). Stress versus traumatic stress: From acute homeostatic reactions to chronic psychopathology. In B. A. van der Kolk, A. C. McFarlane, & L. Weisaeth (Eds.), *Traumatic stress: The effects of overwhelming experience on mind, body, and society* (pp. 77–101). New York: Guilford Press.

Sheppard, C. H. (1998). *Brave Bart: A story for traumatized and grieving children.* Grosse Point Woods, MI: TLC Institute.

Smith, C. (2001, October 29). Facing their fears. *New York, 34*(41), 29–33.

Steele, W. (1998). *Trauma debriefing.* Grosse Pointe Woods, MI: TLC Institute.

Terr, L. C. (1979). Children of Chowchilla. *Psychoanalytic Study of the Child, 34* 547–623.

Terr, L. C. (1991). Childhood traumas: An outline and overview. *American Journal of Psychiatry, 148*(1), 10–20.

Webb, N. B. (Ed.). (1991). *Play therapy with children in crisis: A casebook for practitioners.* New York: Guilford Press.

Webb, N. B. (Ed.). (1993). *Helping bereaved children: A handbook for practitioners.* New York: Guilford Press.

Webb, N. B. (1996). *Social work practice with children.* New York: Guilford Press.

Webb, N. B. (1999a). School-based crisis assessment and intervention with children following urban bombings. In N. B. Webb (Ed.), *Play therapy with children in crisis* (2nd ed.): *Individual, group, and family treatment* (pp. 430–447). New York: Guilford Press.

Webb, N. B. (Ed.). (1999b). *Play therapy with children in crisis* (2nd ed.): *Individual, group, and family treatment.* New York: Guilford Press.

Appendix

Training Programs and Certifications

PLAY THERAPY

A comprehensive directory of play therapy training programs may be obtained for a fee from University of North Texas, Center for Play Therapy, Denton, TX 76203. The programs listed here represent a small selection of those available in different parts of the United States.

Boston University
Postgraduate Certificate Program in Advanced
Child and Adolescent Psychotherapy
School of Social Work
264 Baystate Road
Boston, MA 02215
Phone: (617)353-3756
Fax: (617)353-7262
E-mail: pepssw@bu.edu

California School of Professional Psychology
at Alliant University
Dr. Kevin O'Connor
5130 East Clinton Way
Fresno, CA 93727
Phone: (559)456-2777, ext. 2273
E-mail: admissions@mail.cspp.edu

Center for Play Therapy
Dr. Garry Landreth, Director
University of North Texas
Denton, TX 76203
Phone: (940)565-3864
Fax: (940)565-4461
E-mail: cpt@coefs.coe.unt.edu

Fairleigh Dickinson University
Center for Psychological Services
Dr. Linda Reddy, Director
131 Temple Avenue
Hackensack, NJ 07601
Phone: (201)692-2649
Fax: (209)692-2164
E-mail: Reddy@ Alpha.fdu.edu

Post-Master's Certificate Program in Child and Adolescent Therapy
Dr. Nancy Boyd Webb, Director
Fordham University
Graduate School of Social Service
Tarrytown, NY 10591
Phone: (914)332-6008
Fax: (914)332-7101
E-mail: Nwebb@Fordham.edu

The Theraplay Institute
Dr. Linda Wark, Director
3330 Old Glenview Road, Suite 8
Chicago, IL 60601
Phone: (847)256-7334
Fax: (847)256-7370
Website: www.theraplay.org

GRIEF COUNSELING

Association for Death Education and Counseling
Nickie Meeks, Director
342 Main Street
West Hartford, CT 06117
Phone: (860)586-7550
Website: www.associationresource.com

Certification courses for grief counselors and death counselors. Offered during the 2 days preceding the annual National Conference in March of each year. Contact the Association for Death Education and Counseling (ADEC) Central Office for details.

Children's Hospice International
1101 King Street, Suite 131
Alexandria, VA 22314
Phone: (800)242-CHILD

College of New Rochelle
Certificate Program in Thanatology
Dr. Kenneth Doka, Director
Division of Human Services
29 Castle Place
New Rochelle, NY 10805-2339
Phone: (914)654-5561
(914)654-5418
E-mail: gs@cnr.edu

Dougy Center (for bereaved children)
P.O. Box 86582
Portland, OR 97286
Phone: (503)775-5683
Website: www.dougy.org

Hospice Foundation of America
2001 S Street NE
Washington, DC 20002
Phone: (202)638-5419
E-mail: hfa@hospicefoundation.org
Website: www.hospicefoundation.org

Make-A-Wish Foundation of America
100 West Clarendon, Suite 2200
Pheonix, AZ 85013
Phone: (800)722-9474

National Center for Death Education
Mount Ida College
Carol Wogrin, Executive Director
777 Dedham Street
Newton Center, MA 02459
Phone: (617)928-4649
Fax: (617)928-4713
E-mail: ncde@mountida.edu
Website: www.mountida.edu.officesandservices

Offers 1- and 2-day continuing education programs plus courses to train professional caregivers.

TRAUMA/CRISIS COUNSELING

American Association of Suicidology
4201 Connecticut Avenue NW, Suite 310
Washington, DC 20008
Phone: (202)237-2280

Conducts an examination for Crisis Worker Certification prior to the annual meeting in April. Course work and relevant counseling experience must be verified to determine eligibility to take the exam.

International Association of Trauma Counselors
4131 Spicewood Spring Road, Suite G-6
Austin, TX 78759-0051
Phone: (512)795-0051

Endorses training programs to certify persons engaged in the field of trauma counseling. For further information, contact the International Association of Trauma Counselors (IATC) office.

The National Institute for Trauma and Loss in Children
900 Cook Road
Grosse Pointe Woods, MI 48236
Phone: (313)885-0390
(877)306-5256
Fax: (313)885-1861
Website: www.tlcinst.org

Resources

SUPPLIERS OF PLAY MATERIALS

Chaselle, Inc.
New England School Supply
P.O. Box 1581
Springfield, MA 01101
Phone: (800)628-8608

Childcraft, Inc.
20 Kilmer Road
Edison, NJ 08818
Phone: (800)631-5657

Childswork/Childsplay
135 Dupont Street
P.O. Box 760
Plainview, NY 11803-0760
Phone: (800)962-1141
Fax: (800)262-1886
E-mail: info@Childswork.com

Constructive Playthings
13201 Arrington Road
Grandview, MO 64030
Phone: (800)225-6124
Fax: (816)761-9295

Creative Therapeutics, Inc.
P.O. Box 522
Cresskill, NJ 07626-0522
Phone: (800)544-6162
Fax: (201)567-3036
Email: ct39@erols.com

Kidsrights
10100 Park Cedar Drive
Charlotte, NC 28210
Phone: (800)892-KIDS
Fax: (704)541-0113
Website: www.kidsrights.com

Rose Play Therapy Toys and Travel Kits
102 Foster Ranch Road
Trinidad, TX 75163
Phone: (800)713-2252
Fax: (903)778-2808

School Specialty
100 Paragon Parkway
P.O. Box 1579
Appleton, WI 54913-1579
Phone: (888)388-3224
Fax: (888)388-6344

Self-Esteem Shop
32839 Woodward Avenue
Royal Oak, MI 48073
Phone: (800)251-8336
Fax: (248)459-0442
E-mail: Deanne@self-esteemshop.com
Website: www.self-esteemshop.com

Family Psychological Services, P.C.
1750 25th Avenue, Suite 200
Greeley, CO 80631
Phone: (800)542-9723
Fax: (970)351-6687
Website: www.playtherapy.WS

Toys to Grow On
2695 East Dominguez Street
P.O. Box 17
Long Beach, CA 90801
Phone: (800)542-8338
Fax: (310)537-5403
E-mail: toyinfo@toystogrowon.com
Website: www.lakeshorelearning.com

Western Psychological Services
12031 Wilshire Boulevard
Los Angeles, CA 92005-1251
Phone: (800)648-8857
Fax: (310)478-7838
E-mail: custsvc@wpspublish.com
Website: www.wpspublish.com

BEREAVEMENT RESOURCES

The Rainbow Collection Catalog
477 Hannah Branch Road
Burnsville, NC 28714
Phone: (828)675-5909
Fax: (828)675-9687
E-mail: heal2grow@aol.com

Lists books, films, and tapes for purchase related to bereavement in general, including many focused on children.

The Good Grief Program
Boston Medical Center
Maria Trozzi, MEd, Director
One BMC Place
Maternity, 5th Floor
Boston, MA 02118
Phone: 617-414-4005
Fax: 617-414-7915
Resources e-mail: mtrozzi@bu.edu

Offers consultation to schools and community groups to help children when a friend is terminally ill or dies. Maintains a resource library of films, books, and materials that may be borrowed or purchased.

National Center for Death Education Library
Mount Ida College
777 Dedham Street
Newton Center, MA 02459
Phone: (617)928-4552

Maintains a collection of print and audiovisual materials on all aspects of dying, death, and bereavement. Some may be borrowed on interlibrary loan.
For information, contact the Coordinator of Resources.

BIBLIOGRAPHIES

The following books contain annotated lists of books and videotapes related to bereaved children:

Adams, D. W., & Deveau, E. J. (Eds.). (1995). *Beyond the innocence of childhood: Vol. 2. Helping children and adolescents cope with life-threatening illness and dying.* Amityville, NY: Baywood.

Chapter 17 by Donna R. O'Toole contains 11 pages of annotated references categorized for use by professionals and caregivers, and for reading to young children, and stories about seriously ill or bereaved children, as well as stories and books about feelings.

Doka, K. J. (Ed.). (2000). *Living with grief. Helping children and adolescents adapt to loss.* Washington, DC: Hospice Foundation of America.

An Appendix section by Charles A. Corr contains 17 pages of annotated references for young people and for adults about death, dying, and bereavement.

Goldman, L. (1996). *Breaking the silence: A guide to help children with complicated grief, suicide, homicide, AIDS, violence and abuse.* Washington, DC: Accelerated Development.

Chapter 10 contains more than 30 pages of annotated references of books, videos, guides and curricula to use with adults, children, and teenagers about various types of deaths and other family problems.

Rando, T. A. (1991). *How to go on living when someone you love dies.* New York: Bantam. (Original work published 1988)

Lists references on grief categorized according to type of grief (i.e., pet loss, suicide, murder, chronic and terminal illness; not focused especially on children, but many references apply).

Wofelt, A. (1983). *Helping children cope with grief.* Muncie, IN: Accelerated Development.

Includes separate reference lists of children's literature concerning death; readings for parents, teachers, and counselors; and general texts focused on death and dying. Also includes topics for discussion groups.

References on Religious/Cultural/ Ethnic Practices Related to Death

Berger, A., Badham, P., Kutscher, A. H., Berger, J., Perry, M., & Beloff, J. (Eds.). (1989). *Perspectives on death and dying: Cross cultural and multidisciplinary view.* Philadelphia: Charles Press.

Coles, R. (1990). *The spiritual life of children* (Christian salvation, pp. 202–224; Islamic surrender, pp. 225–248; Jewish righteousness, pp. 249–276). Boston: Houghton Mifflin.

Corr, C. A., Nabe, C. M., & Corr, D. M. (2000). Cultural differences and death. In C. A. Corr & D. M. Corr (Eds.), *Death and dying, life and living* (3rd ed., pp. 103–129). Belmont, CA: Wadsworth.

Grollman, E. A. (Ed.). (1967). *Explaining death to children.* Boston: Beacon Press.

Johnson, C. J., & McGee, M. G. (Eds.). (1991). *How different religions view death and afterlife.* Philadelphia: Charles Press.

McGoldrick, M., Almeida, R., Hines, P. M., Garcia-Preto, N., Rosen, E., & Lee, E. (1991). Mourning in different cultures. In F. Walsh & M. McGoldrick (Eds.), *Living beyond loss: Death in the family* (pp. 176–206). New York: Norton.

A list of references at the end of this chapter cites additional sources related to the following cultural/religious groups: Irish, Indian, African American, Jewish, and Puerto Rican.

Nader, K., Dubrow, N., & Stamm, B. H. (Eds.). (1999). *Honoring differences: Cultural issues in the treatment of trauma and loss.* Philadelphia: Brunner-Routledge.

Ryan, J. A. (1986). *Ethnic, cultural and religious observances at the time of death and dying.* Boston: The Good Grief Program.

Index